HISTORY OF PEDIATRICS 1850–1950

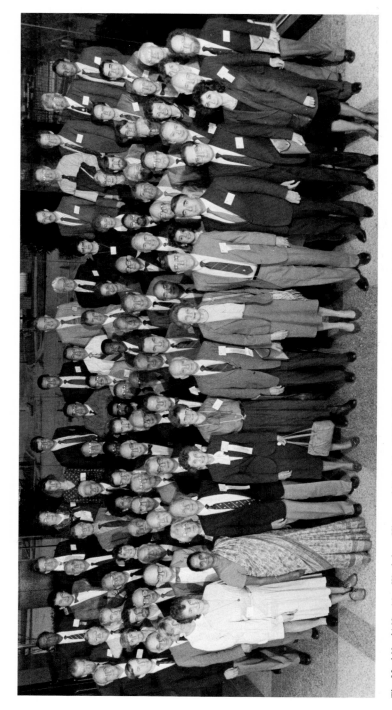

The 22nd Nestlé Nutrition Workshop, History of Pediatrics 1850–1950, was held February 20–22nd, 1989, at the Children's Nutrition Research Center, Baylor College of Medicine, Houston, Texas, USA.

History of Pediatrics
1850–1950

Editors

Buford L. Nichols, Jr., M.D., M.S.
Professor of Pediatrics
Children's Nutrition Research Center
Baylor College of Medicine
Houston, Texas, USA

Angel Ballabriga, M.D.
Professor of Pediatrics
Children's Hospital of the
"Seguridad Social"
Autonomous University
Barcelona, Spain

Norman Kretchmer, M.D., Ph.D.
Professor of Nutritional Sciences
University of California at Berkeley
Berkeley, California and
Professor of Pediatrics and Obstetrics
San Francisco General Hospital
San Francisco, California, USA

Nestlé Nutrition
Workshop Series
Volume 22

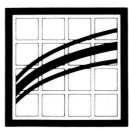

NESTLÉ NUTRITION

RAVEN PRESS ■ NEW YORK

Nestec Ltd., 55 Avenue Nestlé, CH-1800 Vevey, Switzerland
Raven Press, Ltd., 1185 Avenue of the Americas, New York, New York
10036

Made in the United States of America

Library of Congress Cataloging-in-Publication Data

History of pediatrics, 1850–1950 / editors, Buford L. Nichols, Angel
    Ballabriga, Norman Kretchmer.
       p.   cm.—(Nestlé Nutrition workshop series; v. 22)
      Papers presented at the 22nd Nestlé Nutrition workshop held at the
    Children's Nutrition Research Center in Houston, Tex., Feb. 20–22,
    1989.
      Includes bibliographical references.
      Includes index.
      ISBN 0-88167-695-0
    1. Pediatrics—History—Congresses. I. Nichols, Buford Lee,
1931– . II. Ballabriga, Angel. III. Kretchmer, Norman, 1923– .
IV. Nestlé Nutrition S.A. V. Series.
    [DNLM: 1. Pediatrics—history—congresses. W1 NE228 v.22 / WS
11.1 H673 1989]
RJ40.H57 1990
618.92'0009'034—dc20
DNLM/DLC
for Library of Congress   90-8717
                                       CIP

9 8 7 6 5 4 3 2 1

Preface

This volume is a comprehensive exposé on the history of pediatrics in the period 1850–1950. This time span was chosen because of the critical antecedents in biology between 1850–1880 that impacted on the development of pediatrics as a specialty apart from internal medicine. The emergence of an understanding of infectious diseases and their transmission revolutionized pediatric care. Major advances in nutrition were made during the period 1900–1925, and 1925–1950 revealed an abundance of information in metabolism and genetics. We chose the closing date of 1950 because (a) it is contemporary and will be a pivotal year for historians of the 21st Century, and (b) it launched the development of molecular medicine.

Knowledge acquired and applied during these 100 years is overpowering. We have advanced from the simple concepts of cleanliness to the intricacies of complex metabolic pathways. The health of the child in the industrial world has improved beyond all expectation. The development and growth of pediatrics from 1850 to 1950 profoundly improved the condition of children. For example, it was the dedication and discoveries of physicians and scientists working under the rubric of pediatrics during the years 1850–1950 that brought substantial reductions in infant mortality and marked alterations in the causes of infant mortality in the world (1). In 1900 the infant mortality rate in the United States, France, and Germany (2) was approximately 150/1000 live births. By 1987 the infant mortality rate had declined to 10.1/1000 live births.

As we draw near the end of "the Century of the Child" (3), we anticipate even greater contributions from pediatrics and pediatricians to the quality of life for all children. The appalling conditions in child health encountered one hundred years ago persist today in many parts of the world. As pediatricians, our goal is to prevent the debilitating diseases and behavioral disorders of both children and adults throughout the world. We have the responsibility to improve the quality of life for present and future citizens, and we seek through scientific research to accomplish this goal.

The opportunity to evaluate the historical basis for future pediatric development was warmly received by the workshop participants. Their contributions will be evident to the reader. The workshop participants have passed to the next generation the sense of commitment to scientific approach and social concerns that are the hallmarks of pediatrics.

BUFORD L. NICHOLS, JR., M.D., M.S.
ANGEL BALLABRIGA, M.D.
NORMAN KRETCHMER, M.D., PH.D.

REFERENCES

1. Wegman ME. Annual summary of vital statistics—1983. *Pediatrics* 1984;74:981–989.
2. McCormick MC. The contribution of low birthweight to infant mortality and childhood morbidity. *N Engl J Med* 1985;312:82–89.
3. Key E. *The Century of the Child*. New York and London: GP Putnam & Sons, 1909.

Foreword

If the term *history,* as taught to my generation, was defined as a "botanical description" of what happened during the previous century, I do not think the history of pediatrics would have deserved a Nestlé Nutrition Workshop or a book in the Nestlé Nutrition Workshop Series.

If we believe in the modern definition of history, by which the understanding of changing economic, political, and sociological medical factors are used to explain events and to construct models to understand the present and possibly predict the future, then the proposal of Professors Angel Ballabriga, Norman Kretchmer, and Buford Nichols to hold such a meeting was fully justified.

In addition, I think we can accept that certain conditions of nutrition, hygiene and education observed in Europe and North America at the turn of the century are to some extent similar to those conditions observed in developing countries today. Therefore, we can use the knowledge gained from the history of pediatrics to help developing countries reach an optimal level of pediatric development more rapidly.

It may seem strange to emphasize the development of pediatric research and assume it would be useful for developing countries. When those countries have so much to do with so little money, the money they do have could be better used for immunization and better feeding of children and pregnant women. To paraphrase a Mao Tse Tung statement, I would reply, immunizing 100 children is great, helping to train a pediatrician who can then save thousands of children is even better, but to give local doctors the opportunity of learning to analyze their own problems and find readily applicable and acceptable solutions for the whole population, is better still.

I hope that this book, in a very modest way, will enable our colleagues from developing countries to understand better how pediatric research in Europe and North America between 1850 and 1950 has played an important role in improving the health of children, and that they are able to pass on this experience for the good of their own children.

PIERRE R. GUESRY, M.D.
Nestec Ltd.
Vevey, Switzerland

Acknowledgments

The editors express appreciation to Dr. Ernie Strapazon from the Carnation Company; Dr. Pierre R. Guesry, Medical and Scientific Director of Nestec; and Dr. Laila K. Dufour, the coordinator of the Workshop Series. Dr. Ralph Feigin, Chairman of the Department of Pediatrics at Baylor College of Medicine, helped make the workshop possible. We also thank Ms. Patricia A. Williams, CNRC, and Ms. Lila K. Lerner, BCM Office of Continuing Education, for their assistance in organizing the workshop; and Jerry D. Eastman, CNRC Publications/Illustrations, for editorial assistance.

In Memoriam

Dr. Leo Stern was internationally known for his vast knowledge of neonatology and general pediatrics. He was Chairman of the Departments of Pediatrics at Brown University and Rhode Island Hospital, Providence, Rhode Island; these departments gained much fame throughout the United States and the world for their work in perinatology. We all mourn the unexpected demise of Dr. Stern.

Dr. Calvin Woodruff was a quiet man dedicated to good nutrition and healthy development of children. We, in pediatrics, will miss his sage advice.

With deep regrets we learned of the death of Professor Harold E. Harrison. Professor Harrison was a giant in the field of pediatrics, and his contributions hold a significant place in its history. We mourn his passing and the loss to our field and to his family.

Contents

xi

Contributors

Ignacio Avila-Cisneros
Departamento de Investigación
Médico-Social, Instituto Nacional de
  Pediatría
México 04530 D.F., México

Angel Ballabriga
Department of Pediatrics
Children's Hospital of the "Seguridad
  Social"
Universidad Autónoma
Paseo Vall d'Hebron S/N
Barcelona 08035, Spain

Lewis A. Barness
Department of Pediatrics
University of Wisconsin Hospital and
  Clinics
600 Highland Avenue
Madison, Wisconsin 53792, USA

Joseph A. Bellanti
Departments of Pediatrics and
  Microbiology
International Center for Interdisciplinary
  Studies of Immunology
Georgetown University School of
  Medicine
3800 Reservoir Road NW
Washington, D.C. 20007, USA

Wolfgang Braun
Department of Pediatrics
Karl-Marx University
Ost Strasse 21-25
Leipzig 7050, Democratic Republic of
  Germany

Sheldon G. Cohen*
Intramural Research Program
National Institute of Allergy and Infectious
  Diseases
National Institutes of Health
Bethesda, Maryland 20892, USA

*unable to attend

John A. Davis
Department of Pediatrics
Clinical School
University of Cambridge
1 Cambridge Road, Gt. Shelford
Cambridge CB2 5JE, United Kingdom

Samuel J. Fomon
Department of Pediatrics
College of Medicine
University of Iowa
Iowa City, Iowa 52242, USA

Gilbert B. Forbes*
Department of Pediatrics
University of Rochester School of
  Medicine and Dentistry
Box 777
601 Elmwood Avenue
Rochester, New York 14642, USA

Silvestre Frenk
División de Nutrición
Unidad de Investigación Biomédica
Centro Médico Nacional
Instituto Mexicano del Seguro Social
México 06760 DF and
California 160
Parque San Andrés
Delegación Coyoacán
México 04040 D.F., México

Bent Friis-Hansen
Department of Neonatology
Rigshospitalet University Hospital
Blegdamsvej 9
DK-2100 Copenhagen 0, Denmark

John D.L. Hansen
University of the Witwatersrand
Johannesburg, Republic of South Africa
Department of Pediatrics and Child
  Health
Medical School
York Road
Parktown 2193, Republic of South Africa

Harold E. Harrison (deceased)
Department of Pediatrics
Johns Hopkins University School of
   Medicine
600 North Wolfe Street
Baltimore, Maryland 21205, USA

Malcolm A. Holliday
Department of Pediatrics
University of California San Francisco
Room A-276
400 Parnassus Avenue
San Francisco, California 94143, USA

Norman Kretchmer
Department of Nutritional Sciences
University of California at Berkeley
Berkeley, California, USA 94720 and
Departments of Pediatrics and Obstetrics
San Francisco General Hospital
1001 Potrero Avenue
San Francisco, California, USA 94110

Robert Laplane
Faculté de Médecine Saint-Antoine
Hôpital Trousseau
75012 Paris, France

Jack Metcoff
Departments of Pediatrics, Biochemistry,
   and Molecular Biology
University of Oklahoma Health Sciences
   Center/CHO
P.O. Box 26901/CHO 3B 700
Oklahoma City, Oklahoma 73190, USA

Buford L. Nichols, Jr.
Departments of Pediatrics and Physiology
Baylor College of Medicine and
USDA/ARS Children's Nutrition Research
   Center
1100 Bates Street
Houston, Texas 77030-2600, USA

Howard A. Pearson
Department of Pediatrics
Yale University School of Medicine
333 Cedar Street
New Haven, Connecticut 06510, USA

Andrea Prader
Department of Pediatrics
Universitäts-Kinderklinik
Steinwiesstrasse 75
CH-8032 Zürich, Switzerland

Ettore Rossi
Department of Pediatrics
University of Berne, Inselspital
3010 Berne, Switzerland

Selma E. Snyderman
Department of Pediatrics
New York University Medical Center
550 First Avenue
New York City, New York 10016, USA

Paul R. Swyer
Department of Pediatrics
The Hospital for Sick Children
University of Toronto
555 University Avenue
Toronto, Ontario M5G 1X8, Canada

James Mourilyan Tanner
School of Public Health
University of Texas at Houston
Houston, Texas 77225, USA

Jarmo K. Visakorpi
Departments of Clinical Sciences and
   Pediatrics
University Hospital of Tampere
Teiskontie 35
SF-33520 Tampere, Finland

John C. Waterlow
London School of Hygiene and Tropical
   Medicine
Keppel Street
London WC1 E7HT, United Kingdom

Calvin W. Woodruff* (deceased)
Department of Child Health
University of Missouri-Colombia School
   of Medicine
910 Wayne Road
Colombia, Missouri 65203, USA

Invited Attendees

Billy F. Andrews/*Louisville, KY, USA*
Giulio J. Barbero/*Columbia, MO, USA*
Enid Barness/*Madison, WI, USA*
Edward F. Bell/*Iowa City, IA, USA*
D.G. Benakappa/*Bangalor, India*
Betty Bernard/*South Pasadena, CA, USA*
Paul M. Bogan/*Denver, CO, USA*
Carrie Byington/*Houston, TX, USA*
Denise Cabeza/*Fayetteville, NC, USA*
Carlo Catassi/*Ancona, Italy*
William R. Collie/*Little Rock, AR, USA*
Colin Collins-Williams/*Toronto, Canada*
Giovanni V. Coppa/*Ancona, Italy*
William J. Darby/*Nashville, TN, USA*
Teresa A. Davis/*The Woodlands, TX, USA*
Dolores M. Delgadillo/*Dallas, TX, USA*
Murdina M. Desmond/*Houston, TX, USA*
Wieslaw A. Dziedzic-Wisinki/*Porter, TX, USA*
Lelon Edwards/*Memphis, TN, USA*
M.S. Elbualy/*Muscat, Sultanate of Oman*
Frank Falkner/*Berkeley, CA, USA*
Philip M. Farrell/*Madison, WI, USA*
Ralph Feigin/*Houston, TX, USA*
Reinaldo Figueroa/*New Orleans, LA, USA*
Laurence Finberg/*Tarrytown, NY, USA*
Romeo Fortin/*Houston, TX, USA*
Eric A. Fraser/*North Little Rock, AR, USA*
Jeffrey L. Gardner/*Fayetteville, NC, USA*
Francis Gold/*Tours, France*

Harry L. Greene/*Nashville, TN, USA*
José Grünberg/*Montevideo, Uruguay*
Helen Harrison/*Baltimore, MD, USA*
Hans Helge/*Berlin, GDR*
Arturo R. Hervada/*Philadelphia, PA, USA*
Gerald Holman/*Amarillo, TX, USA*
Helmut Huebers/*Houston, TX, USA*
Yolanda Johnson/*Houston, TX, USA*
Michael Katz/*New York, NY, USA*
Herbert S. Kaufman/*San Francisco, CA, USA*
Joel B. Kirkpatrick/*Houston, TX, USA*
Emily Roseland Klein/*Houston, TX, USA*
Nora Klein/*Houston, TX, USA*
Peter D. Klein/*Houston, TX, USA*
William J. Klish/*Houston, TX, USA*
John A. Knapp/*Houston, TX, USA*
Otakar Koldovsky/*Tucson, AZ, USA*
Judith W. Lederhandler/*Miami, FL, USA*
Carlos Lifschitz/*Houston, TX, USA*
Marta Lifschitz/*Houston, TX, USA*
Jean D. Lockhart/*Belvedere, CA, USA*
Horace Long/*Greenville, NC, USA*
A. Harold Lubin/*Winnetka, IL, USA*
Riorita Maano/*Pensacola, FL, USA*
Ameeta M. Martin/*Houston, TX, USA*
Anne Miller/*San Antonio, TX, USA*
Charles E. Mize/*Dallas, TX, USA*
Jai Mohan Dato/*Perak, Malaysia*
Corinne M. Montandon/*Houston, TX, USA*
Christian Morkeberg/*Houston, TX, USA*
Doris M. Moutos/*Oklahoma City, OK, USA*
Veda N. Nichols/*Houston, TX, USA*
Maria Nikolaidis/*Kingwood, TX, USA*
N. Paramaesvaran/*Penang, Malaysia*
Elisabeth Peer/*Wattens, Austria*
Victor Pineiro/*San Antonio, TX, USA*

Bernard Pollara/*Albany, NY, USA*
Marilyn Gregory Porter/*Oklahoma City, OK, USA*
Laurel L. Prestridge/*Bellaire, TX, USA*
Jose Quintanilla/*Killeen, TX, USA*
Enrique Quintero/*San Antonio, TX, USA*
Jesse Reeves-Garcia/*Miami, FL, USA*
Malcolm Rourk/*Durham, NC, USA*
Arnold J. Rudolph/*Houston, TX, USA*
T. Yanuario Sanchez-Burgos/*Houston, TX, USA*
Irene Santos/*Houston, TX, USA*
James R. Smalley/*San Antonio, TX, USA*
Dwi Atmadji Soejoso/*Surabaya, Indonesia*
Gregory Sokol/*Norfolk, VA, USA*
Bozeme Sommer/*Kingwood, TX, USA*
Bonny L. Specker/*Cincinnati, OH, USA*

Leo Stern/*Providence, RI, USA*
Dana L. Suskind/*Kansas City, KS, USA*
Robert Suskind/*New Orleans, LA, USA*
Fred M. Taylor/*Sugar Land, TX, USA*
William Threlkeld/*Memphis, TN, USA*
Paul L. Toubas/*Oklahoma City, OK, USA*
Reginald Tsang/*Cincinnati, OH, USA*
John N. Udall/*Tucson, AZ, USA*
Carlos Vallbona/*Houston, TX, USA*
Jorge H. Vargas/*Los Angeles, CA, USA*
Fernando Velasquez/*Tampa, FL, USA*
David G. Walters/*Miami, FL, USA*
Elizabeth White/*Houston, TX, USA*
Daniel Willard/*Strasbourg, France*

Carnation Participants

Laurie MacDonald/*Los Angeles, CA, USA*
Al Piergallini/*Los Angeles, CA, USA*
Kendall Neal-Schrader/*San Antonio, TX, USA*

Larry Somerville/*Dallas, TX, USA*
Ernie Strapazon/*Los Angeles, CA, USA*
Steve Witherly/*Los Angeles, CA, USA*

Nestec Participants

Pierre R.Guesry
Nestec Ltd.
Vevey, Switzerland

Laila Dufour-Khouri
Nestec Ltd.
Vevey, Switzerland

Nestlé Nutrition Workshop Series

History of Pediatrics 1850–1950, edited by
B.L. Nichols, A. Ballabriga, and N. Kretchmer.
Nestlé Nutrition Workshop Series, Vol. 22. Nestec
Ltd., Vevey/Raven Press, Ltd., New York © 1991.

One Century of Pediatrics in Europe

Angel Ballabriga

Department of Pediatrics, Children's Hospital of the "Seguridad Social,"
Autonomous University, 08035 Barcelona, Spain

To review the development of pediatrics in Europe between 1850 and 1950, it is first necessary to understand the circumstances that influenced the later development of knowledge about diseases of children.

In the nineteenth century, Europe was still under the influence of the consequences of the French Revolution (1789–1815), the various wars of independence, and the fall of the Napoleonic Empire. After the Vienna Congress (1814–1815), a new way of life emerged (1) with the development of national romanticism and a populist sentiment. The French Democratic Revolution in 1848 and the revolutionary movements that happened almost simultaneously in other countries (2) were small, liberal, nationalist "bourgeois" movements that would lead in successive years to the concept of class among workers. With the nineteenth century, the revolutionary proletariat made its appearance in history, and the development of institutions and the concept of *nations* were to be produced during this century; it was the end of the *ancien régime* (3). The middle class had reached its highest status and assumed social power (4), and the period also coincided with the communist manifest (5) of Marx and Engels (1848). The French Revolution made it evident that the concepts of *medicine* and *society* were inseparable and the concept of *charity* was displaced toward that of *social justice*.

In the eighteenth century, the mother, the wet nurse, and the educator were the key figures, not the child, and infancy was considered a time when there was a particular disposition to illness. Disease was considered by some as forming part of a process of moral regeneration. The nineteenth century brought about a greater concern for public hygiene, a better basic education for women, the beginning of their emancipation (6), and new definitions of the concept of city planning. The reigning social injustice and the relationship between poverty and disease had already been bravely brought to light by J.P. Frank (7) in the University of Padua in 1790 and afterward by Villermé (8) in France in 1840, in the English report by Chadwich (9) in 1842, and also by Virchow in 1848, who referred to the situation of the workers in Silesia (10). The Industrial Revolution, beginning in 1815 (11), facilitated the propagation of infectious diseases due to the strong immigration movements that occurred in some countries, and, the abandonment of rural zones and the creation of industrial areas, caused serious housing problems and miserable living conditions.

Likewise, there existed a great collective lack of sensitivity about the living conditions of children. The concept of the sick child, needful of care and special attention, took time to be accepted. Children worked in the textile industry and even in the mines. In 1833, a law in Great Britain created inspectors of work in the textile industry in order to limit the labor of children between 9 and 13 years of age to only 9 hours a day (12), and, in France, the first law limiting the work of children was passed in 1841. It has been calculated that, in 1842, 12% of the work force was under 13 years of age. According to a report in 1843, in the lace industry, children under the age of 6 were working for long hours each day. Little notice was taken of the scanty official regulations that existed. There was an enormous contrast between the bourgeois housing conditions and the workhouses and workers' slums. The novels of Charles Dickens reflected very clearly the living conditions of working-class children. Illegitimate children had only a 10% chance of reaching 20 years (13), passing through the dangers of the orphanage, adoption, and exploitation. It is true that in the nineteenth century an authentic medical revolution had begun that would reach its height in the last 40 years of the century, but there was a notable contrast between this spectacular progress in medical knowledge and the fact that a large section of the working-class population still believed in traditional empiric medicine. In the nineteenth century, the development of scientific hygiene was promoted, for which a door had already been opened by J.P. Frank (1745–1821) when he published *"System einer vollständigen medizinischen Politik"* in 1782 (14). The work of Hufeland (15) in 1799 encouraged the development of social assistance in the care of infants.

MEDICAL THOUGHT IN 1850 AND ITS DEVELOPMENT DURING THE REST OF THE NINETEENTH CENTURY

At the beginning of the nineteenth century, the empiric doctrine of Berhaave (1668–1738), *Comunis Europae Praeceptor,* based on inspection, questioning, and observation, and, in part, on the correlation with patho-anatomic findings, was in opposition to the dogmatic Galenism dominant at that time. Berhaave's disciples, among whom were Haller (1708–1777), who wrote an eight-volume work, *Elementa Physiologiae Corporis Humani,* Van Swieten (1700–1772), founder of the Alte Wiener Schule, and Nils Rosen von Rosenstein (1706–1773), would make important medical contributions. In my opinion, the main impetus for the explosive development of medicine in the nineteenth century was provided by Morgagni (1682–1771), Bichat (1771–1802) and Laënnec (1781–1826). With the work of Morgagni, *De Sedibus et Causis Morborum Per Anatomen Indagatis* (1761), anatomically related clinical empiricism had been created. Fifty years after its first publication, there were 11 editions in Latin and 7 in other languages. The European concept of *clinics* had begun, and with it the idea of the anatomical localization of the "morbid process". With Morgagni, the concept of an organic pathology appeared. Bichat modified existing ideas about organic structure by introducing the concept of *tissu* as a morphologic and physiologic unit of the living being (16,17). His works would substitute some aspects of the theoretical *Naturphilosophie* dominant in Germany, and promoted by Schelling (1775–1858). Later on, Schönlein (1793–1864) and Johannes Müller (1801–1858), among others, would try to replace these philosophical speculations with clinical and experimental facts. Laënnec began a confrontation with classical medicine—his new doctrine being based on the conjunction of exploratory clinical examination with the introduction of clinical auscultation (18) and clinical anatomic method. This was the foundation of semeiology, and it led to a system that would constitute the basis of medical practice until the beginning of our century. Until Bichat and Laënnec, it could be said that medicine had not been a science, but from then on the residues of the dogmatic doctrines of Hippocrates, Galen, and Aristotle could be brushed aside. In Great Britain during the same period, Graves (1796–1853), Bright (1789–1858), Addison (1793–1860), and Hodgkin (1793–1860) all made important contributions to the identification of new types of diseases through clinical anatomic examination.

Leaving the stages of romantic medicine (1830–1850) and the *Naturphilosophie* behind, medicine of the nineteenth century developed into a scientific discipline, substituting the predominance of the botanical influences with those of chemical science. While the patho-anatomic orientation toward the search for the lesion remained, the etiopathologic concept began with the aim of identifying the external cause of the "morbid process". Thus Henle (1809–1885), in his work, *Von den miasmen und von den miasmatisch-contagiosen krankheiten,* published in 1840 (19), tried to establish the genesis of contagious miasmatic diseases.

The so-called Zweiter Wiener Schule, with the clinician, Skoda (1805–1881), the dermatologist, Hebra (1816–1880), the anatomist, Hyltl (1810–1894), and the pathologist, Rokitanski (1804–1879), was to have a great influence on medical evolution. Rokitanski, referred to by Virchow as "Linnaeus of Pathology" because of his book *Handbuch der speziellen Pathologischen Anatomie,* would be the most influential of these men (20). With the Zweiter Wiener Schule, the era of converting diagnosis into a science had arrived; it was the time of the great clinical diagnosticians, not only Skoda, but also the French men, Trousseau (1801–1867) and Charcot (1825–1893). In this second half of the nineteenth century, the theory of evolution, promoted by Darwin (1809–1882) in his work, *On the Origin of Species* published in 1859, also played a very important role. The metaphysical concept of medicine was abandoned, and the influence of physics and organic chemistry facilitated the development of scientific methodology and the change from *Naturphilosophie* to *Naturwissenchaft,* and the new pathophysiologic orientation of men such as Traube (1818–1876), Frerichs (1819–1885), Wunderlich (1815–1878), and Kussmaul (1822–1902). The concept of *Médecine physiologique* of Broussais (1772–1838) (21), which maintained Brownian principles, had also been abandoned. In the meantime, the fundamental facts of physiology and organic chemistry had been established by Ludwig (1816–1895) with his *Lehrbuch der physiologie des Menschen* (1852), and Liebig (1803–1873) (see p. 50, Fig. 1), whose studies are basic for understanding the evolution of biochemistry and nutrition.

We cannot penetrate the specific field of pediatrics without reference to the important roles played by Virchow (1821–1902) (see p. 137, Fig. 2), C. Bernard (1813–1878), Pasteur (1822–1893), Lister (1827–1912) and Koch (1843–1910). A decisive step in the study of tissue was taken by Virchow, disciple of Müller in Berlin, when in 1858 his *Die cellular pathologie* (22) established the concept of *Omnis Cellula e Cellula*. Bichat's concept of *tissu* had passed on to that of Virchow's *zelle*. Later on, the systematization of the cellular composition of tissues was established with the work of Hertwig, *Zelle und Gewebe* (1893). This new knowledge promoted the change of medicine from a speculative science to an experimental science.

With Claude Bernard, the notion of *milieu interne* was introduced and, with his book *Introduction à l'étude de la médecine expérimentale* (1865), the field was opened to analytical experimentation. With Pasteur, the stage of bacteriological pathology was entered and the infectious origin of many diseases was confirmed. Thus, the etiopathogenic doctrine was achieved, shortly to be followed by the work of Koch, especially his identification of the tuberculosis bacillus (23). With Koch and Klebs (1834–1913), a period of bacteriological development occurred that, between 1881 and 1914, resulted in the identification of etiologic agents of more than 30 infectious diseases. All these findings have a special significance for pediatrics, as did the discovery of x-rays by Röentgen (1845–1923) (24), although the practical application of this discovery did not occur in pediatrics for some decades. The step taken by Lister in creating the concept of antisepsis published in his work, *Antiseptic Principles in Practical Surgery* (1867), is also of great importance and superseded the work of Semmelweis (1818–1865) (25) who developed the concept of obstetric antisepsis in Vienna. Even greater progress in this field was made when E. von Bergmann (1836–1907) (26) used steam sterilization in Berlin in 1886. The conjunction of Virchow, Bernard, Pasteur, Koch, and Klebs heralded a total change in the evolution of medicine, and it is not by chance that it also coincided with the start of great developments in scientific pediatrics. Parallel developments in technology made the last part of the nineteenth century the era of measurement. At the same time, experimentation, in the old sense of alchemy, gave way to analytical experimentation according to Bernard (27).

PEDIATRIC THOUGHT IN THE MID-NINETEENTH CENTURY AND ITS EVOLUTION

Pediatric knowledge in 1850 was, in part, the result of work carried out in the first half of the nineteenth century and, in part, the heritage of the eighteenth century. Meissner (1796–1860) points out in his compilation *Grundlage der literatur der Pädiatrik, enthaltend die Monographien über die Kinderkrankheiten* (1850) (28) that, of the nearly 7,000 works collected through 1832 that refer to diseases of childhood, 16 were written before the seventeenth century, 21 during the seventeenth century, 75 during the first half of the eighteenth century before Rosen, and the rest from Rosen to 1832. I shall quote three of the works published in the eighteenth century referring to pediatrics, since their influence would have lasted until well into the nineteenth century. These are the books by Niels Rosen von Rosenstein (1706–1773), *Underrättelser om Barn Sjukdomar och deras Bote-Model,* which appeared in 1764 (29,30), Underwood (1737–1820), *A Treatise on the Disorders of Childhood and Management of Infants from Birth Adapted to Domestic Use,* which appeared in 1784, and in particular the third edition with three volumes that appeared in 1797 (31); and Girtanner (1760–1820), *Abhandlung über die Krankheiten der Kinder und über die Physische Erziehung derselben* (32), which appeared in 1794.

The English edition of Rosen's book appeared in 1776 and the fifth edition in Swedish appeared in 1851 (30). At the beginning of the nineteenth century, the work by Jahn (1771–1831), *Neues system der Kinderkrankheiten nach Erfahrung und Brownischen Grundsätzen,* was published (33). Jahn criticized Girtanner and Rosen but did not mention Underwood. Jahn, who belonged to the school of romantic medicine, was an enthusiast of the Brownian system, quoted in his title, which had been attacked by Girtanner. The work of Billard (1800–1832), *Traité des maladies des enfants nouveau-nés et à la mamelle,* published in 1828 (34), must be quoted. This was dedicated exclusively to the newborn. There was also a good clinical anatomic study (35) with evidence of knowledge of antenatal pathology. Other important works were those by Capuron (*Traité des maladies des enfants jusqu' à la puberté* (36)) and by Barthez (1811–1891) and Rilliet (1814–1861) (*Traité clinique et pratique des maladies des enfants* (37)). *Traité de la difterté* by Bretonneau (1778–1862) (38), published in 1826, must also be mentioned.

In the second half of the nineteenth century, speculative pediatrics had already changed to the anatomic-clinical pediatrics of Billard, Rilliet, Barthez, and Bednar (1816–1888), the latter with his work *Die Krankheiten der Neugeborenen und Säuglinge* (39) published in 1850. The patho-anatomic influence was also notable in Vienna, where Rokitanski collaborated first with Mayr (1814–1863) and later with Widerhofer (1832–1901), both of whom directed the St. Anna Kinderspital (40). However, an exclusively clinical-anatomic approach was not sufficient to solve all pediatric problems of the time, since autopsies did not always reveal the cause of disease. Because of this, pediatrics had to follow the same orientation as internal medicine and move toward pathophysiologic investigation. It is not surprising, therefore, that the directional axis of pediatrics was displaced toward Germany, where the development of medical biochemistry was beginning to exercise a strong influence.

The work of Gerhardt (1833–1902), who was an internist and the successor of Frerichs (1819–1885) as Director of the II Medical Clinic of Berlin, should be specifically mentioned. His monumental book *Handbuch der Kinderkrankheiten* (41), which comprised six volumes with more than 7000 pages, was published in 1887–89 and was translated into Italian in 1893 from the second German edition. The book included contributions from, among others, Baginsky (1843–1919), disciple of Traube, Jacobi (1830–1919), the Russian, Rauchfuss (1835–1915), the Hungarian, Bokay, and the Swiss, Demme (1836–1892). This book constituted a complete handbook of pediatric knowledge at that time. The concepts of Bernard on the *milieu interne* would have a later influence on the care of the seriously ill child, and the bacteriological era that developed rapidly after Pasteur, Koch, and Klebs resulted in the orientation of pediatrics' becoming a clinical-anatomic, pathophysiologic, and etiopathogenic entity.

Pediatrics based on these concepts would be called upon to solve the multiple serious and urgent problems that were the cause of a high infant mortality. The objectives were to contribute to nosographic and semeiological development, with a better classification of diseases and more precise physical exploration, helped by the new technologies that were being established. At the same time, there were dietetic advances with expanding knowledge of nutritional disturbances together with a move toward social and preventive aspects of pediatrics.

THE DEVELOPMENT OF PEDIATRIC HOSPITALS IN EUROPE

The development of pediatric hospitals is linked with the history of pediatrics. Before 1850, 25 pediatric hospitals already existed (41), the most ancient being the Hôpital des Enfants Malades in Paris (1802), followed by the Pediatric Pavillion of the Charité of Berlin (1830), and those of Saint Petersburg (1834), Vienna, and Breslau (1837). From 1850 to 1879, another 67 pediatric hospitals opened in Europe, although many of these were pediatric departments integrated into general hospitals. A chronological list of children's hospitals from 1802 to 1879, with a description of the number of beds and other details of each unit, can be found in Latronico's book (42). Many were enlarged and transformed over the years. Among the directors of the St. Anna Kinderspital of Vienna, I should like specifically to mention Widerhofer and Escherich, whose works receive comment below. Complete data on the first 150 years (1837–1987) of the St. Anna Kinderspital of Vienna can be found in the recent publication of Krepler and Gadner, *Das Kind und sein Arzt* (40). There are also complete historical data on the first 100 years of the Kinderspital in Zurich (1874–1974) (43). I shall make special mention of the time corresponding to Feer (1864–1955) and Fanconi (1892–1979). With Feer, modern pediatrics came to Switzerland. He directed the Kinderspital in Zurich from 1911 to 1929 and, in 1911, the first edition of his book, *Lehrbuch der Kinderheilkunde* (44), was published. It was translated in the same year into Italian and afterward into Spanish. It reached its tenth edition in German in 1930. In line with the times, his work covered the most varied aspects of pediatrics, from infectious diseases such as diphtheria, whooping cough, and chicken pox, to dermatological processes of infancy, infant mortality, and reform of the medical study curriculum. He placed special emphasis on dietetic aspects of childhood. In 1923, he published the paper, *"Eine eigenartige Neurose des vegetativen Systems beim Kleinkinde"* (45) referring to infant acrodynia. In 1929, he was succeeded by Fanconi, who had already been working in the clinic for six years. His first work, *Studien über die Serumlipase* (46), was published in 1923. He remained Professor of Pediatrics for 32 years. His work was the forerunner of what was to become pediatric clinical research in Europe, the basis of the development of modern laboratory and technical methods. For years he studied all aspects of pediatric diseases, from scarlet fever to anemias, from ascariasis to cisternal puncture, from the pathology of the tubulus to dietetics, nutritional disturbances, and alimentation—no disorder escaped his attention. In his work, *Der intestinale Infantilismus and ähnliche Formen der chronischen Verdauungstörung* (47), he defined what later with Uehlinger and Knauer (48) and later still with Botsztejn (49) would come to be known as cystic fibrosis. His study of renal tubular disorders associated his name with the syndrome of de Toni-Debré, and in 1948 his study with Botsztejn on *Feer'sche krankheit . . .* (50) threw new light on a disorder that his teacher, Feer, had considered a vegetative neurosis 25 years earlier. The first edition of the Fanconi-Wallgren textbook (51), which went through many editions in Europe, appeared in 1950. He was a fascinating personality. In time, those of us who had the opportunity of working with him often noted how he became less "Herr Professor" and how his human warmth emerged. His interest in his work never faltered; when he was 73, I had the opportunity of spending an entire day with him, and we spent hours visiting the slums of Hong Kong, so that he might learn more about the situation of the Chinese refugees and their living conditions. He was untiring.

The Kinderspital of Basel is another hospital that deserves mention. Between 1846 and 1857, this hospital, was a small unit of twelve beds. It was later replaced in 1862 by a new children's hospital, which was the first in Switzerland. A complete historical study of this hospital was published by Hottinger (52). I worked there with Freudenberg 1944. With Freudenberg, modern pediatrics came to the Kinderspital in Basel. He had been a disciple of Ibrahim (1877–1953) and Moro (1874–1951) and was Professor of Pediatrics at the University of Marburg. In the 1930s, the problems caused by national socialism forced him to emigrate before the situation worsened. In a list of displaced German scholars edited in London in the autumn of 1937 (53), Freudenberg figures as "unplaced without position." At the beginning of 1933, there were some 6,500 Jewish doctors in Germany, of whom a little more than 300 were pediatricians (54). For many of these, the only alternative was to start life in exile. Eckstein went to Ankara, Engel stayed in London at the Hospital for Sick Children, L. Meyer went to Jerusalem, and Rosenbaum to Tel Aviv. Freudenberg then went to Basel as Director of the Kinderspital and opened the way toward biochemically oriented pediatrics.

At the same time that the new pediatric hospital began in Basel (1862), a small unit called the Foundation Salome Julie von Jenner (55) began to function in Bern, directed by Demme (1836–1892), who was succeeded by Stoos (1855–1939). It was successively enlarged in 1902 and 1941 and became the Jenner Kinderspital of Bern, directed by Glanzmann from 1932. Glanzmann had studied in Zurich and worked with Czerny (see p. 27, Fig. 3) in Berlin in 1916. One day in 1943, newly arrived in Switzerland as a young student, I met Glanzmann. He arrived walking slowly down a corridor in the hospital with a very deformed school-age child clinging to each hand. In that clinic were patients with the strangest cases that pediatric pathology was able to produce. It could be said that its Director was a collector of rarities. Every day he visited the wards, making comments in a very low tone be-cause he had difficulties with his voice. His powers of observation and memory were prodigious. His book *Einführung in die Kinderheilkunde* and his concept of *dysporia* (56), about cystic fibrosis of the pancreas, appeared at this time. He had enormous interest in hematology and had already described hereditary thrombocy-tasthenia, which has been given his name. He continued to give his attention to the many types of alterations that can be present in blood platelets. Dietetics was an im-portant part of the routine in the clinic, using *sauervollmilch* in infants and *linsen-brei* in celiac patients. His knowledge about infectious diseases of childhood was extensive. He paid great attention to the psychosomatic component of disease, and I will always be grateful for this teaching, not only for the knowledge he transmit-ted, but because he also showed me the kindly manner in which children and their families should be treated by their pediatrician.

The opening of the Hospital for Sick Children in Great Ormond Street in London in 1852 (thanks to the efforts of West (1816–1893)), was an important step for the development of pediatrics in Great Britain. From this time onward, there was an ex-pansion of children's hospitals in the country. Important personalities such as Bar-low (1845–1945) and Still (1868–1941), about whom I shall comment later, worked in this hospital. The history of the Hospital for Sick Children in London has been published in works by Higgins (57) and Besser (58).

THE BEGINNING OF THE PROFESSORSHIPS OF PEDIATRICS IN EUROPE

The establishment of pediatric pedagogy at the end of the last century was an im-portant step in the development of the discipline. The first doctor to be named Pro-fessor "Ordinarius" of Diseases of Childhood was Widerhofer in 1884 in Vienna. Official inclusion of pediatrics in the medical curriculum in Austria was not recog-nized until 1899; in Germany this official recognition did not take place until 1918.

Henoch (1820–1910), while working in internal medicine in Berlin, had been in charge of a pediatric ward in the Charité of Berlin since 1872, and in 1883 he be-came the head of what was the blue-print of a pediatric university clinic. The history of pediatrics of Berlin is well described in the publications of Stürzbecher (59) and Dost (60). Henoch had worked with Schönlein and some time later described ab-dominal purpura occurring in association with the cutaneous purpura described by Schönlein (1793–1864) in 1829. Some have considered Henoch to be the founder of clinical pediatrics in Germany. He also published a treatise *"Vorlessungen über Kinderkrankheiten"* in 1881, which reached its seventh edition in 1893 (61). Hen-och was succeeded by Heubner (1843–1936) (see p. 25, Fig. 2), who was a disciple of Wunderlich, in 1894, and in this year Heubner was named Professor of Diseases of Childhood, the first in Germany. He was greatly interested in the prevailing in-fectious diseases, such as diphtheria and syphilis, and he published *Lehrbuch des Kinderheilkunde* in two volumes in 1903–1906 (62).

In various other European countries in the last two decades of the nineteenth century, nominations of Professors of Pediatrics had been made, and Dante Cervesato (1850–1905), who had worked with Widerhofer, received the first University Professorship in pediatrics in Padua in 1882, Fede (1832–1913) in Naples in 1887, and Concetti (1855–1920) in Rome in 1897 as a free Professorship. In 1879, the first *Chaire de Clinique des maladies des enfants* was created in Paris, and Parrot was named; Criado Aguilar in Madrid in 1895; Soltmann in Leipzig in 1896; Czerny in Breslau in 1906, and Pfaundler in Munich in 1912. Between 1919 and 1921 another 14 professorships of pediatrics were established in Germany in different towns, among which were Heidelberg in 1919 with Moro, Marburg in 1920 with Bessau (see p. 27, Fig. 4) and Greifswald in 1921 with Peiper. The basic training of most of the first Professors of Diseases of Childhood was in internal medicine, in contrast to earlier times when obstetricians were mainly interested in diseases of infancy, as in the cases of Tarnier and Budin in France. Some pediatricians took a neonatologic orientation from the start, such as Billard and Bednar (1816–1888), to whom we have already referred, and Reuss who worked in Escherich's clinic between 1904 and 1909 and who worked as a neonatologist in the first obstetric clinic in Vienna with the obstetrician, Professor Schauta. Reuss wrote a book on the newborn, *Die Krankheiten des Neugeborenen,* published in 1914 (63) and was later Professor in Graz. He was named Professor of Pediatrics in Vienna in 1911.

The development of pediatric societies contributed to the progress of scientific propagation and the birth of the pediatric section of the Gesellschaft für Heilkunde in Berlin in 1879. The Deutschen Gesellschaft für Kinderheilkunde was founded in 1883. Information concerning the evolution of this society during its first one hundred years can be found in the publications of Schlossmann (64), Windorfer and Schlenk (65) and in the book, *Lebendige Pädiatrie* (66).

The many treatises on pediatrics published from 1900 onward, for example, that of Pfaundler and Scholssman (67), provided the practicing doctor and the university pediatrician with an abundant literature, even to the extent, as today, of having to select from among the mass of information available.

The historical account of German and Austrian pediatricians in exile after 1933 by Moll (54) is of special interest. Other interesting aspects of the relations between pediatrics and national socialism regarding the problems of social Darwinism and racial hygiene have also been published (68, 69). Of all the countries involved in the Second World War, Germany probably experienced the greatest impact on the status of pediatrics. The first meeting of the German Society of Pediatrics after the war took place in Göttingen in 1948, when an impressive summary of the situation was made by Kleinschmidt (70).

INFLUENCE OF EUROPEAN COUNTRIES ON THE EVOLUTION OF PEDIATRICS

The health problems in other European countries ran parallel to those of Germany and Austria, and were dominated by the high mortality rate, particularly among infants. In France, Parrot (1829–1883) centered his attention on nutrition and hence his classical work, *L'atrepsie* (71), published in 1877, and his studies on syphilis, especially the osseous forms with pseudoparalysis (72), and rickets (73). After Parrot, it could be said that the foundation of modern French pediatrics was in the hands of Marfan (1858–1942), Grancher (1843–1907), and Hutinel (1849–1933) (74). Scientific pediatrics was centered mainly at L'Hôpital des Enfants Malades and L'Hospice des Enfants Assistés. Marfan's work, *Traité de l'allaitement* (75), published in 1899, constituted an extraordinary step forward and was translated into German. Grancher, together with Comby (1853–1947) and Marfan, wrote the *Traité des maladies de l'enfance* (1897–1898) (76) in five volumes, which contributed to better knowledge of nutritional disturbances. Grancher was especially interested in tuberculosis and its prophylaxis and studied a system of isolating infants through the use of cubicles. Hutinel was a disciple of Parrot and successor of Grancher at L'Hôpital des Enfants Malades in 1907, and he published *Les maladies des enfants* (77) in 1909. He occupied the Chair of Pediatrics between 1908 and 1921, and was the initiator of the International Association of Pediatrics in 1913. Of the same generation, one should not forget Tarnier (1828–1898) and his disciple, Budin (1846–1907), both of whom were obstetricians. The latter was interested in questions of feeding and commended the use of the soxhlet apparatus and rules for the use of cow's milk; Tarnier was interested in premature infants and constructed an incubator in 1880. A complete study on the evolution of the incubator can be found in the monograph by Marx (78). The Roussel Law in 1875 for protection in infancy should also be remembered.

Later, the names of Lesné (1871–1962), disciple of Hutinel, Ribadeau-Dumas (1876–1950), Cathala (1891–1969), Lamy (1895–1975), who later became a specialist in medical genetics, Mouriquand (1880–1966), Lelong (1892–1973) and Robert Debré (1882–1978) are among the most prominent. Debré must be considered one of the most important physicians of European medicine in our century, not only for his classes, his treatises, and the new syndromes he discovered, but also because he radiated an enormous enthusiasm in promoting the development of pediatrics. The result has been the formation of the great pleiad of collaborators that has lent so much prestige to French pediatrics.

In Great Britain, West (1816–1898) (see p. 32, Fig. 1) was a true pioneer. His "Lectures on the Diseases of Infancy and Childhood" (79) published in 1848 reached seven editions, and he also published an important study on *Some Disorders of the Nervous System in Childhood* in 1871 (80). West created Great Ormond Street Hospital for Sick Children in 1852. This institution was the starting point for other pediatric hospitals. After West, as described by McNeil (81), came a triumvirate formed by Barlow (1845–1945), Thomson (1856–1926) and Still (1868–1941). Barlow was fundamentally a clinician, not a teacher, and his most important works were on subcutaneous nodules in rheumatic fever and the identification of infantile scurvy. In 1883, he recommended prophylaxis of this disease by the use of fresh foods (82). Thomson was another important clinician who was interested in the general problems of the time, such as meningitis and rickets. He translated Henoch's book and is considered the founder of pediatrics in Scotland. He ultimately developed a particular interest in the problems of children with mental deficiency. For some, Still (see p. 35, Fig. 4) is the founder of modern English pediatrics. He studied the relationship between rickets and scurvy and between rickets and syphilis (83) and he was interested in the problem of epidemic meningitis. In 1896, he published an article about the form of arthritis that would later carry his name (84), and in 1906 he was nominated Honorary Professor of Pediatrics in King's College. In his book, *History of Pediatrics* (85), he collected information from ancient times up to the end of the eighteenth century, and in 1933 he was president of the Third International Congress of Pediatrics in London.

In Scandinavian countries, the situation at the end of the nineteenth century was similar, but there was rapid improvement in infant mortality due to the interest shown in the development of social pediatrics. Jundell (1866–1945) was one of the pioneers in this field. He gave special attention to bacteriological studies and took the initiative for the Second International Congress of Pediatrics to be held in Stockholm in 1930. In 1919 he took part in the founding of *Acta Paediatrica Scandinavica*. In my opinion, the most internationally renowned classical Swedish pediatrician was Arvid Wallgren (1889–1973), who was made Director of the Children's Hospital of Gothenburg, which at that time was the largest in Sweden, at the age of 33 years. His activities were mainly concerned with the problems of tuberculosis, bacille Calmette-Guérin (BCG), and correlations between erythema nodosum and tuberculosis, and with the concept of aseptic meningitis. In 1942 he went to Stockholm as Professor of Pediatrics and stayed there until his retirement in 1956. His *Lehrbuch der Pediatrie* (51) in collaboration with Fanconi was for many years one of the works of art of European pediatric textbooks. His activity in social pediatrics was very important. His clinic enjoyed great international fame, promoting pediatric research and the development of subspecialties in pediatrics. Siwe (?–1966) must also be mentioned. He graduated in 1924 and became Professor of Pediatrics in Lund in 1936. His studies on the pathology of the pancreas and on reticuloendotheliosis, which would later carry his name, were very important, as were his activities in the field of social pediatrics. In Denmark, Hirschsprung (1830–1916) was appointed Professor of Pediatrics in 1877. He published works on rheumatism, diagnosis of pyloric stenosis and congenital megacolon, a disease that is named after him (86). In Finland, nineteenth century pediatrics was mainly the province of obstetricians and surgeons. The great progress in Finnish pediatrics occurred after Ylppö's return from the Kaiserin Auguste Victoria Haus in Berlin in 1921 (87). His works had been on neonatal jaundice, acidosis of the newborn during fasting and dehydration, and on the pathology of the premature infant (88,89). As professor in Helsinki since 1920 and Director of the Children's Hospital between 1925 and 1957, the influence of Ylppö (see p. 264, Fig. 4) on the development of pediatrics in his country was extremely important. Finland had been underdeveloped in the field of child health for a long time. In 1855, the infant mortality rate was 21.7% and in 1900, 15%, dropping to 10% in 1920. Since then, thanks to the public health system developed in Finland, it has fallen to 0.6%, one of the lowest rates in the world. The special dedication of Ylppö to the problems of child health, with the Mannerheim League for Children's Welfare, was one of the main factors in this great progress up to the time of the Second World War.

The history of Spanish pediatrics is well covered in the book by Granjel (90). Among the pioneers were Martinez Vargas and Vidal Solares who had extensive connections with French pediatrics. It is impossible to review all the European countries in this chapter but I should nonetheless like to quote the names of a few pediatricians I consider important: in Italy, apart from those already mentioned, were de Toni (1895–1973) and Frontali (1889–1963); in Belgium, Denys (1903–1969) and Hooft (1910–1980); in the Netherlands, de Lange (1871–1950), Gorter (1881–1954), van Creveld (1894–1971) and Dicke (1905–1962); in Russia, Rauchfuss (1835–1915) and Filatow (1847–1902); in Bulgaria, Vatew; in Greece, Vitsaris, Zinnis and Choremis (1900–1966).

In Portugal, Jaime Salazar de Sousa was the pioneer of Portuguese pediatrics and became the first Professor of Pediatrics in 1916. In 1917 and 1918, Chairs of Pediatrics were created in Coimbra and Porto. Later on, in Lisbon, Carlos Salazar de Sousa occupied the Chair of Pediatrics. He was the father of modern pediatrics in Portugal and had great international renown.

In Hungary, the first Children's Hospital was opened in Pest in 1839 thanks to the efforts of Schoepf. In the first period of this hospital (1839–1842), all clinical records were written entirely in Latin. Later, Schoepf was forced to leave the country because of his political and military participation in the War of Independence. Afterward, J. Bokai became the Deputy Director of the Hospital and was later nominated Professor of Pediatrics *ad personam*. In 1833, a new children's hospital opened with 100 beds, sponsored by the Archduchess Stephanie, the wife of Crown Prince Rudolph, and the old Children's Hospital was closed. Janos Bokai was not Director for long as he died in 1884. He was succeeded by his young son Janos Bokai, Jr., who called attention to the fact that chicken pox and herpes zoster were closely related. Aurel Koós, one of the creators of modern pediatric surgery, worked in the Children's Hospital for almost half a century. Bokai, Jr. became a University Professor in 1907 and remained Chief of the Department until 1929 when he was succeeded by Pal Heim.

In Turkey, when the Sultan Abdulhamit II lost a daughter to diphtheria, he established a children's hospital in Istanbul in 1899. The lack of trained pediatricians was a handicap, but in 1917 a Chair of Child Diseases was established in the University. In the meantime, residents were selected to be sent to Paris for training in pediatrics. Following the establishment of the Turkish Republic in 1923, a second Chair, in Child Health, was established, and, within a few years, children's hospitals were opened in Ankara, Konya, and Kayseri, in addition to new ones in Istanbul. Dr. Albert Eckstein was named head of the new Ankara Numune Hospital children's ward in 1935 and when Ankara University was established in 1946, Prof. Eckstein was made the Chief of Pediatrics.

MAJOR PROBLEMS CONCERNING CHILDREN'S DISEASES EXISTING AT THE END OF THE NINETEENTH CENTURY AND THE BEGINNING OF THE TWENTIETH CENTURY

Infectious Diseases

Infectious diseases and intestinal disorders were the most important contributors to the high mortality rate during this period. After the publication of the *Théorie des Germes* by Pasteur, a whole new field of interest developed, confirming ideas that had been raised in the past by authors such as Fracastoro (1476–1553) (91) and Bassi (1773–1856) (92) concerning epidemic diseases propagated by means of invisible live agents (91).

Europe in the nineteenth century was still subject to epidemic outbreaks of cholera, typhus, and exanthematic typhus. Smallpox outbreaks varied in intensity in different countries according to the levels of vaccination with lymph vaccine. After the Franco-Prussian War in 1871, an epidemic of smallpox with 175,000 cases and more than 100,000 deaths occurred in Germany. As a result, a law making vaccination obligatory was passed in Germany in 1874. Our understanding of the epidemiology of diphtheria is founded on the work of Bretonneau, who published careful observations on epidemic outbreaks observed between 1815 and 1821. He had the vision to realize that the pharyngeal and laryngeal forms of *difterite* were one disease. His disciple Trousseau (1801–1877), in his clinical lectures in the Hôtel Dieu in Paris (93), described the disease in detail, including the paralysis of the soft palate, and he was the original sponsor of tracheotomy (94). It is not certain why Trousseau condemned the *tubage de la glotte* when Bouchut (1818–1891) presented it at the Academy of Sciences in 1858 (95). The earlier descriptions of the disease, such as *soffacatio stridula,* or *angina soffocante, morbus strangulatorius* or *mal del garrotillo* (96,97), as it was called in different countries, corresponded largely to the era around the year 1600 onward and in many cases were mixed or confused with other clinical conditions. The descriptions made by Ghisi (1715–1794) (98) of the presence of pseudomembranes in cases observed during an epidemic in 1749 were the reason why, years later, Bretonneau considered him to be the *"père du croup"*.

Diphtheria was a common cause of death in the nineteenth century. Information from the St. Anna Kinderspital in Vienna shows that, of 395 cases operated for laryngeal stenosis before the introduction of antiserum, 69% died. When antidiphtheric serum was first administered in 1895, the mortality dropped to 18.4%. Zeiss and Bieling (99) stated that, in 1892, there were 50,000 deaths caused by diphtheria in Germany. Proof of the importance of infection at that time is that, among the 263 scientific works published in the Kinderspital of Zurich between 1872 and 1920, 73 were on the subject of infectious disease, and, of these, 16 were related to diphtheria. Tuberculosis was an equally important cause of infant mortality, and the contributions of Parrot and Ranke were very important, as was the cutaneous reaction used by Pirquet (1874–1929), the intradermal reaction used by Mantoux (1877–1947), and the percutaneous test used by Moro (1874–1951). Scarlet fever also constituted a very serious infection with high mortality, as did measles. Data from Vienna in 1855 show the mortality for measles to be 31.4% and for scarlet fever, 22%, in patients admitted to the hospital (40). In 1900, Moser, quoted by Schick (1877–1967) (100), who worked with the Widerhoffer group, used antitoxic anti-streptococcal serum for the treatment of scarlet fever. The serum, prepared by injecting horses with heart blood from patients who had died from scarlet fever, had a spectacular effect. The same procedure was used later by Bokay in Budapest.

With regard to prevention, the obstetrician Crede (1812–1892) established the use of silver nitrate drops for blennorrhagic ophthalmia of the newborn in Leipzig in 1881. Data from Peiper show that between 1874 and 1879 the incidence of gonococcal conjunctivitis in live newborns ranged from 9.2% to 13.6%, and after Crede's prophylactic treatment was introduced these figures dropped to 0.25% to 0.29% (101).

It is evident that in the last quarter of the nineteenth century, the development of hygiene became important, and was promoted by books by Uffelmann in 1881 (102) and particularly Max von Pettenkofer (1818–1901), a disciple of Liebig (1803–1873) and Professor of Hygiene in Munich, in 1882 (103). The next step was social hygiene, which covered those sectors not included in individual hygiene, including bettering of living conditions through adequate feeding, city planning, housing, vaccination, and general hygiene. This aspect of social hygiene is revealed in the work of Grotjahn (1839–1931) and Kaup (104) published in 1912. It could then be said that since the work of J.P. Frank (14), considered the founder of social hygiene at the end of the eighteenth century, a long and positive road had been travelled.

Nutritional Disorders of Childhood

An interest in nutritional disturbances of the infant developed as a result of the high mortality rate still dominant in the last decade of the nineteenth century and the first decades of the twentieth century. In this regard the influence of Escherich in Austria and Czerny (1863–1941) and Finkelstein (1865–1942) in Germany was very important. The French schools with Parrot and Marfan also made important contributions to the subject, to which I have already referred.

The bacterial era of nutritional disturbances was initiated with Escherich. He began working in Vienna in 1902, coming from Graz where he was professor. At that time, Vienna was still influenced by the clinical-anatomic doctrines of Rokitanski, but Escherich understood that anatomical doctrine was not sufficient to explain many disturbances of the digestive tract, and he centered his attention on intestinal flora. Escherich had studied with Gerhardt in Würzburg, with Frobenius, disciple of Koch, and with Widerhofer. His important works in relation to intestinal flora (105,106) were published before he went to Vienna. His identification of *coli* was the precursor of many important later publications including those of Adam in 1923 (107) and Kauffmann in 1943 (108). His time in Vienna until 1911 contributed to the importance of the clinic as a reference center, in which, among others, Pirquet worked for a time (100). During this period the concept of *Ernährungsstörungen* was developing in Germany in the sense of a general and functional disturbance with metabolic repercussions. The terms *dystrophy, atrophy, decomposition, hydrolability, dystrophy of hunger, dystrophy consecutive to quantitative hypoalimentation, mehlnährschaden, milchnährschaden,* and *distrofia da farinace* were widely used. Czerny (1863–1941) (see p. 27, Fig. 3) succeeded Heubner in Berlin in 1913. At this time it was known that there was rivalry between his group and that of Finkelstein. In 1906 Czerny and A. Keller (1862–1934) wrote their famous book *Des Kindes Ernährung, Ernährungsstörungen und Ernährungstherapie* (109). Their basic idea was to consider nutritional disturbance as a general manifestation in itself, independent of other preceding phenomena, highlighting the accompanying disturbances of water, salt, nitrogen, fat and carbohydrate metabolism. Czerny studied and created the concept of exudative diathesis from the clinical and biochemical point of view. Part of the extensive material he collected in infants corresponded to the time he was in Prague working with Epstein. During his time in Breslau he created the concept of *turgor* and studied the interactions between natural immunity and nutrition and the problems of alimentary anemias. He presented this subject at the First International Congress of Pediatrics held in Paris in 1912. He was a great observer, who had an enormous capacity for improvisation in his clinical presentations according to Schiff (110). His contradictory spirit led him into arguments with Heubner about mortality in infants when the latter was in Liepzig. He has been described as very authoritarian, and his relations with Langstein in Berlin were not good (87).

Finkelstein (1865–1942) (see p. 140, Fig. 3) was a disciple of Heubner, whom he called his "venerated teacher," and with whom he worked at the Charité in Berlin for 7 years. Afterward he worked in an orphanage in Berlin until 1918 when he became the director of the Kaiser and Kaiserin Friedrich, also in Berlin, where he remained until 1933. With the uprising of national socialism he emigrated to Chile. He created the concept of *hospitalism,* the result of inadequate alimentation, repeated infections, and psychic inanition, and the concepts of *hydrolability* and *alimentary fever* were of interest to him. He was a good teacher and an enthusiast of anatomic studies, personally carrying out post-mortem studies on occasion. He was more of a clinician than a laboratory man. His book *Lehrbuch der Säuglingskrankheiten* (111) enjoyed great success. The fourth German edition in 1938 was edited in Holland, for political reasons. In 1940, the third Spanish edition appeared, which was expanded from the fourth German edition with two chapters written by Professor Scroggie of Chile (112). At this time Finkelstein was still living in Chile and did so up to his death in 1942. His biographical details have been recorded by his collaborator Rosenstern (113) and by his Chilean friends Cienfuegos, Pascual, and Ariztia (114). The latter had trained with Finkelstein in Berlin in 1925.

The danger of hospitalization for young infants was enormous and the results appalling, as can be understood from the comments of Parrot, the story of Bela Schick (100) concerning Escherich's department, the critical comments of Letamendi about the infant section opened in the hospital of the Niño Jesus of Madrid at the end of the nineteenth century (90), and the discussions of Henoch with Heubner, advising him to close the infant service in the Charité in Berlin because of the high mortality rate.

An institution that also played an important role in pediatrics in Berlin at the beginning of the century was the Kaiserin Auguste Victoria Haus (KAVH), which opened in 1909 under the direction of A. Keller and which from 1911 to 1933 was directed by Langstein (1876–1933). Statistical data published by Ballowitz (115) show that the mortality rate in the institution was 20% in 1911. Referring to the cases catalogued as *enterokatarrh,* the mortality rate between 1911 and 1928 oscillated between 25% and 29% and the cases of *Ernährungsstörung* in the period from 1911 to 1917 had a mortality rate of 14%. Loeschke (116) and Joppich (117) traced a historical profile of this institution covering the period from 1909 until 1959. New forms of feeding for nutritional disturbances were introduced, such as the Keller soup (109), buttermilk (118), *Eiweissmilch* (119), *Eiweissrhammilch* (120), *gärtner'scher Fettmilch* (121), *Bifidusmilch* (118), *Buttermehlnährung* (118) and *karotten Suppe* of Moro in 1902 (118), though Mauthner (122) was the first to publish a work on *Karottenbrei* in 1850. Beikost was also an object of discussion. Lesage (118) and Marfan did not give meat until 18 months of age, and Steffen (1825–1910) recommended a diet of 1.5 liters of cow's milk and 25 g of meat and an egg yolk daily for children of 9 to 12 months.

CONCLUSIONS

The evolution of pediatrics in Europe in the century between 1850 and 1950 followed a course parallel with that of internal medicine, and many of the pioneers in pediatrics entered from the field of internal medicine. Pediatric thinking passed from an earlier, clinical-anatomic doctrine to the functional concept incorporated in a pathophysiological doctrine, combined with the additional concepts of the etiopathology of disease derived from the discoveries of the bacteriologic era. The fundamental concern was to combat the high infant mortality rate, particularly in young infants, and thus pediatrics was oriented toward the disorders that were responsible for this mortality, such as infectious diseases and nutritional disturbances. The development of the teaching of pediatrics and the creation of children's hospitals consolidated clinical knowledge in the discipline, and favored introduction of laboratory methods and new techniques for diagnosis and prevention, leading to deeper involvement in the field of pediatric research and the initiation of subspecialties, which is still ongoing today. The rapid development in pediatrics throughout the period in question has been the fruit of new knowledge in basic disciplines such as physiology, pathophysiology, biochemistry, and the sciences of nutrition and hygiene, which have improved our knowledge of both the healthy and the sick child.

In parallel, the improvement in social and environmental conditions has been dependent on economic development in the different European countries, which has led to resounding success in reducing infant mortality, although the success has varied among different countries.

ACKNOWLEDGMENTS

I thank the following persons for their help in providing data for the preparation of this manuscript: K. Betke (Munich); J. Brines (Valencia); E. Cserhati (Budapest); I. Dogramaci (Ankara); H. Gadner (Vienna); F. Haschke (Vienna); B. Lindquist (Lund); D. Nikolopoulos (Athens); S.H. Ninio (Sofia); P. Pascual (Givona); J. Rey (Paris); E. Rossi (Bern); J. Salazar de Sousa (Lisbon); J. Visakorpi (Helsinki).

REFERENCES

1. Seignobos C. 1815–1915. *Du congrès de Vienne à la guerre de 1914*. Paris: Hachette, 1915.
2. Hobsbawm EJ. *The age of revolution in Europe (1789–1848)*. Lourdes: NAL, 1962.
3. De Tocqueville A. *L'ancien Régime et la Révolution*. Paris: Gallimard, 1952.
4. L'homme J. *La grande bourgeoisie au pouvoir 1830–1880*. Paris: PUF, 1960.
5. Marx K, Engels F. *Kommunistisches Manifest*. London, 1848.
6. Evans RJ. *The feminist women's emancipation movements in Europe, America and Australasia 1840–1920*. London: Croom Helm, 1977.
7. Frank JP. Oratio academica de populorum miseria, morborum genitrice. In: Cid F. *Breve historia de las ciencias medicas*, Barcelona: Espaxs, 1978.
8. Villermè M. Tableau physique et moral des ouvriers employes dans les manufactures de coton, de laine et de soie en 1840. Quoted by Mesliand CL In: *La formacion de un mercado mundial; Historia Universal*, vol 8. Barcelona: Salvat, 1980.
9. Chadwick E. The moral and physical condition of the working classes employed in the cotton manufactures in Manchester. Quoted by F Cid.In: *Breve historia de las ciencias medicas*. Barcelona: Espaxs, 1978.
10. Virchow R. Quoted by P Lain Entralgo. In: *Historia de la medicina*. Barcelona: Salvat, 1978.
11. Kemp T. *Industrialisation in nineteenth century Europe*. London: Longman, 1969.
12. Tudesq AJ. Los cambios sociales y el apogeo de la burguesia. In: *Historia universal*, vol 8. Barcelona: Salvat, 1980.
13. Guillaume P. Las transformaciones sociales y economicas del siglo XIX. In: *Historia universal*, vol 8. Barcelona: Salvat, 1980.
14. Frank JP. *System einer vollständigen medizinischen Polizey*. Mannheim: CF Schwan, 1780.
15. Hufeland CW. Guter Rat an Mütter über die wichtigsten Punkte der physischen Erziehung der Kinder in den ersten Jahren nebst einem Unterricht für junge Eheleute betr. die Vorsorge für Ungeborene. 4te Aufl. Berlin, 1835.
16. Bichat MFX. *Anatomie générale appliquée à la physiologie et à la médecine*. 2 vols. Paris, 1801.
17. Bichat MFX. *Recherches physiologique sur la vie et la mort*. Paris, 1800.
18. Laennec RTH. *De l'auscultation médiate*. 2 vols. Paris, 1819.
19. Henle J. Quoted by P Lain Entralgo In: *Historia de la medicina*. Barcelona: Salvat, 1977.
20. Rokitanski C. *Handbuch der Speziellen Pathologischen Anatomie*. Wien: Braumuller und Seidel, 1842.
21. Broussais FJV. *Examen de la doctrine médicale généralement adoptée*. Paris, 1809.
22. Virchow RLK. *Die Cellularpathologie in ihrer Begründung auf physiologische und pathologische Gewebelehre*. Berlin, 1858.
23. Koch R. Die Aetiologie der Tuberkulose. *Klin Wochenschr* Berlin: 1882;19:221–30.
24. Röntgen WC. Ueber eine neue Art von Strahlen. *SB Phys-Med Ges Würzburg* 1895;132–41.

25. Semmelweis IPh. Quoted by F Cid In: *Breve historia de las ciencias medicas*. Barcelona: ES-PAXS, 1978.
26. Bergmann E von. Quoted by P Lain Entralgo. In: *Historia de la medicina*. Barcelona: Salvat, 1978.
27. Bernard C. *Introduction à l'étude de la médecine expérimentale*. Paris, 1865.
28. Meissner FL. *Grundlage der Literatur der Pädiatrie, enthaltend die Monographien über die Kinderkrankheiten*. Leipzig, 1850.
29. Rosen von Rosenstein N. *Underrättelser om barn sjukdomar och deras bote-model*. Stockholm: Lars Salvius, 1764.
30. Vahlquist B, Wallgren A. Nils Rosen von Rosenstein and his textbook on paediatrics. *Acta Paediatr Scand* (suppl) 156. Uppsala, 1964.
31. Underwood M. *Treatise on the diseases of children*. London, 1784. French Translation Paris-Montpellier: Gabon, 1823.
32. Girtanner Ch. *Abhandlung über die Krankheiten der Kinder und über die physische Erziehung derselben*. Berlin, 1794.
33. Jahn N. Neues System der Kinderkrankheiten nach Erjahrung und brownischen Grundsätzen. 1803. Quoted by B Vahlquist, A Wallgren. In: Nils Rosen von Rosenstein and his textbook on paediatrics. *Acta Paediatr Scand* (suppl)156. Uppsala, 1964.
34. Billard CM. *Traité des maladies des enfants nouveau-nés et à la mamelle*. Paris, 1828.
35. Billard CM. *Atlas d'anatomie pathologique pour servir à l'histoire des maladies des enfants*. Paris, 1828.
36. Capuron J. *Traité des maladies des enfants jusqu'à la puberté*, 2nd edition. Paris: Croullebois, 1813.
37. Barthez E, Rilliet F. *Traité clinique et pratique des maladies des enfants*. Paris: Germer-Baillière, 1843.
38. Bretonneau P. *Traité de la Difterite, angine maligne ou croup épidemique*. Paris, 1826.
39. Bednar A. *Die Krankheiten der Neugeborenen und Säuglinge*. Wien: C Gerold, 1850.
40. Krepler P, Gadner H. *Das Kind und sein Arzt*. Wien: Facultas Universitätsverlag, 1988.
41. Gerhardt C. *Handbuch der Kinderheilkunde*, 1st ed. Tübingen: Verlag d H Lauppschen Buchhandlung, 1877–1880.
42. Latronico N. *Storia della pediatria*. Torino: Edizioni Minerva Medica, 1977.
43. *100 Jahre Kinderspital Zürich 1874–1974*. Zürich: Buchdruckerei Berichthaus, 1974.
44. Feer E. *Lehrbuch der Kinderheilkunde*. 1. Auflage. Jena: Gustav Fischer, 1911.
45. Feer E. Eine eigenartige Neurose des vegetativen Systems beim Kleinkinde. *Ergeb Inn Med Kinderheilk* 1923;24:100–22.
46. Fanconi G. Studien über die Serumlipase. *Fermentforsch* 1923;7:307–48.
47. Fanconi G. Die chronischen Verdauungsstörungen des älteren Kindes (Herter'scher Infantilismus) und ihre Behandlung mit Früchten und Gemüsen. *Schweiz Med Wochenschr* 1928;38:789–99.
48. Fanconi G, Uehlinger E, Knauer C. Das Coeliakiesyndrom bei angeborener zystischer Pankreasfibromatose und Bronchiektasien. *Wien Med Wochenschr* 1936;86:753–6.
49. Fanconi G, Botsztejn A. Die familiäre Pankreasfibrose mit Bronchiektasien. *Schweiz Med Wochenschr* 1944;74:85–93.
50. Fanconi G, Botsztejn A. Die Feer'sche Krankheit (Akrodynie) und Quecksilbermedikation. *Helv Paediatr Acta* 1948;3:264–71.
51. Fanconi G, Wallgren A. *Lehrbuch der Pädiatrie*. 1.Auflage. Basel, Stuttgart: Schwabe, 1950.
52. Hottinger A von. Das Kinderspital Basel. Historische Studie. *Ann Paediatr* 1962;199:1–26.
53. List of displaced German scholars. London, Autumn 1936. In: *Lebendige Pädiatrie*. Munich: Marseille Verlag, 1983.
54. Moll H. Pädiater im Exil. In: *Lebendige Pädiatrie*. Munich: Marseille Verlag, 1983.
55. Sommer P, Leu F. *Das Jenner Kinderspital in Bern, 1862–1962*. Bern: Buchbinderarbeit Stämpfli, 1978.
56. Glanzmann E. Dysporia entero-broncho-pancreatica congenita familiaris. Cystische Pankreasfibrose. *Ann Paediatr* 1946;166:289–313.
57. Higgins TT. *Great Ormond Street, 1852–1952*. London: Odhams Press, 1952.
58. Besser FS. 125 Jahre hospital for sick children London. *Med Welt* 1978;29:645–50.
59. Stürzbecher M. Die Geschichte der Kinderheilkunde in Berlin. *Med Mittlg Schering* AG 20, 1959;2:2–6.
60. Dost FH. *Geschichte der Universitätskinderklinik der Charité zu Berlin*. Giessen, 1960.

61. Henoch E. *Vorlesungen über Kinderkrankheiten.* 7 Aufl. Berlin, 1893.
62. Heubner O. *Lehrbuch der Kinderheilkunde.* 2 Bde. Leipzig, 1903–1906.
63. Reuss A. *Die Krankheiten des Neugeborenen.* Berlin: Springer, 1914.
64. Schlossmann A. Die Geschichte der Gesellschaft für Kinderheilkunde in Beziehung zur Entwicklung der Kinderheilkunde in den letzten 25 Jahren. Verhandlg 25, Vers Ges für Kinderheilk. Cologne-Wiesbaden, 1908.
65. Windorfer A, Schlenk R. *Die Deutsche Gesellschaft für Kinderheilkunde.* Berlin: Springer, 1978.
66. Schweier P, Seidler E. *Lebendige Pädiatrie.* Verlag: Marseille, 1983.
67. Pfaundler M, Schlossmann A. *Handbuch der Kinderheilkunde.* 1st ed. Leipzig: FWC Vogel, 1906.
68. Baader G. Psychiatrie, Psychotherapie, Psychosomatik. In: Ev Akad Bad Boll (Hrsg); *Medizin im Nationalsozialismus.* Bad Boll, 1982.
69. Winau R. Euthanasie und Sterilisation. In: Ev Akad Bad Boll (Hrsg): *Medizin im Nationalsozialismus.* Bad Boll, 1982.
70. Kleinschmidt H. Eröffnungsansprache der 48. Vers der Dtsch Ges für Kinderheilk. Göttingen, 1948. *Mschr Kinderheilk* 1949;97:97–101.
71. Parrot J. *L'athrepsie.* Paris: Masson, 1877.
72. Parrot MJ. Sur une pseudo-paralysie causée par une altération du système osseux chez les nouveau-nés atteints de syphilis héréditaire. *Arch de Phys,* 1872.
73. Parrot MJ. La syphilis héréditaire et le rachitisme. *Progres Medical,* 1880.
74. Huard P, Laplane R, Imbault-Huart MJ. *Histoire illustrée de la pédiatrie,* vol 3. Paris: Editions Roger Dacosta, 1983.
75. Marfan AB. *Traité de l'allaitement.* Paris: G. Steinhell, 1981.
76. Grancher J, Comby J, Marfan AB. *Traité des maladies de l'enfance.* 5 vol. Paris: Masson 1897–1898.
77. Hutinel V. *Les maladies des enfants.* Paris: Asselin et Houzeau, 1909.
78. Marx FF. *Die Entwicklung der Säuglingsinkubatoren.* Bonn: Verlag Siering KG, 1968.
79. West C. *Lectures on the diseases of infancy and childhood.* London: Longman, 1848.
80. West C. *On some disorders of the nervous system in childhood.* London: Longman, 1871.
81. McNeil C. John Thomson. In: Veeder BS. *Pediatric profiles.* St Louis: Mosby Co, 1957.
82. Barlow A. Sir Thomas Barlow. In: Veeder BS. *Pediatric profiles.* St Louis: Mosby Co, 1957.
83. Sheldon W. George Frederic Still. In: Veeder BS. *Pediatric profiles.* St Louis: Mosby Co, 1957.
84. Still GF. On a form of chronic joint disease in children. *Med chir Trans* 1897;80:47.
85. Still GF. *The history of pediatrics.* London: Oxford University Press, 1931.
86. Hirschsprung H. Stuhlträgheit Neugeborener infolge von Dilatation und Hypertrophie des Colons. *Jahrb Kinderh* 1887;27:1–8.
87. Ballowitz L. Arvo Ylppö der Archiater Finnlands ein Sohn des kavh. Schriftenreihe zur Geschichte der Kinderheilkunde aus dem Archiv des Kaiserin Auguste Victoria Hauses (KAVH) Berlin. Humana Milchwerke Westfalen, Heft 3, 1987.
88. Ylppö A. Neugeborenen. Hunger und Intoxikationsacidosis in ihren Beziehungen zueinander. *Z Kinderheilk* 1916;14:268.
89. Ylppö A. Pathologische-anatomische Studien bei Frühgeburten. *Z Kinderheilk* 1919;20:211.
90. Granjel LS. *Historia de la pediatria española.* Cuadernos de historia de la medicina española, Universidad de Salamanca. Salamanca, *Ediciones del Seminario de Historia de la Medicina Española.* 1965.
91. Fracastoro G. *De contagione et contagiosis morbis.* Venice, 1546.
92. Bassi A. *Sui contagi in generale e segnatamente su quelli che affliggono l'umana specie.* Lodi, 1844.
93. Trousseau A. Clinique médicale de l'Hôtel Dieu de Paris. Paris: JB Baillière, 2 vol, 1861.
94. Trousseau A. *Du tubage de la glotte et de la tracheotomie.* Paris: Ballière, 1859.
95. Bouchut E. Mémoire sur une nouvelle méthode de traitement de l'asphyxie du croup par le tubage du larynx. *Compte rendus de l'Académie des sciences,* 1858.
96. Casales P. *De morbo Garrotillo appellato.* Madrid, 1611.
97. Mancebo Aguado P. *De essentia signis, causis, prognostico et curatione Anginae, vulgo Garrotillo.* Sevilla, 1618.
98. Ghisi M. Quoted by Latronico N. In: *Storia della pediatria.* Torino: Edizioni Minerva Medica, 1977.
99. Zeiss H, Bieling R. *Behring, Gestalt und Werk.* Berlin: Bruno Schultz, 1940.

100. Schick B. Pediatrics in Vienna at the beginning of the century. In: Veeder BS. *Pediatric profiles*. St Louis: Mosby Co, 1957.
101. Peiper A. Historia de la pediatria. In: Opitz H, Schmid F. *Enciclopedia pediatrica* vol I/1. Madrid: Ediciones Morata, 1973.
102. Uffelmann J. *Handbuch der privaten und öffentlichen Hygiene des Kindes*. Leipzig, 1881.
103. Pettenkofer M, Ziemssen H. *Handbuch der Hygiene und der Gewerbekrankheiten*. Leipzig: FC Vogel, 1882.
104. Grotjahn A, Kaup J. Handwörterbuch der sozialen Hygiene. Leipzig: FC Vogel, 1912.
105. Escherich T. Die Darmbakterien des Neugeborenen und Säuglings. *Fortschr Med* 1885;3:515.
106. Escherich T. *Die Darmbakterien des Säuglings und ihre Beziehungen zur Physiologie der Verdauung*. Stuttgart: Ferdinand Enke, 1886.
107. Adam A. Biology of colon bacillus dyspepsia and its relation to pathogenesis and to intoxication. *Jahrbuch Kinderheilk* 1923;101:295.
108. Kauffman F. Über neue thermolabile Körper-antigene der Coli-bakterien. *Acta Pathol Mikrobiol Scand* 1943;20:21.
109. Czerny A, Keller A. *Des Kindes Ernährung, Ernährungsstörungen und Ernährungstherapie*. 2 Bde. Leipzig, 1906–1917.
110. Schiff E. Adalbert Czerny In: Veeder BS. *Pediatric profiles*. St. Louis: Mosby Co, 1957.
111. Finkelstein H. *Lehrbuch der Säuglingskrankheiten*. Berlin: Buchhandlung H Kornfeld, 1912.
112. Finkelstein H. *Tratado de las enfermedades del lactante*, 3rd ed, Barcelona: Labor, 1941.
113. Rosenstern I. Heinrich Finkelstein. In: Veeder BS. *Pediatric profiles*. St. Louis: Mosby Co, 1957.
114. Ariztia A. El Profesor Finkelstein y la personalidad del maestro. *Rev Chilena de Pediatria* 1942;13:485–91.
115. Ballowitz L. Aufnahmefrequenz, Diagnosen und Letalität im KAVH 1909–1947. Schriftenreihe zur Geschichte der Kinderheilkunde aus dem Archiv des Kaiserin Auguste Victoria Hauses (KAVH). Berlin: Humana Milchwerke Westfalen, 1986.
116. Loeschke A. Das Kaiserin Auguste Victoria Haus 1909 bis 1959. *Berliner Medizin* 1959, 5–8.
117. Joppich G. Das Kaiserin Auguste Victoria Haus und die Anfänge der Sozialpädiatrie in Deutschland. *Der Kinderarzt* 1975;5.
118. Teixeira de Mattos. Quoted by Schreier In: Säuglingsernährung In: *Lebendige Pädiatrie*. Munich: Marseille Verlag, 1983.
119. Finkelstein H, Myere LF. *Ueber Eiweissmilch. Ein Beitrag zum Problem der künstlichen Ernährung*. Berlin: Karger, 1910.
120. Feer E. Säuglingsernährung mit einer einfachen Eiweiss-Rahmmilch. *Jahrb Kinderheilk* 1913; 78:1–46.
121. Chasin-Sobol NJ. *Über die Ernährung kranker Säuglinge mit Gartner'scher Fettmilch*. Zürich: Diss, 1909.
122. Mauthner LW. Karottenbrei zur künstlichen Ernährung von Säuglingen. *J Kinderkr* 1850;14:316.

DISCUSSION

Dr. Stern: You opened your paper with Goethe. Goethe was in fact the main supporter of *Naturphilosophie* and he waged a running battle with Thomas Huxley. He believed the world would remember him as a scientist rather than as the author of *Wilhelm Meister*. He believed in the pantheistic theory of light, arguing that it could not be broken up into its component parts because it was created by God as a single color. However, his quotations about science were wonderful. In particular he argued that where there is little knowledge there is much discussion.

I was also interested in what you said about the Kaiserin Auguste Victoria Haus. The Kaiser was so enamored of the Kaiserin that when he took her to Jerusalem he had the main gate to the old city widened so that her carriage could pass through it. The Arab Children's Hospital on Mount Scopus is still called the Auguste Victoria Hospital after her.

Ylppö's work in the Kaiserin Auguste Victoria Haus in Berlin was of extreme importance.

In 1903, three years before Van den Berg described his bilirubin reaction, he wrote in a monograph that there was something unusual about the umbilical cord because it appeared yellow. He speculated that it contained an unidentified pigment.

Dr. Ballabriga: Medicine represented an important part of the intellectual expression of romanticism, and was promoted by figures from the German Idealism movement such as Hegel and Schnelling. These were called *naturphilosphers.* The heyday of this period was 1800 to 1850, and particularly until 1830 with the rediscovery of Paracelsus. Romanticism later diminished, passing through an intermediate phase to *Naturwissenschaft,* with supporters such as Müller and Liebig, and finally toward a pathophysiological doctrine with Traube, Frerichs, and Wunderlich, among others.

With regard to the Kaiserin Auguste Victoria Haus in Berlin: it was directed by Leo Langstein at the time of Ylppö's most important work (on acidosis of the newborn, necropsy examinations of premature infants, and Salvarsan treatment of congenital syphilis). This was in the period 1912 to 1920, before he returned to Helsinki. The history of the Augusta Victoria Haus is very well covered in a publication by Leonore Ballowitz.

Dr. Kaufman: It is correct that the problem of the membrane in whooping cough produced a great diagnostic dilemma, particularly in relation to other non-infectious diseases. However, long before the 1850s it was an American, Benjamin Rush, the man who started the first medical school in the United States and who signed the Declaration of Independence, who first described (in a letter to John Millar in 1759) the difference between wheezing from the membrane of diphtheria and wheezing due to asthma.

Dr. Ballabriga: Rush lived before the time we are dealing with. I know of his publication of 1773 on the *Cause and Cure of Cholera Infantum;* however I do not know what he had to say about the differences between diphtheria and whooping cough. He surely must have referred to these, since he also studied scarlet fever. But the clinical individuality of diphtheria as a "malignant angina" was described by Bretonneau under the name *difterité* in 1826. The epidemic character of diphtheria had already been described by Martino Ghisi in Cremona in 1749, based on the observation of epidemic outbreaks, and he called attention to the presence of pseudomembranes.

Dr. Guesry: Do you know what led to the creation in Paris of the first children's hospital in 1802? Was it to prevent cross-infection between children and adults, or was it in order to have more specialized physicians and nurses? Was room for lactating mothers provided, or was the hospital only for older children?

Dr. Ballabriga: The first children's hospitals were dedicated only to children beyond the period of lactation because of the high mortality that could be caused by cross-infection in infants. Bela Schick recounts how, when Escherich opened an infant ward in Vienna, all the children including the son of the wet nurse died in a short space of time.

Dr. Laplane: There were two reasons for building children's hospitals. In the first place, physicians were convinced that it was necessary to separate children from adults. Secondly, it became necessary to differentiate between a hospice—a place of refuge for children—and a hospital, which was devoted to the care of children with disease.

History of Pediatrics 1850–1950, edited by
B.L. Nichols, A. Ballabriga, and N. Kretchmer.
Nestlé Nutrition Workshop Series, Vol. 22. Nestec
Ltd., Vevey/Raven Press, Ltd., New York © 1991.

German Pediatrics

Wolfgang Braun

*Department of Pediatrics, Karl-Marx-University, Leipzig 7050, Democratic Republic of
Germany*

In dealing with this topic I shall concentrate on German countries only and exclude German-speaking countries such as Austria and the German-speaking part of Switzerland, although the pediatric relationships between these countries and Germany are of great importance for the development of pediatrics and child health. The term *school* needs explanation, since different definitions are used.

For our purposes it is sufficient to formulate some practical criteria characterizing a school. In my opinion these are: the leadership of an outstanding personality; the study of common and important scientific problems; uniform methods of investigation and interpretation; major dissemination of scientific ideas; and an institution as a basis for collaborative work (this may be a hospital, an institute, or a laboratory).

The leading personality ranks first. This does not only mean that he or she has the best ideas. Of equal importance is the ability to create and lead a team able to continue the work of the master creatively in the future. Preservation of a tradition is not sufficient in itself. I shall consider the development of pediatrics in Germany in this light.

SOCIOECONOMIC AND POLITICAL BACKGROUND

Infant mortality rate in the nineteenth century was about 20%, latterly tending to increase (1). At the same time, the birth rate decreased. The connection between industrialization and the changing social situation was obvious: an enlarging working class, bad living conditions in overcrowded cities, industrial work by women, low rates of breast feeding, lack of artificial food, and a high incidence of infectious diseases in overcrowded homes. In this situation the child became the great social challenge for pediatrics as well as for the government and the local health authorities. Czerny knew this when he wrote that there had always been a great demand for pediatrics when a disproportion between mortality and birth rate developed (2). This phenomenon was observed at the end of the World War I. Within a few years, 14 of 19 German universities founded chairs of pediatrics (3). This development was initiated by a resolution of the 31st assembly of the German Pediatric Society, held on

September 22, 1917, at the Leipzig Children's Hospital. In his memorable speech *"Kinderkrankheiten und Krieg"* ("Children's Diseases and War"), A. Schlossmann proved the need for medical education to include pediatrics (3). The memorandum with the title *"Unterricht in der Pädiatrie und seine Bedeutung für die Bevölkerungspolitik"* ("Teaching in Pediatrics and Its Importance for Population Policy") resulted in the establishment of new chairs within two years.

THE SCIENTIFIC BASIS FOR THE DEVELOPMENT OF PEDIATRIC SCHOOLS

By the middle of the eighteenth century, some books on diseases of children had already been published, mainly nosological descriptions of diseases or combinations of symptoms with a practical orientation. In the nineteenth century, scientific interest in the child became dominant. Rudolf Virchow's book, *Cellularpathologie,* (1858) became the scientific morphological basis for pediatrics and many other medical disciplines in research and practice. The professor of internal medicine Carl Gerhardt (1833–1902) (Fig. 1), like Virchow, worked at the University of Würzburg, and promoted clinical work based on the local morphological diagnosis of clinical symptoms (4). New methods of clinical investigation, including percussion and auscultation, microscopic examination and chemical methods, were introduced into clinical medicine. Doctors of internal medicine such as Otto Heubner (1843–1926) in Leipzig and Gerhardt in Würzburg, for scientific or practical considerations, promoted the view that pediatrics should be an independent teaching subject at the universities. The traditional medical faculties, however, tried to inhibit the formation of pediatric chairs. When Heubner (Fig. 2) opened the modern Town Hospital for Children in Leipzig, the faculty refused to appoint him Professor and Chairman of Pediatrics. Two years later he was appointed Chairman of Pediatrics at Berlin University, also against the vote of the faculty. However their decision was overruled by Althoff, director at the Ministry of Culture, who was an important promoter of pediatrics in Prussia. Another example occurred in Jena, where Jussuf Ibrahim became Chairman of Pediatrics in 1917. The faculty decided that infectious disease was a branch of internal medicine and restricted the pediatricians' care to children with such diseases.

The foundation of scientific pediatrics in Germany was largely due to the work of C. Gerhardt. His important speech at the Pediatric Section of the Society for Medicine *(Gesellschaft für Heilkunde)* in Berlin on April 24th, 1879, is worthy of mention (4,5). The study of the pathology of childhood, he said, was a challenge of the time. He referred to the great schools of pediatrics in Paris and Vienna, which promoted pediatrics with their morphologically oriented clinical work. Gerhardt not only demanded microscopic research, but also stressed the physiologic aspects of pediatrics, because "differences between the developing and the developed body are less a question of structure than of function." He felt that it was important to study diseases in the growing and developing body, and to make scientific general-

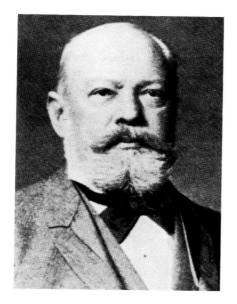 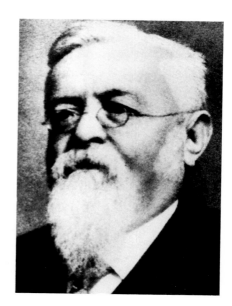

FIG. 1. Carl Gerhardt (1833–1902).   **FIG. 2.** Otto Heubner (1843–1926).

izations from the results of many individual studies. E. Seidler (6) called Gerhardt's speech the hour of birth of German scientific pediatrics. With his great manual of diseases in children (7), the first in the German language and edited between 1877 and 1896, Gerhardt became the most important promoter of pediatrics in science and practice.

THE FOUNDATION OF THE GERMAN PEDIATRIC SOCIETY

This was a very important event in the process of establishing pediatrics in German universities. The society developed from the Section *für Pädiatrie* of the *Gesellschaft für Naturforscher und Ärzte* (Society of German Natural Scientists and Physicians). The majority of medical societies had originated in this way. The initiator of the Section for Pediatrics was August Steffen, who was not a member of a university faculty but organized summer courses in pediatrics for students and young physicians. He held that the basis of practical pediatrics should be the study of physiology of children; that university hospitals with necessary pediatric teaching personnel should be founded; and that outpatient departments should be opened to allow children to be treated within their families (Seidler, in 3). Steffen and Rudolf Demme, a pharmacologist and pediatrician in Bern, later proposed that the Section for Pediatrics should be replaced by an independent Society for Pediatrics. This aim was achieved at the 56th meeting of the Gesellschaft Deutscher Naturforscher und Ärzte in September, 1883, in Freiburg.

THE SCHOOL OF PEDIATRICS AT BERLIN

When Otto Heubner was called from Leipzig to Berlin, he found a pediatric tradition already established. The Friedrich-Wilhelm University was the first university to appoint pediatricians to lecture in pediatrics. The first such lecturer was Stephan Barenz, and the first extraordinary professor of pediatrics was Eduard Henoch, founder of the children's hospital at the Charité, a hospital with all the problems of the time. The clinical mortality rate of infants was 76%, and Henoch advised Heubner to close the infant ward (2).

In Leipzig Heubner had already shown his talent for scientific work. He was also a splendid organizer and architect. Heubner's children's hospital in Leipzig was the most modern of the time. The situation in Berlin was extremely unsatisfactory, but Heubner forced through the establishment of a new hospital, which was opened in 1903. This provided a base for his scientific work. Collaborating with Julius Cohnheim, pathologist in Leipzig, Heubner had already proved his ability to do scientific work. However he found the morphologic approach insufficient and turned to physiologic methods. In close collaboration with the physiologist Rubner he did important work on energy metabolism in infancy. The term respiratory *quotient* goes back to Heubner. Celiac disease is called Heubner disease or Heubner-Herter disease in Germany. As a scientist and teacher, later chairmen of pediatrics in other universities, and with numerous co-workers and scientific disciples, Heubner became the founder of the first school of pediatrics in Germany.

Heinrich Finkelstein (see p. 140, Fig. 3) must be especially mentioned as Heubner's disciple. His textbook (8) of diseases of infants is worth reading even in our time. He received special acknowledgment for his research work on infant nutrition, and he created the so-called *Eiweissmilch* (casein-enriched milk). This milk was being used as recently as 1960 at the children's hospital in Jena, with quite good results with dystrophic and enteritic infants. I have been told by a former patient of Finkelstein, living in London, that he was an excellent physician and family doctor.

When Heubner retired in 1913 he left not only a highly regarded department and a hospital of the same high standard as the hospital for internal medicine; he was also responsible for a general appreciation of the importance of pediatrics in the whole of Germany. Heubner's successor was Adalbert Czerny (Fig. 3). Many years earlier in Prague, Heubner called the young pediatric scientist Czerny to the attention of the Culture Minister Althoff. After studies in morphology and training in internal medicine and physiological chemistry, Czerny joined the staff of the Epstein Hospital, where he was able to study diseases of infants. He was called to Breslau, Strassburg and in 1913 to Berlin. Like Heubner he turned his interest from structure to function, and carried out important research on metabolism. He published his work in a textbook that he edited with Arthur Keller: *Des Kindes Ernährung, Ernährungsstörungen und Ernährungstherapie (Child Nutrition, Nutritional Disorders and Nutritional Therapy)* (9). Czerny introduced the terms for nutritional disorders: *ex alimentatione, ex infectione,* and *ex constitutione.* These have been used didactically in pediatric education up to the present. Czerny's *Lectures on Pediatrics* (10), giv-

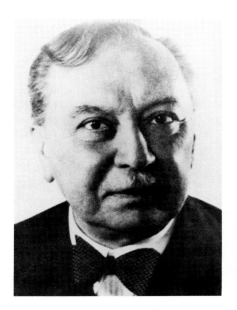 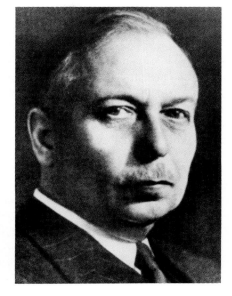

FIG. 3. Adalbert Czerny (1863–1941).   **FIG. 4.** Georg Bessau (1884–1944).

ing his personal view of pediatric diseases and children's problems, still make good reading today. It has been said that Czerny taught more on scientific questions (and this at a very high level), than on diseases as such. F.H. Dost (2) emphasized that Czerny's work led to international appreciation of German pediatrics. Of Czerny's numerous disciples, Arthur Keller, head of the Kaiserin Auguste Victoria Haus, and H. Kleinschmidt deserve first mention. The doctrines of the Czerny school and their applications contributed to an improvement of child health and to a diminution of infant mortality. Without doubt, the pediatric school at Berlin had its heyday in the Czerny era.

Georg Bessau (Fig. 4), another pediatrician from Leipzig, was appointed at Berlin as Czerny's successor. After studies in bacteriology and immunology he turned to pediatrics. He introduced clinical bacteriology in Leipzig, and this is still a recognized speciality in my hospital. His plasma therapy of toxic shock is well known. However, Bessau's time in Berlin was the time of fascism in Germany, with all its consequences.

THE PEDIATRIC SCHOOL OF MUNICH

The Munich school of pediatrics is also of special importance for the development of pediatrics in Germany. This is mainly due to the von Haunersche Kinderspital, (11,12), which was founded in 1848 and which became a university hospital in 1886. A particular attribute of Munich is the existence of a separate clinical institute of pediatrics. One of the important heads of this institute was H. von Ranke. After studies in London with Sir William Jenner and Charles West, (see p. 32, Fig. 1) he became at first prosector, and later head of the clinical institute and, in 1887, director of the von Hauner Hospital. Ranke's successor was Meinhardt von Pfaundler, an Austrian from Graz. With M. von Pfaundler, Munich became a great pediatric center. The personality and life of Pfaundler show the factors involved in the successful development of a school—scientific ability, powers of communication, and an extraordinary talent for organization. Pfaundler organized the financial support needed for a new pediatric hospital from official and private sponsors. His handbook of pediatrics (4 volumes) edited in conjunction with Schlossmann in 1906, shows the high level achieved by Pfaundler and his school. With various collaborators, Pfaundler worked in nearly all pediatric fields. Today his explanations on growth and differentiation are still valid. He pointed out: "Growth stimulates and produces differentiation but differentiation inhibits growth; in this way a self-control of growth can be recognized" (13). His studies on growth (1916) show his mathematical talent. The condition *dysostosis multiplex* is known as Pfaundler-Hurler disease.

The child was the important factor in Pfaundler's Hospital. He is quoted as saying, "the patients are not here for us, we are here for the patients" (11). This tradition is taught and maintained by Klaus Betke, one of the scientific descendants of Pfaundler (14). Meinhard von Pfaundler worked for 33 years as director and chairman of the Munich University Children's Hospital, and during this time an important pediatric school developed. Many hospitals and pediatric chairs founded after the World War I were managed by Pfaundler's academic disciples.

PEDIATRICS BETWEEN 1933 AND 1945

It is impossible to talk about the highlights of pediatrics in Germany without examining the darkest chapter of German history, the time of fascism, which ended with World War II. But the war was only the culmination of this period. It began with the development of fascist ideology, with the Nürnberg laws and the ideas of worthless life, with sterilization of men and women, and killing of malformed and handicapped children. There were some pediatricians who, infected with fascist ideology, were willing to put these ideas into practice, men such as Catel. The banishment of many Jewish colleagues, and later the Holocaust, caused great damage to pediatrics. About 15% of German physicians were Jews, a great number of them pediatricians (15). Such famous names as Albert Eckstein, Stefan Engel, Heinrich Finkelstein, Ernst Freudenberg, Siegfried Rosenbaum, and Erwin Schiff had to leave their native country—an immeasurable loss for German pediatrics.

A NEW BEGINNING

In 1945, at the end of the war, German pediatrics was in ruins. But this became a challenge and also an opportunity for all pediatricians. The needs of children were boundless, morbidity and mortality had increased, hospitals were destroyed. Care for the children was the first duty immediately after war. Everything was lacking: food, medical facilities, medical personnel. But the most important thing to overcome was the ideologic burden of fascism. At the end of the 100-year period from 1850 to 1950, we find two German states, the Federal Republic of Germany and the German Democratic Republic, each with different political and socioeconomic circumstances. The effects of this on the future development of pediatrics are another chapter of pediatric history.

REFERENCES

1. Peiper A. *Chronik der Kinderheilkunde*. Leipzig: G Thieme, 1951.
2. Dost FH. Geschichte der Universitäts-Kinderklinik der Charitè zu Berlin: *Kinderarzt* 1980;11:99–103, 249–56, 409–15.
3. Schweier P, Seidler E. *Lebendige Pädiatrie*. Munich: H Marseille, 1983.
4. Seidler E. Carl Gerhardt und seine Rede: "dis Aufgaben und Ziele der Kinderheilkunde." *Monatsschr Kinderheilkd* 1983;131:545.
5. Gerhardt C. Uber die Aufgaben und Ziele der Kinderheilkunde. *Dtsch Med Wochenscht* 1879; 5:215–8.
6. Seidler E. Daten zur Geschichte der Deutschen Gessellschaft für Kinderheilkunde. *Monatsschr Kinderheilk* 1983;131:544.
7. Gerhardt C. *Handbuch der Kinderkrankheiten*. Tübingen, 1877.
8. Finkelstein H. *Lehrbuch der Säuglingskrankheiten*. Berlin, 1912.
9. Czerny A, Keller A. *Des Kindes Ernährung, Ernährungsstörungen und Ernährungstherapie*. Leipzig and Vienna, 1906–1918.
10. Czerny A. *Sammlung klinischer Vorlesungen über Kinderheilkunde*. Leipzig: G Thieme, 1948.
11. Betke K. In: *Berichte aus der Universitätskinderklinik im Dr. von Haunerschen Kinderspital*. Munich, 1972.
12. Betke K. Das Dr. von Haunersche Kinderspital im Wandel der Zeit. *Kinderarzt* 1982;13:1090–6.
13. Pfaundler M, von Schlossmann A. *Handbuch der Kinderheilkunde*. Berlin: FCW Vogel, 1931.
14. Wiedemann HR. Pfaundler-Deszendenz. *Kinderarzt* 1985;167:1599–2001.
15. Thom A. Das Schicksal der jüdischen Ärzte unter dem Faschismus. *Humanitas* 1988;28 (No 23):8.

DISCUSSION

Dr. Waterlow: It would be appropriate to add to the list of pediatricians who had to emigrate from Germany the name of Paul Gyorgy, who became Professor of pediatrics at Philadelphia. At a personal level, he was an important link between European and Third World pediatrics. He took an intense interest in the Third World and showed great hospitality to all people working in pediatrics in those countries.

Dr. Ballabriga: In 1933, there were around 6,500 Jewish doctors in Germany of whom rather more than 300 were pediatricians. For political reasons many of them emigrated. Thirty well-known pediatricians previously working in Germany featured in a list of displaced German scholars published in London in 1936, many of whom had held university appointments. Some, such as L. Meyer, went to Jerusalem. Eckstein went to Ankara and later became the director of the Children's Hospital. Freudenberg went to Switzerland and became director of the Kinderspital in Basel, where I had personal dealings with him in 1944. With a few exceptions, it must be said that the European contribution toward harboring these highly qualified persons was poor.

Dr. Stern: Brown University, where I come from, has a special relationship with the medical school of the University of Rostock in the German Democratic Republic. We have an exchange program, both for students and faculty. Some Brown students get all their training there and vice versa. Would you tell us something about Rostock, which has a long pediatric tradition, and also about Jena, which you mentioned in your paper? How is it that the children's hospital in Jena is named the *Youssef Ibrahim*?

Dr. Braun: I was a student in Jena so I am familiar with the situation there. Jussuf Ibrahim was the first Professor of pediatrics in 1917. His main interest was pediatric clinical care rather than research. He was followed by E. Hässler from Leipzig, and then W. Plenert from Rostock, who reorganized research work in nutrition and hematology.

A few important pediatricians worked in Rostock. These include Stolte, known for a diabetes diet called *freie Kost,* and after the second World War, Kirchmayer and Liebe.

History of Pediatrics 1850–1950, edited by
B.L. Nichols, A. Ballabriga, and N. Kretchmer.
Nestlé Nutrition Workshop Series, Vol. 22. Nestec
Ltd., Vevey/Raven Press, Ltd., New York © 1991.

British Pediatrics

John A. Davis

Department of Pediatrics, Clinical School, University of Cambridge, Cambridge CB2 5JE, United Kingdom

Although the period to be covered in this workshop is the century beginning in 1850, the history of pediatrics in Britain since then cannot be understood except in relation to movements and events in the century before, i.e., approximately from 1750 to 1850. It was then that the foundations not only of British, but to some extent of European and American pediatrics, were laid by men such as George Armstrong (1) and my namesake, John Bunnel Davis (2)—a Scot and an East Anglian who were among the pioneers who established dispensaries for the children of the poor that were the embryos of our children's hospitals (although at the time Armstrong did not contemplate this development, stating, in an often-quoted letter, "if you separate an infant from its mother or nurse . . . you will break its heart immediately"). The dispensary movement coincided in time and spirit with the establishment of the Foundlings Hospital by Captain Coram, a good-hearted seaman whose associates included the musician Handel and the founder of the State of Georgia, General Oglethorpe. Sadly the dispensaries more or less died out in the United Kingdom—the demagogue Wilkes taking some part in scotching the movement— although the pediatric concept was exported to the continent and led to the creation of departments of pediatric medicine in a number of major European centers. The discipline was reimported after the 1848 revolutions—notably in Manchester (3,4) by the Prussian, Louis Borchandt, and the Hungarian, Josef Schopfer-Merei, (whose office has been preserved and can still be visited in Budapest). However, the Hospital for Sick Children, Great Ormond Street can trace its origins back to Davis's dispensaries via the leading spirit in its foundation, Dr. Charles West (5) (Fig. 1). From about the turn of the nineteenth century onwards, quite a large number of charitably founded "voluntary" children's hospitals were established in large British cities (6–12): that in Norwich, for instance, being mainly funded by the exertions of the singer, Jenny Lind. These hospitals recruited to their staff men and later women who earned their livings in general or consultant practice in surgery as well as medicine, acquired a certain know-how in the recognition and management of the diseases of childhood, and often worked as honorary consultants in the large general hospitals as well. They were essentially general physicians interested in children and their interests tended to be focused on diseases peculiar to children, as

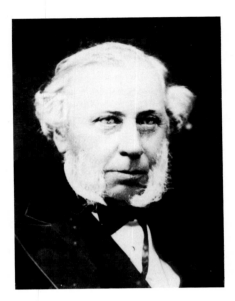

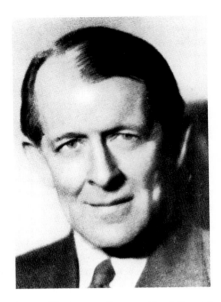

FIG. 1. Charles West, founder of Hospital for Sick Children, Great Ormond Street, London. (Courtesy of the British Pediatric Association.)

FIG. 2. Sir James Spence, the father of British social pediatrics. (Courtesy of the British Pediatric Association.)

others of their kind might have been interested in diseases of the heart or of women. It was by such men and women with essential clinical expertise that the first academic pediatric departments were to be established in Britain after the First, and particularly the Second World Wars, that in Newcastle being particularly noticeable because of the concern of its head, Sir James Spence (Fig. 2), with the social aspects of disease in childhood.

But British pediatrics did not grow entirely from one taproot (13–15). Around the turn of the century there was increasing governmental concern about the health of the poor, which in many cases was so precarious that children were not able to take advantage of their schooling, and which resulted in the rejection of a large proportion of recruits volunteering for army service. This led to the passage of enabling legislation authorizing local authorities to set up medical services for school children, and later for pregnant women and infants. Their brief was essentially surveillance and prevention but later they were to take on the task of immunization against infectious diseases and screening for mental and physical defects—the children so discovered being placed in appropriate special schools or excluded from education as being unable to take advantage of it. In time, enlightened authorities established institutions for the (then) long term management of children with chronic diseases such as tuberculosis (especially of bones and joints), osteomyelitis and rheumatic fever, while the longer established community fever hospitals catered to those with the known infectious fevers such as diphtheria, spotted fever (meningococemia), whooping cough, severe measles, etc. The purposes of these services were essentially social—to meet the needs of the community rather than of individuals—and they led to a rapid fall in infant mortality, from 150 per 1,000 at the turn of the century to less than a third of that figure in 1950, despite the two wars in between (16).

A third root must also be mentioned, i.e., access to general practitioners provided for by the extension of national health insurance from working men to their wives and children. But these developments came relatively late, and some of the poor continued to use hospital casualty departments as purveyors of primary care long after the establishment of the National Health Service (NHS) in 1946, almost at the end of the period under review. And, indeed, until comparatively recently, the original "voluntary" hospital services—sometimes extending their work into the so-called community—continued to run in tandem with the previous local authority services also taken over by the NHS—rather as the muddy Arve and the clear Rhone run in the same bed without mingling below Lake Leman.

So far I have said little about academic pediatrics in Britain. This is at least partly because the first (in Scotland) academic departments were founded only after the First World War and most after the Second (that in Manchester with the help of the Czech emigré, Aron Holzel), but it also stems from the fact that although British basic biological research and British clinical practice have always been of high quality, the middle ground—clinical science—developed relatively late in the United Kingdom and very late in the pediatric field, where English pragmatism tended to reign supreme. I well remember Professor Odon Kerpel-Fronius saying to me when I first visited Hungary in 1957 how impressed he was with British clinical expertise and how relatively he was disappointed in our science. There were notable exceptions—for instance, the distinguished pediatric hematologist, Sir Leonard Parsons (Fig. 3) in Birmingham, the first pediatric Fellow of the Royal Society and the first

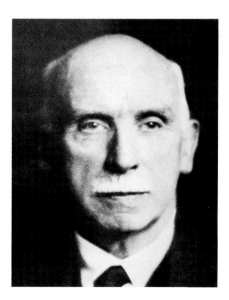

FIG. 3. Sir Leonard Parsons FRS, the father of English academic pediatrics. (Courtesy of the British Pediatric Association.)

worker to recognize that so-called erythroblastosis fetalis was a hemolytic disease—but they were exceptions to the rule. This situation was to be transformed in the 1950s by the connections forged between British and American Pediatric departments on the one hand and between British Pediatric and Physiology departments on the other—notably, in the latter case, the Nuffield Institute in Oxford, the Department of Experimental Medicine in Cambridge, and Huggett's group at St. Mary's, all interested in adaptation to extra-uterine life, and complementing the work of early neonatologists such as Dr. Mary Crosse in Birmingham.

One important academic landmark was the foundation of the British Pediatric Association (BPA) in 1928 on the model of Osler's Association of Physicians. The BPA initially provided a forum for the exchange of knowledge and opinion between the small number of physicians, surgeons, pathologists and public health doctors interested in children, but later, as it expanded its membership, it became concerned with child health in all its aspects. This came in time to include some child psychiatrists, their subject being actively explored at the time by analytically oriented psychiatrists such as Anna Freud, Melanie Klein, and, particularly, in this context, because of their peculiarly British points of view, Margaret Lowenfield and Donald Winnicott, who made London the world center in this field at that time (17). One consequence of this concern for the child as a person (which was reinforced by the experience of evacuation of children from major cities in the World War II) was a humanization of hospital practice leading to all-day visiting, rooming in, and home care—changes that would have pleased George Armstrong.

SUMMARY

British pediatrics was a late developer after a premature birth and a period of fostering abroad. This—with the tendency in British medicine for scientists not to be clinicians and vice versa—led to a certain weakness in clinical science. On the other hand, Britain may have led the world in the art of pediatric medicine, notable contributions to the natural history of children's diseases being made by men such as West (infantile spasms—*Blick Nick* and *Salaam krämpfe* or BNS fits), Gee (celiac disease), Still (Fig. 4) (juvenile arthritis), Little (cerebral palsy), Poynton and Coombes (rheumatic fever), Gauvaigne and Jones (bone and joint tuberculosis), Barlow (scurvy), Parsons (rickets), and, a bit later, Moncrieff and Dent, Schwarz, Holzel and Komrower (inborn errors of metabolism) and Cicely Williams (see p. 34, Fig. 1) (kwashiorkor), and also in the application of medical knowledge to child care in the community. A noticeable weakness was in the study of infectious disease and immunity—the result of the hiving off of children with acute infections to fever hospitals run by infectious disease physicians—and of electrolyte physiology in the context of gastroenteritis.

Both the strengths and weaknesses of British pediatricians in the period under review were at least due in part to the way in which British medicine was organized, as well as perhaps to the commonly noted indifference of English families to the

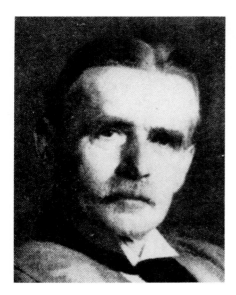

FIG. 4. Sir Frederick Still, the father of British clinical pediatrics.

well-being of their children. Certainly private pediatric practice has never flourished in the United Kingdom as it has elsewhere. But the advent of so-called socialized medicine, with the establishment of an NHS in 1946, changed both attitudes and organization, especially with the recent demonstration that the well-being of a cohort in infancy is the best predictor of its well-being up to old age.

REFERENCES

1. Maloney WJ. *George and John Armstrong of Castleton.* Edinburgh: E & S Livingstone, 1954.
2. Davis JB. *Annals historical and medical during the first four years of the universal dispensary for children.* London: Simkin & Marshall, 1821.
3. Wilkinson P. *The story of the Children's Hospital, Pendlebury, Manchester.* The Gutenberg Words, 1889.
4. Young JH. *St. Mary's Hospitals, Manchester 1790–1963.* Edinburgh: E & S Livingstone, 1964.
5. Higgins T. *Great Ormond Street 1852–1952.* London: Odhams Press, 1957.
6. Franklin AW. Children's hospitals. In: Poynter, ed. *The evolution of hospitals in Britain.* London: F.N.L Pitman Medical, 1964.
7. Hugo T. *The history of the Hospital of St Margaret, Taunton.* London, 1960.
8. Hunter RH. The Belfast Hospital for Sick Children. *Ulster Med J* 1937;No 6:46–50.
9. Ridley U. *The Babies Hospital, Newcastle upon Tyne.* Newcastle: Andrew Reid & Co, 1956.
10. Stanton BN. Title of the East London Hospital for Children. London, 1920.
11. Guthrie D. *The Royal Edinburgh Hospital for Sick Children 1860–1960.* Edinburgh: E & S Livingstone, 1960.
12. Waterhouse R. *Children in hospital: 100 years of child care in Birmingham.* London: Hutchinson, 1962.
13. Back EH, Levin S. Paediatrics of the past. A note on practice over the past 60 years in the Queen Elizabeth Hospital for Children. *Br Med J* 1954;ii:406–8.

14. Still GF. *A history of paediatrics*. Oxford: Oxford University Press, 1965.
15. Nicoll JH. The surgery of infancy. *Br Med J* 1909;II:753–4.
16. Frazer WM. *A history of English public health 1834–1939*. London: Balliere, Tindall and Cox, 1950.
17. Urwin C. Introduction. In: *Child psychotherapy: war and the normal child* (selected papers of Margaret Lowenfield). London: Association Books, 1988.

Further Reading

Armstrong G. *An essay on diseases most fatal to infants*. London, 1767.

Barker DJP, Osmond C. Inequalities in health in Britain: Specific explanations in three Lancashire towns. *Br Med J* 1987;294:749–52.

Brownslow J. *The history and design of the Foundling Hospital with a memoir of the founder*. London: Warr, 1858.

Cameron H. *The British Paediatric Association 1928–52*. London: Pitman, 1970.

Pinchbeck I, Hewitt M. Children in English society, vol. 2. Routledge/Kegan Paul: University of Toronto Press, 1969.

The Yorkhill story—the history of the Royal Hospital for Sick Children, Glasgow. Edna Robertson, Robert Maclehose and Cox Ltd: The University Press Glasgow, 1972.

DISCUSSION

Dr. Swyer: One of the themes that one could examine in studying the history of pediatrics is the interaction between the science of pediatrics, pediatric practice in general, and art. I should like to ask Professor Davis for a comment on the influence of Charles Dickens in arousing the social conscience of the British public in his novels, many of which have pediatric connotations.

Dr. Davis: Charles Dickens was one of the people who was involved in the establishment of the Hospital for Sick Children at Great Ormond Street. In his novel, *Bleak House*, Joe, the crossing sweeper, dies in Great Ormond Streeet.

Dr. Friis-Hansen: You mentioned that the study of the relationship between disease and social conditions was pioneered in England. Why do you think this has been the case? Is it because of the greater class differences, poor nutrition, poor heating in the winter, overcrowding, drinking, or smoking? What is the background? I ask this particularly because it was stated by an English pediatrician that premature infants from an upper-social-class background only appeared to do better than their peers from a lower-social-class background because they were more often looked after by their own mothers. When they were compared with lower-class infants who were looked after by their own mothers there was no difference.

Dr. Davis: You have hit the nail on the head. In the study of the three Lancashire towns I was discussing, one of the main differences was in the proportion of mothers who looked after their children themselves, in comparison with those who sought work outside the home and had their children looked after by a child-minder.

Dr. Tanner: Could I add a supplementary answer? One reason why it was in England that what has been called *social pediatrics* first appeaed is simply that England was the first country to embrace the Industrial Revolution. Conditions of children in the industrial centers were so appallingly bad that something had to be done.

Dr. Darby: Since this is a nutrition workshop on the history of pediatrics and you have been describing the contribution of the British to pediatrics, the enormous contribution made in the twentieth century by figures such as Harriet Chick, Cicely Williams, Trowell, and others, who were working at least in part abroad, should be mentioned.

Dr. Davis: You are quite right, although these were mostly not pediatricians. While working for the Colonial Medical Service, Cicely Williams gave the first and perhaps the best description of kwashiorkor back in 1931. It is also right to mention the contribution of Elsie Widdowson in Germany after the war. She went to study malnutrition in German orphanages in Wuppertal and found, rather to her surprise, that a diet consisting essentially of bread and pulses was quite enough for them to grow on provided that the matron of the home where they were being looked after was a sympathetic person.

Dr. Banakappa: The social aspects of treating disease are very important. The free distribution of milk and vitamins that occurred in Britain after the introduction of socialized medicine was a major factor in improving the nutrition of British children. I have recently learned that the present administration in the UK is not favorably disposed toward socialized medicine. If this is the case, you may see an increase in nutritional disorders over the coming years.

Dr. Davis: In the last year or two, infant mortality rates in England have stopped falling as they had been for the previous 20 to 30 years. Quite clearly this has a great deal to do with the quality of life of the poor.

Dr. Guesry: At the end of the 1940s in the UK there was a program for distributing milk to babies and this of course probably prevented malnutrition. However it also caused quite a number of cases of hypernatremic dehydration. This raises the question of the influence of pediatricians in the organization of such social programs.

Dr. Davis: You are right. Not only did the way in which we prepared our dried milk probably result in the development of hypernatremic dehydration in babies with gastroenteritis, but the way in which we tried to prevent rickets also resulted in quite a large number of babies developing hypercalcemia. I don't think science can advance in any other way. You have to try things out and there will be errors that must be recognized and corrected.

Dr. Holliday: This points to the importance of doing some kind of control study before releasing a new program onto the population at large.

Dr. Davis: I absolutely agree. One of the problems of so-called socialized medicine is that when something is decided on the bureaucracy is inclined to introduce it universally, rather than trying it out first. This is the disadvantage of having a tightly controlled unified system. The concept of the controlled trial was, of course, developed in England after the war by Mark Daniel.

Dr. Visakorpi: British pediatricians have made a very special contribution by producing textbooks that are small in size and suitable for undergraduate students, whereas the Germans produce huge textbooks, *Kurtze Einleitung in Kinderheilkunde in 12 Bänden*. Was this tradition already established before the Second World War or is it a new trend?

Dr. Davis: We have always rather envied the Germans their immense tomes, but maybe it's something to do with the fact that if you look at notices on the London Underground saying the same thing in German, French, and English, they take about half the number of words in English!

History of Pediatrics 1850–1950, edited by
B.L. Nichols, A. Ballabriga, and N. Kretchmer.
Nestlé Nutrition Workshop Series, Vol. 22. Nestec
Ltd., Vevey/Raven Press, Ltd., New York © 1991.

French Pediatrics

Robert Laplane

Faculté de Médecine Saint-Antoine, Hopital Trousseau, 75012 Paris, France

Throughout the period 1850–1950, pediatrics progressed on two parallel courses: child welfare, which we call in French *Puériculture,* and pediatrics, dealing with disease. I shall underline the contributions made by the major French pediatricians to both these branches and then discuss some of our main schools of pediatrics.

Infant mortality was the major concern of French physicians during the nineteenth century. Despite all efforts, it had remained almost unchanged since the eighteenth century, at around 25% to 27%. It was still 20% in 1850 and remained between 15% and 20% until the end of the century. Infanticide was common at that time, as indeed it was in the rest of Europe. The official figure was 5,591 cases between 1832 and 1862 but it certainly must have been higher. Newborn abandonment increased greatly during the nineteenth century to the point of becoming a major problem, especially in towns, the victims being mainly illegitimate children born into a poverty-stricken population. These children, usually left at church doors, were inevitably fated to die. As a palliative, a *tour d'abandon* (turning wheel) was installed near the doors of convents; they increased and in 1811 they had become a state institution. There were 269 in 1830 but after that their number diminished, the last one's being closed in 1868. During this period, the number of abandonments decreased from 13,000 in 1833 to 5,200 in 1864.

In spite of the *tours,* the death rate among the newborns remained unchanged; progress in that field could be gained only through improving maternal assistance and child welfare. This was to be the aim of nineteenth century medicine, and its doctrine, laws, and structures were the first step toward the development of what was to be the pediatrics of today.

As early as 1821, a law had fixed the distinction between a *hospice,* a place of refuge, and a children's hospital, a place for the treatment of diseases. The first pediatric hospital, Les Enfants Malades of Paris, dates back to 1802. Others followed between 1850 and 1900. Once this distinction was made, eminent physicians working in hospitals were able to make valuable progress in the field of pediatrics.

The work of Friedlander, based on 7,000 cases, proved, as early as 1815, the importance of weighing the newborn. Experience has subsequently shown that weight is a reliable guide to prematurity. The first days of life were soon to become a fruitful field of research. The first incubator was devised by Stéphane Tarnier at the Maternité de Port-Royal in 1880, and was soon improved upon by Pierre Budin. Tarnier was the first to state that the survival of premature infants required isolation, faultless hygiene, appropriate feeding through nasal intubation and a humid, warm atmosphere. Thanks to such measures, infant mortality at Maternité de Port-Royal declined from 66% to 38% between 1879 and 1882. Tarnier established the main principles of neonatal intensive care, thus paving the way for future progress (1).

Hospitals created solely for children were an important factor in improving medical care. However, mortality caused by infection remained a serious problem until it became obvious that infectious diseases were due to contagion. Thereafter infected patients were isolated. In 1877, special wards were provided for such diseases as scarlet fever, diphtheria and measles. Joseph Grancher, a disciple of Pasteur, fought to impose proper regulation to prevent intra-hospital contamination: isolation of the children, cubicles, compulsory uniforms for nurses, and hand washing. Medical antisepsis was obtained by 1889 and, as a result, morbidity and mortality in hospitals decreased considerably.

Pediatric hospitals are but one of many structures that were established between 1850 and 1900 to promote maternal and child welfare. The role played by dispensaries was equally important and due to Budin, whose influence spread throughout Europe (2), their numbers increased rapidly. By 1890 their value was clearly established through the decreased mortality among infants who benefited from such care. A day nursery for the children of working mothers was opened in Paris in 1848. By 1873 there were 27 of them and, by 1946, 360. The first nursery for short-term infant care was opened in 1875.

It soon became obvious that the care of the mother could not be separated from child welfare. As early as 1850, institutions were founded to help mothers at home, to promote breastfeeding, to make gifts of money and in kind, and to provide work at home. Later, institutions were created that gave shelter and care to young mothers in distress after delivery. It was the task of the twentieth century to enlarge and diversify these structures.

Several laws were to regulate this welfare activity. In 1849, a government agency, *l'Assistance Publique,* was created to deal with abandoned children and orphans. In 1874, the Roussel law required that the condition of children sent into the provinces for wet-nursing be supervised. National Health Insurance was established by law and became compulsory in 1936. It was officially termed *National Health and Retirement Insurance* in 1941. The next step was the institution of Social Aid to Children: l'Aide sociale à l'enfance. All this was the achievement of work that had started one century earlier.

One important cause of infant mortality had long been gastroenteritis, and by the middle of the eighteenth century it was known that food played a major part in this. Stimulated by J.J. Rousseau and Beaumarchais, the medical community engaged in a crusade in favor of breastfeeding in the first half of the nineteenth century. During this period agreement was reached on various questions that had long been controversial: the benefits of early feeding of the newborn, the schedule of feedings, the age and management of weaning. However, wet-nurses and bottle or spoon feeding remained in favor with the public, and the high incidence of severe gastroenteritis and the poor health of children persisted. During the last part of the nineteenth century, research mainly involved the study and improvement of bottle feeding.

It finally became obvious that ill-kept cow sheds, contamination during the milking process and by unclean cans, and the time required for delivery of milk to the home were the major causes of milk contamination. Many measures were tried. Parrot and Tarnier even raised asses inside the *Hôpital des Enfants Trouvés* so that infants could feed directly from the udder, as was practiced in some mountain regions. Various techniques were introduced to improve the preservation of milk—cooling; boiling (the efficacy of which had long been proved by the chemist Gay-Lussac) oversweetening, drying, addition of various ingredients. But these experiments were done on a laboratory scale and child morbidity was not affected. Deviller, at the Académie de Médecine in 1877, stated: "No progress has been made in the last 25 years." Infant mortality was between 35% and 45% with bottle feeding.

Things were to change with Pasteur's discovery that milk contamination is brought about by microbes; to avoid contamination, microbes must be destroyed by sterilization. His theory was quickly accepted by pediatricians who understood its importance. Among the first to apply and to promote the method was Pierre Budin (3). By 1905, the mortality rate of bottle-fed infants was practically the same as for those who were breast-fed.

Research was also carried out to determine the various physico-chemical characteristics of human milk compared to animal milk. This work was initiated by Donné, Vernois and Becquerel. Experiments were conducted to try to make cow's milk better tolerated by infants. The simple techniques of diluting and sweetening it, proposed by Budin, Marfan, and Hutinel came into general use. This led to the development of more and more complex formulas. Louis Ribadeau-Dumas, Edmond Lesne, Robert Debré and Marcel Lelong were pioneers in the promotion of these artificial milks.

The first research on nutrition began around 1850. Budin showed that milk intake must be proportional to the weight of the child. Natalis Guyot in 1852 stressed the importance of weighing the infant before and after feeding. Following German biologists, more and more importance was given to the study of energy balance, calorie requirements, and basal metabolism. The role of *diastases,* today called *enzymes,* was shown by Emile Duclaux, a chemist, and the role of amino acids, by Lucie Randoin.

The study of mental problems in childhood was for long quite limited. An early worker in child psychiatry seems to have been Paul Moreau, of Tours, who published a major work, *Mental disorders in children,* in 1888. Some time before this, such pioneers as Ferrus, Fabret, and Voisin had studied the care of backward children. Edouard Seguin continued their work, first in France then in the United States, where his influence was considerable as early as 1850. Bourneville applied his theory to the school for retarded children founded at the Hospice de Bicêtre. Alfred Binet and Théodore Simon were the first to measure in retarded children what they called *le quotient intellectuel* or "Q.I." (4). They developed a series of tests that opened the way for many more to come. The first school for the mentally retarded was created in 1909. Child psychiatry developed after 1920 under the influence of Georges Heuyer, for whom the first European Professorship in Child Psychiatry was created in 1948.

Pediatricians take advantage of progress in adult medicine and adapt new discoveries to the idiosyncrasies of children. In the nineteenth century, they applied the now well known *Méthode anatomo-clinique* that did away with the dogmatic theories that had prevailed too long. It was the first scientific approach to medicine. This new mode of thought was introduced by Corvisart, Bichat, Bayle, and Laënnec in adult medicine. Thanks to Billard it had established some order in the rather chaotic approach to infant's diseases as early as 1828 (5). It was particularly stressed and clearly defined in the famous work of E. Barthez and F. Rilliet (1843) which was republished several times in succeeding years (6).

The *Méthode anatomo-clinique* is based upon accurate and thorough clinical examination of the patient with scrupulous noting of all functional and physical data. Thanks to such strict discipline, Trousseau, in his famed *Clinique de l'Hôtel-Dieu,* dispelled all confusion between an epileptic and an hysterical attack and gave a striking description of "Summer cholera" (7). In the same way, Henri Roger characterized ventricular septal defect clinically, and Bouveret, in 1889, did the same for paroxysmal tachycardia. It was also through strict clinical observation that H. Roger showed the importance of measuring body temperature in children.

Barthez and Rilliet insisted upon clinical signs being checked by anatomic examination of the lesions found at autopsy. They would note all clinical-anatomic data on a preprepared document. Analysis of the case histories enabled them to establish a coherent classification of diseases.

This strict method was successfully applied by numerous clinicians. Here are a few examples.

Fallot in 1885 described and characterized the cardiac disease that bears his name (Fallot's tetralogy). In 1876, Parrot made clear that in tuberculosis an alveolar lesion of the lung precedes the presence of mediastinal glands. In 1877, Hutinel described the various types of meningeal hemorrhage. In 1868, Hayem characterized acute encephalitis and, a few years later, Bourneville did the same for chronic encephalopathy. It was also thanks to the clinical-anatomic method, helped by histology and neurophysiology, that Charcot, Dejerine, and Babinski laid the foundations of neurology that still today remain valid.

Interest in these methods was renewed by developments in microscopic examination, which advanced rapidly after Virchow. Clinical biopsy, named by Bernier, allowed the clinical-anatomic method to do away with some of the justified criticisms of postmortem examination, and showed that lesions originally thought to be hallmarks of the disease, could be absent, non-specific, or the result of postmortem change.

A new door was to be opened.

In the wake of German studies, French physicians and scientists such as Fourcroy, Magendie, Tanret, Andral, and Potain understood the potential importance of physico-chemical research. The well-known works of Claude Bernard and his disciple Brown-Sequard were to show clearly the importance of metabolic disorders of the *milieu intérieur*. This was the birth of biology.

Henceforth, diseases of the gastrointestional tract, for instance, could be approached by new methods. The terms *gastritis* or *enteritis* were replaced by *dyspepsia:* the functional disturbance appeared more important than the anatomical lesion. Trousseau in 1873 blamed dyspepsia for imbalance between motility and secretion in the digestive tract. Parrot characterized *athrepsia* by its pathophysiology in 1877. Diarrhea is the *primum movens:* it brings in its wake digestive disturbances responsible for nutritional disorders named *toxicosis* or *marasmus* by German authors (8). Marfan was of the same mind when describing intolerances to cow's milk, human milk, and starch, or *"periodic vomiting and acetonemia in infancy"* (9). Much later, around 1925, L. Ribadeau-Dumas suspected the essential part played by electrolytic disorders in acute dehydration of the infant and the importance of correcting them by intravenous infusion.

These studies were not concerned with the problems of disease etiology. These problems were to be dealt with for the first time in relation to contagious diseases.

As early as 1820, Bretonneau was aware of the importance of epidemiology in pediatrics and had asserted that diseases such as typhoid fever have a specificity related to a particular agent. He had also established that pharyngeal diphtheria (a name he created) was the same disease as croup and that both were contagious. Trousseau, expressing the same ideas in 1861, defended the notion of "disease specificity." Germain See, in 1859, had seen the connection between chorea and rheumatic fever, which he treated with sodium salicylate.

There were many who denied that illnesses such as scrofula were really tuberculosis. However, Laënnec, Louis, Barthez, and Rilliet had based their convictions about the various clinical presentations of tuberculosis on clinical as well as epidemiologic and anatomic grounds. In 1872, Villemin, following the work of Langhans and Friedlander, confirmed their findings using histologic data. He also showed, 15 years before Koch's discoveries, that tuberculosis is infectious, contagious, and can be inoculated into an animal.

In the meantime, microorganisms had been demonstrated in various diseases but their role was not certain. The time was ripe for Pasteur's revolution and for the identification of most bacteria from 1878. Pediatric medicine as a whole was transformed with regard to classification of diseases, food hygiene in infancy, and prevention of infection in hospitals.

The French contributions in the field of infectious diseases included Fernand Widal's agglutinin reaction in typhoid fever (1896), Charles Mantoux's intradermal test for tuberculosis (1908), and the concept of sub-clinical infections introduced by Charles Nicolle, winner of the Nobel prize (1909).

Claude Bernard believed, contrary to Pasteur's assertions, that individual idiosyncrasy was more important than microbes in the causation of disease. In fact the two theories were not incompatible, as modern medicine has shown.

Men are not equal in the face of illness; some are affected by specific hypersensitivity, as shown by Nobel prize winners Charles Richet and Paul Portier in 1902. The concepts of "allergy" and "auto-immune disease" have extended the field of diseases related to sensitization considerably. The discovery of the HLA antigens in 1964 by Jean Dausset, Nobel prize winner in 1980, has opened entirely new prospects in immunology.

The emergence of bacteriology has completely changed the prophylaxis and treatment of infectious diseases in childhood. Earlier, the only possibility of defense was to improve hygiene and to use symptomatic drugs. The unique exception, thanks to Jenner, was vaccination against smallpox. With the successful vaccination against rabies of young Joseph Meister in 1885, Pasteur opened a new era in the specific prevention of infectious diseases.

Among the many applications of the method, I shall mention two that brought renown to French scientists.

E. Roux, C. Martin, and A. Chaillou showed, at the Budapest International Congress in 1894, the spectacular curative value of antidiphtheric serum therapy in pharyngeal diphtheria as well as in croup. Mortality fell at once from 73% to 14%.

After many years, another discovery was to banish diphtheria definitively from the array of child diseases: in 1925, Gaston Ramon utilized "Anatoxin" with total success for prophylaxis (10). Some time later, he was able to prevent tetanus, thanks to a specific Anatoxin prepared using the same technology. Since 1940, vaccination against diphtheria and tetanus has been compulsory in France.

The story of the bacille Calmette-Guérin (BCG) vaccine is a good example of the triumph of tenacity. Since 1885, vaccination against the Koch bacillus had been tried repeatedly without success. A. Calmette and C. Guerin devoted themselves to the problem in 1905. Using a faultless experimental process, they worked 16 years to achieve their goal. In 1921, they were able to vaccinate neonates with full success (11). By 1962, despite the drama at Lübeck in 1930, more than 400,000 children had been vaccinated in 46 countries. Thanks to the dissemination of BCG that was to follow, there was a dramatic change in tuberculosis among children. BCG is compulsory in France, as in many countries.

Although sulphonamides have been relegated to the background by the ever increasing numbers of antibiotics that have emerged since Sir Alexander Fleming's discovery of penicillin, it is worth mentioning that Fournier, Trefouel, Bovet, and Nitti, of the Institute Pasteur, established in 1936 that sulfonamide is the active fraction of chrysoido-sulfonamide, discovered by Domagk.

My short review of French pediatrics has given but a fragmentary sketch of the men who worked and fought for its development. I shall therefore end with a brief study of the medical schools of which they were the leaders.

Paris has always been the center of French pediatrics. Two medical centers have shared special distinction due to the quality of the physicians who worked there and the historical importance of their contribution to pediatrics.

It was in the Hôpital des Enfants Malades that Antoine Barthez and Frédéric Rilliet conducted their comprehensive study of pediatric diseases. Ernest Bouchut (1818–1891) practiced intubation in croup, 30 years before O'Dwyer. He was also a pioneer in ophthalmoscopy.

Armand Trousseau (1801–1867), the follower of Bretonneau and well known for his brilliant teaching, was the most famous representative of the Clinique française.

Joseph Grancher (1843–1907) greatly improved the rules of hospital hygiene and was most effective in fighting tuberculosis. Eugène Apert (1868–1940) characterized *Acrocephalosyndactyly* and established in 1910 that pseudo-hermaphroditism could be related to an alteration of the adrenal glands.

Nearer to our time, Maurice Lamy (1895–1975), an early geneticist, founded the first chair in the world in this discipline in 1951. Raymond Turpin (1895–1988) was involved in the first BCG vaccinations of infants, collaborating with Benjamin Weill-Hallé (1875–1958), but his fame was mainly due to his identification, with Jérôme Lejeune, of the chromosome 21 anomaly in Down syndrome.

The Hospice des Enfants Trouvés, founded in 1814, which was to become Hospice des Enfants Assistés in 1838, and then Hôpital Saint-Vincent de Paul, attained in the nineteenth century a reputation equal to that of the Hôpital des Enfants Malades.

Henri Roger (1809–1891) pursued his highly original research there for 15 years. Jules-Joseph Parrot (1829–1883), a man with an independent, innovative but disciplined mind, described *athrepsie,* and characterized *achondroplasia* and syphilitic *pseudo-paralysis* of the hip. Among his followers, foremost were Victor Hutinel (1849–1933) and Antonin Marfan (1858–1942), who, together with Joseph Grancher (1843–1907), were the founders of modern French pediatrics (12). In our times, Marcel Lelong (1892–1973) was an important figure in the development of child welfare in France.

Other medical centers shared in the widespread influence of Parisian pediatrics. Among the physicians who worked at the Hôpital Trousseau, founded in 1880, were Arnold Netter (1855–1936), who deserves special mention. Endowed with an encyclopedic mind, he had a worldwide reputation based largely on his achievements in the field of infectious diseases, where he was one of the first to apply bacteriology to pediatrics.

Edmond Lesné (1871–1962) used his training as a physiologist to deal with nutritional problems that had hardly been studied at that time. He was convinced that clinical activities should be supported by experimentation and conducted important laboratory research on the pathogenesis and treatment of rickets.

Jean Cathala (1891–1969), although he was well-read in biology, insisted on keeping himself in the clinical field. Thus his fame rested as a first-rate physician.

The Maternité de Port-Royal was famous in the nineteenth century, because of two obstetricians who played a leading part in neonatal pediatrics. Stéphane Tarnier (1828–1893) was the first to establish principles for the management of premature infants. His follower Pierre Budin (1848–1907) devoted himself to the encouragement of breastfeeding and to promoting infant hygiene.

At the Hôpital de la Salpétrière, Louis Ribadeau-Dumas (1876–1950) shed light on some infant diseases that were poorly understood at the time. He introduced into France the infant rehydration techniques that had been defined in the United States by Schick and Karelitz, as well as the use of soya flour.

The fame attached to Parisian schools of pediatrics should not be allowed to overshadow the part played since the First World War by some provincial schools such as Lyon with Maurice Pehu (1875–1945) and Georges Mouriquand (1880–1966),

Strasbourg with Paul Rohmer (1878–1977), Bordeaux, Toulouse, and Marseilles.

The men I have written about are responsible for the leading role long played by France in world pediatrics. Their clinics attracted many foreign physicians who were able to become, in their turns, heads of medical schools in their own countries. However, after 1920, some of those who were responsible for French pediatrics were not fully aware of impending changes and of the increasing importance of biology, especially in research in the United States. French pediatrics ran the risk of being left behind. To meet the challenge, new doors had to be opened. Robert Debré (1882–1978) was the soul of this renovation. His scientific achievements were so extensive that they cannot be summarized here. A few items can be highlighted. Very early he took an interest in contagious diseases. He collaborated with Gaston Ramon in the first trial of diphtheria anatoxin. He explored aspects of skin testing, immunity, transmission of infection, and BCG vaccination in the field of child tuberculosis. At the same time as Lee Fosty, Mollaret, and Reilly he described cat-scratch disease. Several syndromes are named after him: muscular hypertrophy of hypothyroidism (Debré-Semelaigne syndrome, 1924), congenital adrenal hyperplasia with salt loss (Debré-Fibiger syndrome, 1925), idiopathic proximal tubulopathy with hypophosphatemia (Toni-Debré-Fanconi syndrome, (1934). He was also a pioneer in child welfare on an international as well as a national scale: he founded UNICEF with J. Rajschman and the Centre International de l'Enfance in Paris.

The status of Robert Debré makes him the equal of the greatest pediatricians of any time. It was mainly due to his efforts and achievements that French pediatrics is what it is today.

REFERENCES

1. Tarnier S, Chantreuil J, Budin P. *Allaitement et hygiène du nouveau-né*. Paris: G Steinheil, 1888.
2. Budin P. *Hommage à*. Paris: PUF, 1930.
3. Budin P. *Manuel pratique de l'allaitement*. Paris: Doin, 1907.
4. Binet A. *Etude expérimentale de l'intelligence*. Paris: Retz, CEPL, 1974.
5. Billard CM. *Traité des maladies des enfants nouveau-nés et à la mamelle*. Paris: Baillière, 1828.
6. Rilliet JL, Barthez CE. *Traité clinique et pratique des maladies des enfants*. Paris: Germer Baillière, 1843.
7. Trousseau A. *Clinique médicale de l'Hôtel-Dieu*. Paris: JB Baillière, 1861.
8. Parrot J. *L'athrepsie*. Paris: Masson, 1877.
9. Marfan AB. *Traité de l'allaitement*. Paris: G. Steinheil, 1899.
10. Ramon G. Sur le pouvoir floculant et sur les propriétés immunitaires d'une toxine diphtérique rendue anatoxique. *Bull Acad Méd* 1923;177:1333–40.
11. Calmette A. *La vaccination préventive contre la tuberculose par le BCG*. Paris: Masson, 1927.
12. Grancher A, Comby J, Marfan AB. *Traité des maladies de l'enfance*. Paris: Masson, 1897.

DISCUSSION

Dr. Stern: I was fascinated by your account of Tarnier and Budin. Tarnier was Budin's teacher. He was also a distinguished physiologist as well as an obstetrician. Together they built the first incubator, but the French medical establishment looked upon it with the same degree of disdain they originally awarded Laennec's stethoscope, as a gimmick without much practical value. The first use of the incubator was in fact for Budin's brother-in-law who was the director of the Paris zoo, where infant monkeys tended to die of cold soon after birth. This story is important for American neonatology because it was Budin's pupil Cooney who brought the idea to the United States and established an entire series of incubators that were displayed at all the traveling circuses. Budin was also the first to propose the use of gavage feeding for premature infants.

Dr. Laplane: Budin was a very influential figure in Europe in the field of child welfare. He fought for clean milk and took a great interest in the care of the newborn. It is quite true that with Tarnier he proposed that premature infants should be fed through a nasogastric tube.

Dr. Suskind: Can we hear something about the interaction that has occurred between the various schools of pediatrics in Europe since the 1850s? Was there an interchange of ideas or were each of these schools really bound by language and geography?

Dr. Davis: After the revolution of 1848, Louis Borchhart from Prussia came to Manchester as a fully equipped pediatrician, introduced pediatrics to Manchester where until then it had not previously been practiced and set about the founding of the Royal Manchester Children's Hospital. Dr. Shöffer-Merei from Budapest, who fled from Hungary after having been involved in revolutionary activities, came to Manchester as well and started another Manchester children's service.

There was also a time when English physicians had to learn German in order to study their subject seriously.

Dr. Laplane: The problem of language has limited the exchanges between France and European countries. However they were aware of the work that was carried out abroad. As early as the middle of the nineteenth century, they used to visit the main schools of pediatrics of Great Britain, Austria, and Germany.

Dr. Ballabriga: Although language difficulties have certainly limited communication between the French, English, Austrian, and German schools, pediatric knowledge can also be widely diffused by translations. For example the *Treatise on Pediatrics* by the Russian, Filatow, was translated into Italian and edited in Naples in 1890 from the third German edition, and a new edition in Italian translated from the third Russian edition appeared in 1907. In Spain one of Gerhardt's books was translated under the title *Tratado completo de las enfermedades de los niños* in 1897, and before that the three volumes by Rilliet and Barthez had been translated under the title *Tratado clinico y práctico de las enfermedades de los niños* (1866). There was also an exchange of scholars. Russian pediatricians followed the Viennese school. Filatow studied in Vienna during Widerhofer's era and Meyerhofer studied with Escherich and later became Professor of pediatrics. The Viennese pediatric school in Widerhofer's time, based on the St. Anna Kinderspital, was much influenced by the great prestige of the *Zweiter Wiener Schule,* and particularly the pathologist Rokitanski and the clinician Skoda. Later, at the beginning of this century, Escherich was devoting his attention to diarrheal pathogens, while at the same time Pirquet introduced the term *allergy* following his work on serum sickness. Bela Schick recounts an anecdote to the effect that the scientific referee who reviewed Pirquet's paper in 1906 considered that "the introduction of a new and useless term such as *allergy* was superfluous."

Dr. Willard and *Dr. Schneegans:* In the mid-nineteenth century, conditions were unfavorable for childbirth in Alsace. The illegitimacy rate was high, working women were in poor health, salaries were low and food was scarce. Traditional practices, especially in the rural areas, precluded progress. Some social advance occurred in the second part of the nineteenth century, for example, wages increased faster than the price of food, and the introduction of German civil law around the turn of the century meant that the fathers of illegitimate children were obliged to provide for them. There were also improvements in sanitation in Strasbourg, and better communications were established in rural areas. However there was little concern with perinatology among Strasbourg physicians during this period.

In 1900, a Local Orphan Board was established to look after the well-being of illegitimate children. House inspections were instituted, which showed gross dietary malpractices accounting in part for the very high mortality. Subsequent legislation made it compulsory for infants to be given regular medical examinations, and food grants came into being.

In 1901, a nursing home for 10 infants was established outside the city, and in 1904 this was moved to larger premises, where 20 infants could be treated. The Local Orphan Board made it a priority to provide lodging for mothers of illegitimate children, and a mother's home was eventually established in 1910. This later became the Infant Care Institute and its premises can still be seen on the corner of quai Fustel de Coulanges and rue de la porte de l'hôpital.

The new Pediatric Nursing Home was built in the same year, with Professor Czerny as Director. Czerny did not, however, show any interest in neonatal medicine, nor did his successor, Salge. It was only when Alsace was returned to France after the First World War that progress was made, with the founding by the new Director, Professor Rohmer, of the Alsace and Lorraine Infant Care Association in 1920. This association was instrumental in developing mother and infant care in Alsace long before such care was available in the rest of the country. Rohmer was particularly interested in the management of underweight babies, using cotton wool wrappings and hot water bottles to achieve an adequate thermal environment, and feeding the smallest infants with a mixture of human milk and cow's milk given through droppers. Although priority was given to combating infection, neonates were not separated from other infants. Mortality between 1927 and 1939 was around 40%.

Rohmer was succeeded by Professor Sacrez, who was responsible for separating neonates and premature infants from older babies, and who introduced the first incubators as well as the practice of exchange transfusion for severe jaundice, as recommended by Diamond.

During this period, neonatology was making progress in the other large Alsatian cities, such as Mulhouse and Colmar, and the Strasbourg obstetric school also made a decisive contribution to improvement in perinatal care. This progress was due to Professor Schikelé, whose inaugural lecture (1), published in January 1920, is worth reading to this day. He explained why extraperitoneal cesarean section was the safest method and he laid the foundations of controlled childbirth whereby uterine contractions were controlled pharmacodynamically. He objected to anesthesia during childbirth because of the risks for the infant. He wrote, "Our twentieth century should be the century of the child. Physicians and lawmakers will have to cooperate to initiate and ensure child protection. . . . A child is alive before he is born. Care is demanded before birth."

Schikelé was succeeded by Professor Keller, who maintained strong ties with pediatricians, to whose care he entrusted neonates immediately after birth. Such cooperation was not usual in France at that time. It was Gandar, working under Keller, who first cleaned the pharynxes of cyanotic newborns by aspirating mucus obstructions, and then gave oxygen. From then on, perinatal care became modern. It came of age with the holding of the first European Congress on Perinatology in Berlin in 1968 and the creation of the European Society for Perinatal Medicine.

REFERENCES

1. Schikelé G. Leçon d'ouverture. *Presse Medicale*, 24 Jan 1920;61–3.

History of Pediatrics 1850–1950, edited by
B.L. Nichols, A. Ballabriga, and N. Kretchmer.
Nestlé Nutrition Workshop Series, Vol. 22. Nestec
Ltd., Vevey/Raven Press, Ltd., New York © 1991.

The European Roots of American Pediatrics

Buford L. Nichols, Jr.

USDA/ARS Children's Nutrition Research Center, Departments of Pediatrics and Physiology, Baylor College of Medicine, Houston, Texas 77030, USA

Although modern scientific methods were first applied to medicine at the dawn of the eighteenth century, pediatric medicine as a science did not develop until a century later. Subtle shifts in attitude began to emerge after Rousseau (1712–1778) questioned the philosophic concept of the time, i.e., that man was naturally evil, and proposed that children were born naturally good. Rousseau believed that children were the future of a civilization and should be preserved, nurtured, developed, and educated (1). After Rousseau's revolutionary insight, children became a social issue and the basis for professional specialization in medicine, education, and law. The philosophic assumption of the intrinsic value of the child opened doors to the development of the art and science of pediatric medicine.

The origins of pediatric medical practice are within the broader development of medicine in the late eighteenth century. After the French revolution, French surgeons entered the mainstream of medical education bringing with them bold empirical methods that included direct observation of the patient and post-mortem anatomical confirmation of the cause of death (2). These innovations replaced the theoretical medical practices of the time. During the first third of the nineteenth century, leading American physicians studied in Paris where bedside observations and post-mortem examinations by Louis (1787–1872) and Laënnec (1781–1826) shaped medical education in the new world (3). Although the practice of pediatric medicine did not develop in this environment, Laënnec was a member of the Paris commission that emphasized the need for such a speciality (3).

The Battle of Waterloo (1815) marked the beginning of the eclipse of French influence in medicine and a reorientation of American medical education toward German universities and clinics. The German university flourished under the leadership of the Humboldt brothers. The universities emphasized *wissenschaft,* or knowledge for its own sake, and *bildung,* intellectual self-development. This intellectual revolution was waged against a theoretical view of the universe characterized by *naturphilosophie.* This new concept of higher education was characterized by the development of faculty research subsidized by the governments of German-speaking states (4). One such development occurred at Giessen when Justus Liebig (1803–1873) (Fig. 1) returned from study in Paris in 1825. Humboldt had recruited

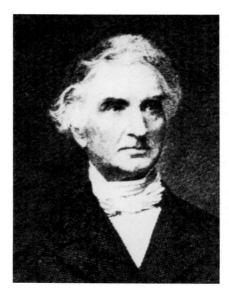

FIG. 1.   Justus von Liebig (1803–1873).

him to occupy a chair of chemistry. Liebig introduced quantitative organic chemical analysis into all areas of biology including pharmacy, medicine, and agriculture. He founded a school of experimental chemistry in which his scientific progeny received more than 30 Nobel prizes. He appeared to recognize the practical impact of chemical investigations and published extensively (5). In 1866, he published the first article on the modification of cow's milk for infant feeding in which he described the use of dextrins *(maltsuppe)* (6).

The first children's hospital, the Hôpital des Enfants Malades, was founded in 1802 in response to a critical study of hospitals in Paris by a committee that included Laënnec. The next children's hospital was formed at the Charité in Berlin in 1830, followed by Vienna and Breslau in 1837, Budapest (1839), Prague (1842), London (1852), Stockholm (1854), and Boston (1869). The early development of hospital pediatric practice was restricted by high mortality rates among hospitalized infants. Grancher (1843–1907), a French pediatrician closely associated with Pasteur, conceived the idea of cubicle construction to isolate infants and children in the wards of hospitals. His work was continued by Hutinel (1849–1933), his successor at the Hôpital des Enfants Malades in 1907. Heubner implemented this construction in the new Kinderklinik in Berlin in 1900, Escherich in Vienna in 1902, Schlossmann in Dresden in 1904, and Pirquet in Baltimore in 1908. On the basis of the isolation technique, infant mortality rates were reduced from 73% to 14% of all admissions at the Charité in Berlin (3).

Preventive hygiene was extended to outpatient care in France when Boudin (1846–1907) established well-child clinics. During his lifetime, Boudin observed a decrease in infant mortality rates from 178 per 1,000 to 46 per 1,000. His work was extended by Variot (1855–1930) who convened a congress in 1905 of *Gouttes de lait* that had a marked influence on the infant welfare movement. The emphasis of the congress was the importance of breast feeding, the need for adequate alternate nutrition with sterilized artificial feedings, and the need to teach the principles of hygiene to mothers. Koplik (1858–1927) of New York was a leader in this international movement (3).

The basic sciences that formed the foundation of child care were developed in Vienna when, under the influence of Rokitansky and Skoda, the work of the French medical scientists was extended to infant diseases. The next stage of development, the physiological science of child care, occurred in Berlin and was guided by Max Rubner (1854–1932) (see p. 274, Fig. 2). Rubner was a student of Karl Voit (1831–1908), who was a student of Liebig. Rubner collaborated with Heubner (1834–1926) (see p. 25, Fig. 2) in studies of infant energy metabolism and they reported their observations in 1898 and 1899. Their studies were the forerunners of modern research on developmental biology and infant metabolism and set a precedent for the teamwork of clinicians and basic scientists. Many of the pioneers in pediatric metabolic and nutrition research, such as Salge, Noeggerath, Finkelstein, Langstein, Bendex, and Niemann were trained by Heubner (3).

Although departments of chemistry existed at Yale and Harvard, the influence or impact of the German university system on the American educational system was epitomized in the founding of Johns Hopkins University. Earlier roots had existed, however, in the founding of the chemistry department at Yale by a student of Liebig, S.W. Johnson. Voit's school was vigorously represented by W.O. Atwater (1844–1907) and Graham Lusk (1866–1932). Lusk (Fig. 2) collaborated with John Howland (1873–1926) on the construction of an infant calorimeter at Bellevue Hospital in a department chaired by L. Emmett Holt (1855–1924) (Fig. 3). Howland spent the year, 1910, in Germany training with Czerny. Howland has been called the pioneer who launched the era of chemistry in American pediatrics. Howland subsequently succeeded Pirquet (1874–1929) as the first full-time chairman of pediatrics at Johns Hopkins University in 1912.

The evolution of pediatric medicine in the Americas reflected a belief in the value of children and the implementation of Rousseau's dictum *"il faut considérer . . . l'enfant dans l'enfant"* in hygiene, immunology, and metabolism. Underlying the development of pediatric medicine in the United States was a revolution in medical education led by William Welch. Welch had trained extensively in Germany and Austria and had championed the transplantation of the German university system to the Americas. It was he who imported the concepts of laboratory-based pathology, microbiology, and biochemistry in the clinical setting that characterized the Johns Hopkins Medical School, founded in 1888 (6). With support from the Rockefeller Foundation, Welch introduced the concept of the full-time clinical scientist to the university scene in North America (7). Funds from The Rockefeller Foundation enabled L. Emmett Holt to begin pediatric metabolic studies in New York and enabled John Howland to implement physical and chemical measurements on children at the Harriet Lane Home of the Johns Hopkins University Hospital. During the middle of the twentieth century, almost all pediatric scientists in North America could trace their genealogy to Howland, the pioneer of quantitative research in pediatric medi-

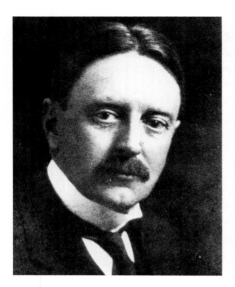

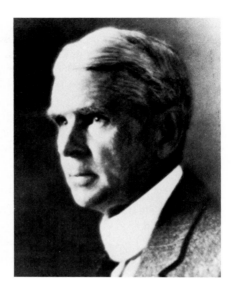

FIG. 2. Graham Lusk (1866–1932). (Light AE. Graham Lusk. *Yale J of Biol and Med* 1934; 6:487–506.)

FIG. 3. L. Emmett Holt, Sr. (1855–1924). (Duffus RL, Holt LE, Jr. *L. Emmett Holt: Pioneer of a Children's Century.* New York: 2. Appleton-Century Co., 1940., frontispiece.)

cine. Included were Gamble in Boston, Tisdall in Toronto, Marriott in St. Louis, Casparis in Nashville, Kramer in Brooklyn, Powers and Shohl in New Haven, and Park in Baltimore (8). My scientific heritage is through Powers, although I met Park when I was in residency training at the Harriet Lane Home of the Johns Hopkins Hospital.

The themes of modern medicine in the nineteenth century that contributed to the development of pediatric medicine in the United States were (1) direct observations at the bedside, (2) autopsy techniques to confirm bedside evaluations, (3) microbiological laboratory observations, and (4) physiological laboratory measurements associated with clinical observations. The early leaders of the American Pediatric Society (APS) were influenced by these innovations from the Viennese and Berlin schools.

A measure of European influence can be determined by a review of the APS. The Society was founded in 1888, 5 years after the founding of the Association for Diseases of Children in Germany. Of the 43 founding members of the APS, 18 had emigrated from, trained in, or traveled extensively in Europe. Of these, 11 had been trained in the most influential European medical centers: 2 in England, 7 in Vienna, and the remainder in Berlin or other German-speaking centers. Of the first 25 presidents of the APS, one had emigrated from, 11 had received training in, and three had traveled extensively in Europe. Vienna (6) and Berlin (3) were regarded at the time as Europe's most influential centers of medical development and training (9).

During the early days of the American Pediatric Society, the social implications of improved child health were recognized and discussed frequently. In the twenty-first meeting of the society held in 1909, Rotch (1849–1914) (see p. 59, Fig. 3) of Boston spoke on "the position and work of the American Pediatric Society toward public questions." In his objection, Holt of New York stated, "I should feel sorry to see a large part of the work of this society devoted to subjects of this kind, which, though of sociologic interest, are not so much along the line of work of most of us on other matters most strictly medical. I believe we can do our best work along the lines of research. We have a duty toward the public, but that should not be the most important side of our work" (10). Regardless of these comments, American children have been the beneficiaries during the past century. Schlossmann (1867–1932) of Dusseldorf referred to the twentieth century as the "Century of the Child." During the twentieth century, infant mortality rates in the United states have fallen from 150 per 1,000 to less than 8 per 1,000, a twenty-fold reduction (11). Our progress in pediatric medicine is the culmination of biological and sociological improvements in prenatal and postnatal care, infant hygiene, and clinical management, areas of research that originated in French- and German-speaking universities.

ACKNOWLEDGMENTS

This work is a publication of the USDA/ARS Children's Nutrition Research Center, Department of Pediatrics, Baylor College of Medicine and Texas Children's Hospital, Houston, Texas. This project has been funded in part with federal funds from the US Department of Agriculture, Agricultural Research Service under Cooperative Agreement number 58-7MN1-6-100. The contents of this publication do not necessarily reflect the views or policies of the US Department of Agriculture, nor does mention of trade names, commercial products, or organizations imply endorsements by the US Government.

REFERENCES

1. Rousseau, JJ. *The social contract and discourse on the origin of inequality.* Crocker LG, ed. New York: Washington Square Press, 1967.
2. Lesch JE. *Science and medicine in France: The emergence of experimental physiology, 1790–1855.* Cambridge, MA: Harvard University Press, 1984.
3. Abt IA. History of pediatrics. In: McQuarrie I, ed. *Brennemann's practice of pediatrics.* 1948; vol 1 WF Prior Co, Inc. Hagerstown, Md: 1–154.
4. Herbst J. *The German historical school in American scholarship. A study in the transfer of culture.* Ithaca, New York: Cornell University Press, 1965.
5. Ackerknecht EH. Metabolism from Liebig to the present. Ciba Foundation Symposium no 6. Amsterdam: Elsevier, 1944;1825–1833.
6. Liebig, J von. *Suppe für Säuglinge,* 2nd edition. Braunschweig: Druck und Verlag von Friedrich Boeweg und Sohn, 1866:5–11.
7. Fleming, D. *William H. Welch and the rise of modern medicine.* Oscar Handlin, ed. Boston: Little, Brown and Company, 1954.
8. Park EA. John Howland 1873–1926. *Science* 1926;64:80–83.
9. Sherman DH, Aldrich CA, Bonar BE, Carr WL, McCulloch H. (American Pediatric Society Committee). Semi-centennial volume of the American Pediatric Society 1888–1938. Menasha, WI: George Banta Publishing Company, 1938.

10. Faber HK, McIntosh R. *History of the American Pediatric Society.* New York: McGraw-Hill Book Company, 1966;76,77.
11. Bremner RH, Barnard J, Hareven TK, Mennel RM. Infant and maternal mortality. In: *Children and youth in America—a documentary history,*vol 2:1866–1932. Cambridge Massachusetts: Harvard University Press, 1971.

DISCUSSION

Dr. Katz: I wonder whether some of the differences between American pediatrics and central European pediatrics derive from the fact that the Americans were not so much disciples of their illuminaries as students, and, as students, they thought independently and often questioned their teachers. Professor Ballabriga commented on the differences he found when he came to my institution and discovered that the residents questioned what the professor said. Perhaps in central Europe the majesty of the professor has sometimes been too great to overcome.

Dr. Nichols: The distinction between disciple and student is an interesting one. Although I never met Dr Howland, we have descriptions by Davison about making rounds with him, and I understand that one never argued with him, at least not at the Harriet Lane Hospital.

Dr. Ballabriga: In one of your slides, Dr Nichols, you placed Finkelstein and Leo Langstein in a similar category to Rubner. I do not think this is entirely justifiable. Rubner was primarily a scientist while Finkelstein and Langstein were primarily clinicians. I do not believe that Finkelstein was interested in laboratory work at all, and if you look at his publications you see that they were not in the main stream of modern scientific developments, quite unlike Rubner.

Dr. Nichols: However, both Finkelstein and Langstein had PhD degrees before acquiring their medical degrees. Finkelstein's PhD was in geo-sciences—his thesis was on the geology of the Jura mountains—and he applied systematic thought to his investigations. His experimental work on diets resulted in the concept of food tolerances, a scientific innovation at the time.

Langstein had a PhD in protein chemistry. He had studied with Fisher and was involved with work on amino acid metabolism. He was the first to study energy expenditure in a premature (1). There was a very strong chemical group at the time at the Kaiserin Auguste Victoria Haus. There was a research laboratory beside the wards and his student Ylppö learned to do chemical investigations on premature infants. So there is a heritage of quantitative chemistry, in the Langstein school.

Dr. Suskind: If there was such a strong influence of European pediatrics on American pediatrics, why is there such a difference between the two schools of pediatrics at the present time?

Dr. Nichols: I think this goes back to the nature of the American university, which has long been more casual than the Germanic or French university systems. It is perhaps even more casual than the English system. This originates from the founding of Harvard and Yale by churches with different theological perspectives. But when Welch chose to import the Germanic school and Germanic standards as described in the Flexner Report, he grafted them onto the original tap root of American academic freedom. Thus we now have a hybrid; and the professor still has to earn his academic wings every day in this environment.

REFERENCES

1. Rubner M, Langstein L. *Arch Anat Physiol* 1915;39:39–70.

History of Pediatrics 1850–1950, edited by
B.L. Nichols, A. Ballabriga, and N. Kretchmer.
Nestlé Nutrition Workshop Series, Vol. 22. Nestec
Ltd., Vevey/Raven Press, Ltd., New York © 1991.

Pediatrics in the United States

Howard A. Pearson

Department of Pediatrics, Yale University School of Medicine, New Haven, Connecticut 06510, USA

The embryonic beginnings of pediatrics in the United States can be traced back to shortly after the founding of the English colonies in the early seventeenth century. For 200 years medical care of children was largely handled by parents, midwives, and nurses. However, a few colonial "physicians" interested in children's diseases can be identified. Part-time pediatrics was practiced by pastor-physicians exemplified by Thomas Thacher of Boston who championed smallpox vaccination and who, in 1677, wrote the first medical publication in the English colonies, a broadside on smallpox (1). Governor-physicians, notably John Winthrop, Jr., of Connecticut, conducted an extensive practice through the colonial mails (Fig. 1). The scarcity of physicians and Winthrop's willingness to prescribe free of charge led to his frequently being consulted. Winthrop's medical records, many of which are preserved in Boston's Countway Medical Library, describe a wide range of pediatric problems, such as rashes, jaundice, seizures, and diarrhea (2). There is even a clear de-

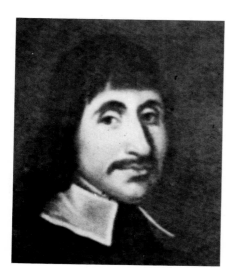

FIG. 1. Governor John Winthrop, Jr., of Connecticut (1606–1676). (Courtesy of the Countway Library of Medicine.)

scription of child abuse. Cotton Mather, the great Massachusetts Puritan preacher, wrote of Winthrop's medical prowess:

> Wherever he came the diseased flocked about him as if the healing angel of Bethesda had appeared in the place.

These part-time, non-physician healers, as well as other colonial physicians who were usually uneducated, poorly trained practitioners, plied a variety of ineffective remedies and anecdotal treatments against the formidable assaults of disease and death. These were perilous times for children. As Ernest Caulfield, an important American pediatric historian wrote:

> In addition to diphtheria, dysentery, measles, and scarlet fever, smallpox, influenza and tuberculosis should certainly be included in the list of common diseases of colonial children. A surprisingly large proportion of them had worms. Death from falls, burns, and poisonings were frequent. It seems a little surprising that any of them survived (3).

Although universities and colleges were founded early in the Americas, they emphasized classical and theological curricula. Training in secular subjects such as medicine came much later with the establishment of colleges of medicine. The first American Medical School opened at the University of Pennsylvania in Philadelphia in 1765.

Teaching of the diseases of children at most of the early medical schools was done sporadically, if at all, and then under the aegis of Physic (Medicine) or Midwifery (Obstetrics). At the University of Pennsylvania, Dr. Benjamin Rush, a preeminent American patriot-physician, a signer of the Declaration of Independence and a prodigious "bleeder", was professor of Medicine between 1789 and 1813. His medical lectures included a section on "Diseases Peculiar to Children." He published articles describing pediatric diseases including spasmodic asthma, diseases of the mind and diphtheria (4). He also coined the term *cholera infantum* to describe the lethal summer diarrhea that killed thousands of American children well into the mid-twentieth century (5).

Dr. William Potts Dewees, a professor of Midwifery at Pennsylvania, published a *Treatise on the Physical and Medical Treatment of Children* in 1825. This text had eight subsequent editions and was arguably the first formal American textbook of pediatrics (6). Dr. John Eberle, Professor of Medicine at Jefferson Medical College, also published a pediatric textbook in 1833 (7).

The first formal medical school course on diseases of children was given at Yale University by Dr. Eli Ives, who held the first faculty appointment in the subject in the United States. For nearly 40 years, between 1813 and 1852, Ives lectured on the diseases of children to an estimated 1,500 Yale medical students (8). His lectures, recorded by hand in student notebooks of the time, are preserved in Yale Sterling Library archives (Fig. 2). They consisted of lectures on subjects ranging from angina to worms. Ives ascribed many medical illnesses to offending substances in the gastrointestinal tract. These had to be removed by inducing vomiting or by purging. Dentition caused or aggravated many diseases during the first 2 years of life and lancing of the gums was considered essential. Ives firmly subscribed to Benjamin

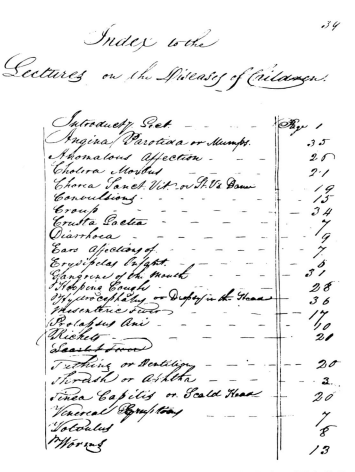

FIG. 2. Index of a medical student's lecture notes. Medical Institution of Yale College, 1821.

Rush's theories that all diseases were "fevers" brought on by over-stimulation of the arteries and so had to be treated by "depletion" by bloodletting, vomiting, or purging. Although Ives used phlebotomy sparingly, his therapeutic sheet anchors were calomel (mercury) and ipecac. Ives' teachings received little attention elsewhere, and formal instruction in diseases of children at Yale ceased after his retirement in 1852.

It was nearly 25 years after Ives that pediatrics in the United States began to take on a more defined presence. Children's hospitals were established, the first being the Children's Hospital of Pennsylvania, which opened in Philadelphia in 1855. The second was the Boston Children's Hospital (1869). Pediatric progress was perhaps most evident in New York City where Abraham Jacobi and Job Lewis Smith were contemporaries in the latter part of the nineteenth century.

Jacobi received his medical training at the University of Bonn, Germany. After graduation he was imprisoned for 2 years as a suspected revolutionist. He emigrated to New York City in 1853. Although he was a general practitioner, he devoted most of his time to the care of children and their diseases. In 1860 he established a children's clinic at the New York Medical College, where his appointment as Professor of Infantile Pathology and Therapeutics is believed to have been the first academic appointment in pediatrics in the United States.

Jacobi's most important contributions to pediatrics were his establishment of pediatric services in several New York hospitals and his involvement in a number of early pediatric societies. He also effectively championed causes that promoted the welfare of children. Although undoubtedly a superior clinician and medical politician, Jacobi made relatively few original contributions to the pediatric literature. However, his drive and enthusiasm were instrumental in establishing pediatrics as a separate discipline in the United States (9).

Job Lewis Smith, who entered practice in Manhattan about the same time as Jacobi, also played a major role in early American pediatrics. Smith worked primarily at the Bellevue Medical School, where he was appointed Clinical Professor of Morbid Anatomy in 1861 and Clinical Professor of Diseases of Children in 1876 (10). Smith was a prolific writer, publishing papers on infectious disease, rickets, and neonatal tetanus. He was very concerned with the dangers of bottle feeding and vigorously promoted milk sterilization. The appalling consequences of hand (artificial) feeding of foundlings in New York were poignantly described by Smith at the 1889 meeting of the American Pediatric Society.

> The steamboat every morning brought foundlings to (Randall's) Island and every afternoon removed an equal number for burial in Potters' Field.

Between 1869 and 1896 Smith also published 8 editions of *A Treatise on the Diseases of Infancy and Childhood* (11), an important resource for medical students and practitioners for 30 years.

One of Smith's signal accomplishments was the organization and founding of the American Pediatric Society. In 1887, following the Pediatric Section of the Ninth International Medical Congress held in Washington, D.C., Smith invited a group of physicians whom he knew to be interested in the diseases of children to join him in establishing the American Pediatric Society, an aim that was achieved in the following year. Forty-three physicians who were interested and involved in pediatrics were elected as the founding members. For fully 50 years the American Pediatric Society was the premier pediatric society in the United States. The presentations and discussions at the annual meetings, as recorded in the Society Transactions, documented striking progress and advances in the specialty (12,13).

Concern for safe, pure milk for infant feeding was an overriding concern in the early days of pediatrics in the United States. Although breastfeeding was strongly advocated, it was recognized that societal pressures and a very high rate of abandonment and orphaning of infants caused artificial feeding to be widely used. In U.S. cities, much of the milk supply was dangerously contaminated and disgustingly adulterated (14). Between 1870 and 1920, the need for safe milk for infant feeding became a crusade for leaders of U.S. pediatrics including Jacobi, Smith, Rotch, La-Fetra, Schick, Abt and many others.

Application of the principles of the burgeoning science of bacteriology to infant nutrition in the early twentieth century provided a scientific basis for safe infant feeding. That pasteurization of milk could prevent milk-transmitted diseases was first appreciated about 1895. However, it was not until 1908 that Chicago became the first U.S. city to make pasteurization of milk mandatory. Soon thereafter, pasteurization became nearly universal, and the lives of many children were saved.

In Boston, pediatrics was taught at Harvard Medical School as early as 1871. In 1893, Thomas Morgan Rotch (Fig. 3) was appointed full Professor of Diseases of Children with a chair on the faculty. Rotch is best remembered for his "percentage method" of infant feeding (15,16). This system was based upon the concept that cow's milk was relatively indigestible and so had to be diluted before feeding. Because dilution reduced fat and carbohydrate content, cream and sugar were added to approximate what was found in human milk. However, this surprisingly modern concept became exquisitely convoluted in Rotch's hands. His system mandated complex formulations with varying percentages of protein, fat, and carbohydrates and changes were frequently made on a day-to-day basis.

The system required

almost the equivalence of an advanced degree in higher mathematics employing algebraic equations to compute the food mixture of a baby (17).

It has been suggested that Rotch's successes were due more to his insistence on pure milk than to his percentage system. This system was widely accepted and employed by most U.S. physicians during the first decade of the twentieth century, but had little acceptance in Europe. Ultimately, the system collapsed under its own complexity. As Oliver Wendell Holmes quipped,

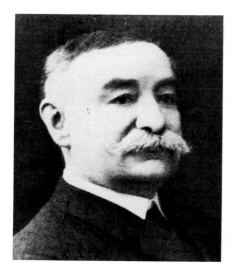

FIG. 3. Thomas Morgan Rotch, M.D. (1849–1914), Professor of Diseases of Children, Harvard Medical School, 1893.

A pair of substantial mammary glands has the advantage over the two hemispheres of the most learned professor's brain in the art of compounding a nutritious fluid for infants (18).

By the end of the first decade of the twentieth century, physicians in the United States developed and employed much more simplified feeding techniques based on the changing caloric needs of growing infants (calorimetric method).

Coincident with the development of the science of bacteriology, chemistry became increasingly incorporated into U.S. pediatrics. L. Emmett Holt, Sr., of New York (see p. 52, Fig. 3) can be credited with establishing a scientific base for pediatrics in the United States. Following his graduation from the College of Physicians and Surgeons in 1878, and a surgical internship, Holt entered private practice in midtown Manhattan. In 1889 he became the medical director of the New York Babies Hospital. This was said to be the first U.S. hospital (as opposed to a foundling asylum) devoted entirely to the care of infants and, at the time, was in danger of closing because of financial and staffing problems. Holt threw himself into the task of rebuilding and reshaping the hospital. His efforts culminated in the opening of a new, modern hospital in 1910. In addition to outpatient facilities and 70 inpatient beds, the new hospital had a dedicated research laboratory. Holt had no formal biochemical training; he therefore appointed experienced chemists to his staff. Holt also played a major role in the founding of the Rockefeller Institute. He worked with Rockefeller scientists and published a score of collaborative papers dealing with the chemical analysis of milk and milk proteins, salt and water balance, and absorption of nutrients and electrolytes in diarrheal diseases (19).

In 1901, Holt succeeded Jacobi as Professor of Pediatrics at Columbia School of Physicians and Surgeons. One of his greatest accomplishments was the authorship of the classic pediatric textbook, *The Diseases of Infancy and Childhood* (20). First published in 1897, it had 11 subsequent editions during Holt's lifetime. It became the standard pediatric textbook in the United States and was considered the equal of Osler's pre-eminent *Textbook of Internal Medicine*.

John Howland (see p. 268, Fig. 1), one of the greatest figures of U.S. pediatrics, graduated from the Cornell Medical School and trained in Europe. He assumed the position of full-time head of the Pediatric Department at Johns Hopkins Hospital in 1912, and during the next 14 years he built and directed the first modern, scientifically based, full-time pediatric department in the United States. The Harriet Lane Home opened in 1912 and Howland ensured that there were well-equipped biochemistry laboratories and a staff of full-time physicians. Howland recognized the importance of biochemical investigations of the diseases of children. He and a group of talented clinician-investigators published a series of classical studies on acidosis, rickets, and tetany (21). The men Howland trained became leaders in U.S. pediatrics for the next quarter of a century (see p. 270, Fig. 6), and included Edwards Park, Kenneth Blackfan, Grover Powers, William McKin Marriott, and James Gamble.

Following the model of Johns Hopkins and encouraged by the Flexner Report in 1912, full-time departments of pediatrics began to be established across the country. In addition to the scientific advances of U.S. pediatrics, psychosocial and humanistic aspects also received attention. This focus was perhaps best exemplified by Grover Powers of Yale (Fig. 4). Powers was educated and trained at Johns Hopkins School of Medicine under John Howland. In 1921 he accompanied Edwards Park to New Haven, Connecticut, where a new department of pediatrics had been established at Yale. When Park returned to Johns Hopkins in 1926 to become Professor and Chairman after Howland's death, Powers was appointed chairman of pediatrics at Yale—a position he was to hold for the next 30 years. Among Powers' unique contributions to U.S. pediatrics were his clear definition and articulation of the humanistic and social aspects of pediatrics and a description of the myriad problems associated with mental retardation. As Powers' colleague at Yale, Daniel Darrow, emphasized, the decreasing mortality and morbidity of infectious diseases made possible by microbiology and fluid and electrolyte therapy during the 1930s and 1940s resulted in an apparent emergence of the importance of childhood emotional disorders and mental retardation. Powers did much to address these issues (22). He imprinted his humanistic philosophy of patient care into the minds and practices of hundreds of Yale pediatric house officers over a quarter of a century. Powers' department also conducted clinical investigation in many areas of pediatric care. These included the contributions of James Trask in the field of bacteriology, and the exemplary work of Daniel Darrow on electrolyte therapy. A number of physicians who trained under Powers at Yale became leaders of U.S. pediatrics.

By 1938, research in nutrition and biochemistry had progressed rapidly, led initially by Holt, Howland, and Hess, and later by Gamble, Darrow, Butler, and others. Quantitative measurements were increasingly applied to pediatric problems. Fluid and electrolyte therapy was largely perfected. Antibiotics were introduced into pediatric practice, permitting control of many of the traditional infectious scourges of childhood.

Following a slowdown during World War II, a post-war boom in pediatrics oc-

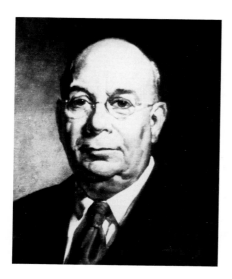

FIG. 4. Grover F. Powers (1887–1968), Professor of Pediatrics, Yale University School of Medicine, 1921. (Courtesy of Yale University Art Gallery.)

curred, particularly in research, largely fueled by federal funds. However, with expansion came subspecialization, compartmentalization and even fragmentation. Intercommunication became more difficult not only between general and academic pediatricians, but also among pediatric specialties. It became increasingly difficult, if not impossible, for the academic pediatrician of the late twentieth century to remain a competent clinician, teacher, and role model and also do fundamental investigation. One of the great challenges of U.S. pediatrics today is to decide whether the art, empathy, and concern for the whole child that have characterized this discipline over the last 100 years can be preserved as technologies become ever more complex and the body of scientific knowledge becomes ever larger.

REFERENCES

1. Viets HR. Thomas Thacher and his influence on American medicine. *Va Med Mon* 1949;76:384–397.
2. Steiner WR. Governor John Winthrop Jr of Connecticut as a physician. *Bull Johns Hopkins Hosp* 1903;14:294–312; 1906;17:357–369.
3. Caulfield E. Some common diseases of colonial children. *Trans Colonial Soc Mass* 1951;35:4–13.
4. Ruhräh J. *Pediatrics of the past: An anthology.* New York: Hoeber, 1925.
5. Rush B. An inquiry into the cause of cholera infantum. In: *Medical inquiries and observations,* vol 1. Philadelphia: Prichard and Hall, 1789;112.
6. Dewees WP. *Treatise on the physical and medical treatment of children.* Philadelphia: Carey and Lea, 1825.
7. Eberle J. *Treatise on the diseases and physical education in children.* Cincinnati: Corey and Fairbank, 1833.
8. Pearson HA. Lectures on the diseases of children by Eli Ives, M.D. of Yale and New Haven. America's first academic pediatrician. *Pediatrics* 1986;77:680–6.
9. Leopold JS. Abraham Jacobi. In: *Pediatric profiles.* St. Louis: CV Mosby, 1957;13.
10. Faber HK. Job Lewis Smith, forgotten pioneer. *J Pediatr* 1961;63:794–802.
11. Smith JL. *A treatise on the diseases of infancy and childhood.* Philadelphia: Lea, 1869.
12. Faber HH, and McIntosh R. *History of the American Pediatric Society* 1887–1965. New York: McGraw Hill, 1966.
13. Pearson HA. *The centennial history of the American Pediatric Society, 1888–1988.* New Haven: American Pediatric Society, 1988.
14. Cone TE Jr. *History of American pediatrics.* Boston: Little Brown, 1979;106.
15. Morse JL. The history of pediatrics in Massachusetts. *N Engl J Med* 1931;205:169–180.
16. Rotch TM. A historical sketch of the development of percentage feeding. *NY Med J* 1907;85:532–540.
17. Meyer JF. *Essentials of infant feeding for physicians.* Springfield, IL: Thomas, 1952.
18. Holmes OW. Scholastic and bedside teaching. In: *Medical essays.* Boston: Houghton Mifflen, 1911.
19. Park EA, Mason HH. Luther Emmett Holt. In: *Pediatric profiles.* St Louis: CV Mosby, 1957;33.
20. Holt LE. *The diseases of infancy and childhood.* New York: Appleton, 1987.
21. Davison WC. John Howland. In: *Pediatric profiles.* St Louis: CV Mosby, 1957;161.
22. Darrow D. Presentation of the John F Howland Award to Grover F Powers. *Pediatrics* 1953;12:217–226.

DISCUSSION

Dr. Collins-Williams: I should like to add something about pediatrics in Canada, which goes back a long way. The Hospital for Sick Children in Toronto was founded in 1875 and started off as a house. It ended up as a hospital with over 800 beds, although there are fewer now since we are treating more patients on an outpatient basis. I think the greatest event that happened there in the time we are talking about was in 1921, when Frederick Banting and Gladys Best, one of our most famous Canadian woman pediatricians, first used insulin for the treatment of juvenile diabetes. We have had many famous staff at this institution but I shall not list their names.

Montreal also started pediatrics very early. Although the Montreal Children's Hospital was not opened until 1904, Blackadder had been lecturer in diseases of children since 1881 and was the first physician-in-chief. He eventually became President of the American Pediatric Society and later of the Canadian Pediatric Society on its formation.

Winnipeg founded its children's hospital in 1909, and of course we now have a children's hospital at every medical school across the country. Generally speaking, pediatrics in Canada is practiced very much as it is in the United States, with a lot of full-timers, and many pediatricians doing only consulting work.

Dr. Pearson: Thank you. I was not being intentionally nationalistic or chauvinistic in omitting Canada.

Dr. Stern: I should point out that people like me who were born and brought up in Montreal never considered Ontario to be part of Canada! The first Canadian medical school was actually founded in 1636 by Bishop Laval, who had been sent by Cardinal Richelieu to be the spiritual leader of French Canada. Richelieu also appointed Jean Talon as Governor, and Talon and Laval struck a deal whereby the Bishop would build a university with a medical school if Talon would build a hospital. This is the origin of the Hotel Dieu Hospital in Montreal, which is situated within the original city of Ville Marie. Thus the French had a medical school before the British took the colony over.

By the mid 1820s the only physicians left in English-speaking Canada were either British Army officers, Hessian mercenaries or United Empire Loyalists, and these were becoming too old or too exhausted to carry on. With nowhere to train their sons to become physicians, four Montreal doctors got together and founded McGill University as a medical school with medicine as its first faculty. James McGill was actually a dishonest Scottish fur merchant and the land he gave for the university did not even belong to him, but to a farmer called Simon McTavish. McGill was originally buried on the campus but in the later 1870s his body was removed for reasons of propriety.

Dr. Farrell: I was interested in the percentage method of Thomas Morgan Rotch for calculating infant feeds. Was there any scientific basis for this system?

Dr. Barness: The system was absolute nonsense. It mandated frequent changes in the diet, for example, you had to give a certain amount of carbohydrate for scarlet fever but an entirely different amount for measles. Day-to-day changes of as little as one-fourth of one percent of the protein intake of a baby were prescribed. The system was almost gibberish.

Europeans have often wondered why Americans call a milk mixture for babies a "formula". This comes from the formulas of Dr Rotch. Abraham Jacobi was quoted as saying to Rotch, "You can't raise a baby by mathematics!"

Dr. Suskind: The deep south of the United States is often forgotten about in discussions of American medicine, although it has a very interesting medical history. The Charity Hospital in New Orleans was founded in the early 1700s and is the hospital with the longest period of continuous use of any in the United States. There was also a children's hospital, built in 1898 but demolished in 1955 when Louisiana State University decided to expand the medical school. The ninth floor of the Charity Hospital then became the Children's Hospital of New Orleans.

There was also a Louisiana State Medical School founded over 150 years ago, which was later renamed Tulane.

History of Pediatrics 1850–1950, edited by
B.L. Nichols, A. Ballabriga, and N. Kretchmer.
Nestlé Nutrition Workshop Series, Vol. 22. Nestec
Ltd., Vevey/Raven Press, Ltd., New York © 1991.

Mexican Pediatrics

Silvestre Frenk and *Ignacio Avila-Cisneros

*División de Nutrición, Unidad de Investigación Biomédica, Centro Médico Nacional Instituto Mexicano del Seguro Social, México, 06760 Distrito Federal; *Departamento de Investigación Médico-Social, Instituto Nacional de Pediatría. México, 04530 Distrito Federal*

In the year 1850, virtually no schools remained in Mexico, the land that, in 1551, had seen the birth of the first university on the American continent. The Establecimiento de Ciencias Médicas, the forerunner of the present-day faculty of medicine of the Universidad Nacional, had just been put into operation by Valentin Gómez Farías in 1833, when a continuous internal and international state of war broke out. A strong tradition, a rich cultural heritage, and an indomitable patriotic spirit, kept the nation alive through 25 years of incessant warfare, a foreign invasion, and the establishment of a spurious empire.

Despite these chaotic conditions, there were some early attempts at organizing maternal and child health care (1,2). In 1861, President Benito Juárez decreed the foundation of a maternity hospital, which had a short life because of the political conditions of the time, and also of a children's hospital, which did not materialize at all.

Almost immediately after its inception in 1864, the empire of Ferdinand Joseph Maximilian of Hapsburg established a council for general welfare, which, under the aegis of the hapless and childless empress Charlotte Amalie, soon dedicated a 20-bed Casa de Maternidad e Infancia. In honor of such august patronage this soon became known as Hospital de San Carlos, a name it lost in 1867, upon the restoration of the Republic. Possibly the first formal institution devoted to providing medical care to small children after independence from Spain (3), it also became the seat of a chair of obstetrics, but not of pediatrics. The first Mexican obstetric treatise, under the title *Guía clínica del arte de los partos* (Clinical Guide to the Art of Childbirth Care), written by Juan María Rodríguez, was published in 1885.

Soon afterwards, the Hospital de Maternidad e Infancia incorporated the children's wards of the venerable Hospital de San Andrés (3), and thus came under the directorship of Professor Eduardo Liceaga, the most prominent medical figure of those years, and the first physician to obtain his tenure through competitive appointment. In 1905 it became part of the new Hospital General, whose creator and founding director was Liceaga. Built in the French style popular in those years, this huge hospital was fitted with a pavillion for children with infectious diseases and one for pediatric orthopedics, as well as a maternity department, but only as recently as 1950 was a building for general pediatric medicine provided.

The first establishment built exclusively for the care of sick children was opened in 1877 in the city of Puebla (4). The little patients in this Hospital de la Caridad para Niños were described as suffering from "loose stools, cough, fevers, pot bellies, and thin limbs; almost all of them were brown-skinned and of small height; a great majority soon perished." In 1917 this institution merged with the general hospital of Puebla.

The above-mentioned clinical condition had been superbly described by F. Hinojosa in volume 1 (1864) of *Gaceta Médica de México,* presently in its 126th volume. This brief article of a mere two pages (5) that was followed by a long commentary (6) has become a classic on the nutritional ailment nowadays known as kwashiorkor; its academic value lies well above the often-quoted paper on *culebrilla* by José Patrón-Correa, which appeared in 1908 (7).

The historical credit for being the first true children's hospital in Mexico belongs to the Hospital de la Infancia, later named Hospital Infantil, in the city of San Luis Potosí (8). Dedicated in 1893, it was the result of purposeful planning and was the brainchild of Dr. Miguel Otero-Arce, who also supported it, mostly out of his own purse. He was the first physician in the country to occupy an official teaching post in child care, and to practice pediatric surgery. In 1896, he started the publication of the *Anales del Hospital Infantil de San Luis Potosí,* the first pediatric journal in Mexico, and one of the first in Latin America. The hospital operated as such until 1900, when Otero moved to the capital to devote himself to research on rabies and on typhus, a disease that he eventually contracted in the laboratory and succumbed to at the age of 70.

In 1899, Dr. Roque Macouzet, who had graduated in Paris, was appointed to the Escuela Nacional de Medicina as Associate Professor in the clinic for children's diseases, first holding the post in the Hospital de San Andrés and later at the new Hospital General. His *Arte de criar y de curar á los niños* (The Art of Rearing and Curing Children) (1910), edited in Barcelona, is the first known textbook of pediatrics written by a Mexican author (Fig. 1). In 1907, Joaquín Cosío, professor of medical clinics, had initiated his courses on medical and surgical clinics in pediatrics. Other general hospitals were opening new pediatric wards, and soon the Academia Nacional de Medicina established a section of pediatrics, with three chairs.

However, the care of sick children and the teaching of pediatrics remained mostly in the charge of general practitioners and obstetricians, who developed a special interest in nutrition and infectious diseases.

During the second and third decades of this century, Mexico was once more torn apart by civil war. In search for more just social conditions, a vital new national spirit emerged. This was attested to by vigorous and innovative literary, musical, and mural painting movements, and in tune with it, a growing number of physicians sought specialization in postwar Europe. As the first pediatricians were being

FIG. 1.   Title page of the first Mexican textbook on pediatrics.

ARTE

DE

CRIAR Y DE CURAR

Á LOS NIÑOS

POR EL

DR. ROQUE MACOUZET

CATEDRÁTICO, POR OPOSICIÓN, DE CLÍNICA DE ENFERMEDADES DE LOS NIÑOS
EN LA ESCUELA DE MEDICINA DE MÉXICO

BARCELONA
FIDEL GIRÓ, IMPRESOR: VALENCIA, 233
1910

trained in French, German, and Austrian schools, the "undifferentiated" stage of Mexican pediatrics was reaching its end (9).

In the year 1922, an obstetrician, Professor Isidro Espinosa y de los Reyes, a modern Soranus of Ephesus, organized the first Centro de Higiene Infantil, which soon expanded into a network of centers, the forerunners of present-day services for primary maternal and child health care. Its aim was to provide free medical and hygienic care to pregnant women and infants under 2 years (10). The success of these initial programs resulted in the creation, in 1929, of the Asociación Nacional de Protección a la Infancia, which since then and under different names, styles, and financial means, has been headed by the wife of the President of the Republic. Over the years, several private foundations followed suit (11).

Formal teaching in pediatrics began as a result of this improved climate. The first professor at the Escuela Nacional de Medicina was Mario A. Torroella, who had been trained by Bernard Marfan, and who successfully adapted Parisian teaching programs to Mexican needs (Fig. 2) (9,11). His methods were also adopted by many of his followers, as they gradually returned from their European training periods; the success of Torroella, Manuel Cárdenas de la Vega, and other pediatricians in private practice helped to make the discipline attractive and popular.

In the mid-1920s, political circumstances led a young military physician to seek an internship with Professor William McKim Marriott (see p. 141, Fig. 4) at the Children's Hospital in Saint Louis, Missouri. Thus started the academic career of Federico Gómez-Santos. His subsequent flair for the metabolic aspects of child diseases was due in no small measure to his having received his pediatric training from such a renowned biochemist.

Upon his return, Gómez became a staff member of one of the new Centros de Higiene Infantil, and, despite frequent differences with his European-trained colleagues, out of the creative amalgamation of the two schools grew modern Mexican pediatrics.

In 1930 a group of young pediatricians founded the Sociedad Mexicana de Puericultura, a decade later renamed Sociedad Mexicana de Pediatría. The society was one of the first academic medical specialist associations in the country. In the same year, publication of its official journal, the *Revista Mexicana de Puericultura,* began. Later *Puericultura* became *Pediatría* and it is now publishing its 57th volume. The dynamic nature of the Society stimulated the creation of other Mexican societies in related disciplines, as well as the first pediatric societies in provincial Mexico. Out of these pioneer groups, grew the idea that the time had come for the creation of a modern children's hospital in the capital city.

In 1932, the old Casa de Cuna (Foundlings home), where material conditions were such that any epidemic caused appalling mortality (2,12), was moved to a new and more adequate building, which would be remodeled to serve as a hospital for sick chidren and was fitted for auxiliary services, including morbid anatomy. A modern organization, inspired by Federico Gómez, provided for the first time an acceptable environment for the care of sick children (13). It started the publication of its medical journal, the *Boletín Médico de la Casa de Cuna,* and became the main pediatric teaching institution for the medical students of the university and the Es-

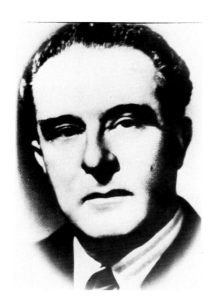

FIG. 2. Professor Mario A. Torroella.

cuela Médico Militar, to which Gómez had recently been appointed Professor of child health. The Casa de Cuna served as the only center for pediatric instruction for general practitioners wanting to improve their pediatric skills. With the intellectual support of a growing number of visiting professors from abroad, who were astonished by the level of care that could be provided for sick children under somewhat primitive working conditions, together with pressure from the Sociedad Mexicana de Pediatría, the inspiration of the staff, and a favorable attitude of the President of the Republic, the construction of a new hospital was begun in 1933. It took 10 years to complete and equip the building, and the new Hospital Infantil de México was finally dedicated on April 30, 1943 (Fig. 3) (14).

In keeping with its role as a teaching hospital, the first premises to be finished were the lecture rooms, which were promptly put to use by the department heads for teaching future medical, nursing, and support personnel. Many of them, particularly the young ones seeking a subspecialty, had previously been sent abroad for training in other children's hospitals.

In his inaugural speech, Professor Gómez (Fig. 4), the director of the new institution, said: "Our goal will be to make out of this hospital an institution with three main functions: an excellent service to society, a propitious field for pediatric teaching, and a fertile environment for research on the pathology of childhood. . . . However, in order to fulfill this commitment with the meticulousness and the efficiency imposed by science and society, we shall need the help of the community, and deep understanding and sympathy" (14).

The building of just one more hospital may seem no special feat. However, to sense the epic nature of the achievement, one needs to place oneself into the context of the times, in a country still recovering from revolution, while, at the same time,

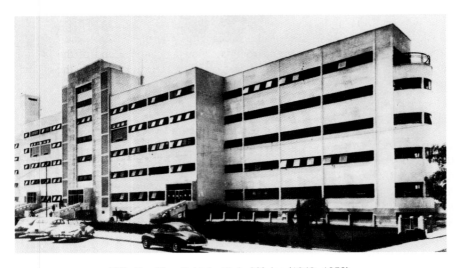

FIG. 3. *Hospital Infantil de México* (1943–1959).

struggling for worldwide recognition of its efforts to become a modern nation (13).

The *Hospital Infantil de México* was modern in the full sense of the term: revolutionary in its organization and in its teaching practices, unique in its relative independence of the health authorities, excellently staffed, well equipped, and up-to-date in medical and surgical procedures. It was the first hospital in Mexico and one of the first in Latin America to adopt the North American model of internship and

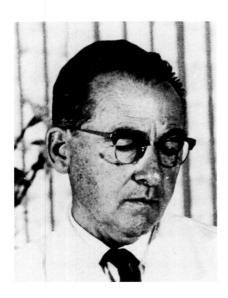

FIG. 4. Professor Federico Gómez-Santos.

residency, and the main postulates of the intellectual revolution initiated by the Flexner report, adapted to the social and academic circumstances of the country. It pioneered clinico-pathologic grand rounds, which meant the end of the infallible magister and his "clinical eye". The first staff member to submit to the ordeal of discussing a "closed" case was Federico Gómez himself; he was also the only one of the leading professors of the time to give up his prosperous private practice in order to devote himself entirely to the Hospital.

New didactic technologies were put into practice. Internship and residency became university postgraduate courses in their own right. Three- and ten-month-long training courses for general practitioners, as well as courses in subspecialties, were also offered. One year after its start, the Hospital was publishing a journal, the *Boletín Médico del Hospital Infantil,* now in its 46th volume, and currently one of the most important pediatric journals in the Spanish language. Its editorial office now also publishes an average of 10 books per year. The Hospital Infantil eventually became one of the main pediatric training grounds in Latin America, attracting scores of young, foreign physicians eager to learn about modern pediatrics.

By the end of the 1940s, the Hospital was contributing to original scientific work. As many young clinical investigators returned from their training abroad, research laboratories started up, mostly attached to hospital wards. Even before the various study groups materialized and before the first formal biochemical and physiological laboratories were put into operation, major scientific achievements were emerging: the discovery, in 1946, of *Escherichia coli Gómez* (presently known as *E. coli* 0 111 B_4), showing that coliform bacilli could be pathogenic (15); and, in the same year, the proposal of the Gómez classification of malnutrition, still widely used (16). Henceforth, the dyad of infection–malnutrition was to become one of the main academic leitmotifs of the institution, and some years later led to the creation of a rural research unit in the central region of the country.

The Mexican school of pediatrics was thus forged: inspired by the outstanding personality of a genuine leader, based on a solid medical institution that was to become the alma mater of almost all professionals henceforth involved in child care in Mexico, sustained by strong ideals, centered on concrete scientific problems, and endowed with a well-defined social and academic role and a deep humanistic spirit.

In 1951, the Academia Mexicana de Pediatría was founded and, in 1955, the Asociación de Investigación Pediátrica. Both were societies that were to exert a powerful influence on academic pediatrics, within and beyond the national borders. The Hospital Infantil soon inspired the construction of children's hospitals in the cities of Bogotá, Guatemala, La Paz, Panamá, and San José. It steered the development of child care in all the Latin American countries and gave a new competitive impulse to those with long-established schools of pediatrics.

In 1957, a severe earthquake shook the capital city and damaged the beautiful hospital buildings. Although it was rebuilt, the institution had to be moved to nearby premises in 1959, and its 500 beds were reduced to 300. This mishap severely curtailed the services provided by the hospital, although its vast research and teaching activities soon recovered their usual pace.

By that time, Mexico City had started its phenomenal growth. The Hospital Infantil promoted the development of small peripheral units, so that, by the end of the 1950s, the city contained a unique network of twelve 100- to 120-bed children's hospitals managed by the city government, together with several others run by the Ministry of Health and by private foundations. They soon became training institutions in their own right.

In 1963, Professor Gómez retired from the Hospital Infantil de México, after directing it for 20 years. But further commitments immediately awaited him: the organization of a second main nucleus for Mexican pediatrics. The Instituto Mexicano del Seguro Social (IMSS) had been founded in March 1943, one month before the inauguration of the Hospital Infantil. By the middle of the 1950s its main pediatric services consisted of two departments, one medical and one surgical, within a big general hospital in the northern part of the city. Headed by Professor Rogelio H. Valenzuela, these departments also trained residents and carried out research. The main textbook for medical students, still in use, came from there. Comparable organizations were later created at the Instituto de Seguridad y Servicios Sociales de los Trabajadores del Estado (ISSSTE), and in the medical services of the armed forces.

The IMSS authorities quickly grasped the need for a modern children's hospital. The ambitious name Hospital de Pediatría was proposed, to symbolize the broad scope of the new hospital, covering all ages from the neonatal period to the end of adolescence. The recently purchased Centro Médico Nacional was remodeled to house the new institution (Fig. 5), which was put into operation on March 15, 1963,

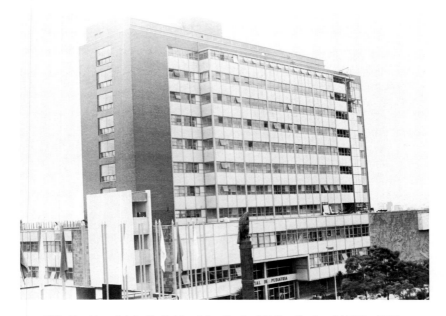

FIG. 5. Hospital de Pediatría of the Centro Médico Nacional (1963–1985).

again under the direction of Federico Gómez (17). Initially most of its medical, nursing, social work, and laboratory personnel came from the ranks of the still young but now mature staff of the Hospital Infantil.

A working continuity was thus provided between the new and the 20-year-old institutions, with the same spirit and discipline, albeit within the framework of the huge machinery of the Mexican Institute of Social Security.

The well-proved system of specialized wards with attached research laboratories was maintained at the Hospital de Pediatría. The institution was provided with an unprecedented number of lecture theaters and seminar rooms. Thus, in a matter of few months, this new center of Mexican pediatrics began a most ambitious teaching, lecturing, and research program. It was the first hospital unit to have its own preventive medicine service. It boosted the child care services in the IMSS, and soon its alumni were staffing other units, mostly second-level general zonal hospitals, which today carry out most of the hospital pediatric care, and share the training of the new generations of pediatricians with the large third-level hospitals. Among these is the Hospital de Gineco-Pediatría in Guadalajara, which functions as an operational unit with a gynecological and obstetric hospital, with shared diagnostic and support facilities.

Strangely, the fate of the Hospital de Pediatría was the same as that of its parent institution, the Hospital Infantil de México: it succumbed to the 1985 earthquake and had to be demolished. A new building, in effect a brand new institution, again with revolutionary clinical, teaching, and research programs, will open shortly.

A third pole of pediatric development was the Hospital del Niño, originally part of the Institución Mexicana de Asistencia a la Niñez. This beautiful hospital, which was designed, built, and equipped with the most advanced technology then available, was opened in 1970. Its scope and programs have been expanded since its transformation into the present Instituto Nacional de Pediatría, and its sister institution, the Instituto Nacional de Perinatología. This unique complex was somewhat later completed with the main research facility in pediatrics, mostly in matters of growth, development, and behavior, the Instituto Nacional de Ciencias y Tecnología de la Salud del Niño.

New children's hospitals are still being opened in most of the main cities of the country. Their technical and educational excellence is such that only a small and dwindling number of young pediatricians from the provinces have to come to the capital city for specialized training.

In this long-lasting process of continuous expansion of hospital care for children, we should note the fact that, as the era of the illustrious giants appears to be fading out, the cohesion of thought and action underlying the schools of medical practice may be disrupted. As the academic spirit and the institutional framework of actively shared ideas, ideals, and ideologies yields to the advance of complex technology and to fragmentation into small groups of super-experts, the scholastic essence of academe runs the risk of getting lost. According to the great Uruguayan writer, Juan Carlos Onetti, the existence of the past depends on how much of the present we are willing to grant it, and this may be a little, may be none.

REFERENCES

1. Alvarez-Amézquita J, Bustamante ME, López-Picazos A, Fernández-del Castillo F. *Historia de la Salubridad y de la Asistencia en México.* vol. 3, México: Secretaría de Salubridad y Asistencia. 1960;450–451.
2. Velasco-Ceballos R. *El niño mexicano ante la caridad y el Estado.* México: Edic de la Beneficiencia Pública en el D F, 1935;103–130.
3. Saavedra AM. Apuntes para la historia de los orígenes del primer hospital de niños en México. *Rev Mex Pueric* 1935;5:991–1007.
4. Fajardo-Ortiz G. *México en sus hospitales. Historia, realidades, leyendas y tragedias.* México: Academia Nacional de Medicina, 1990.
5. Hinojosa F. Apuntes sobre una enfermedad del pueblo de La Magdalena. *Gac Med Mex* 1865;1: 137–9.
6. Coindet L. Rapport sur une épidémie observée a La Magdalena. *Gac Med Mex* 1865;1:139–144.
7. Patrón-Correa J. ¿Qué es la culebrilla? *Rev Med Yuc* 1908;3:89–92.
8. Padrón-Puyou F. Ensayo sobre la historia de los hospitales en San Luis Potosí. *Rev Med Hosp Centr San Luis Potosí* 1948;1:5–25.
9. Martínez PD. Notas sobre la pediatría en México en la primera mitad del siglo XX. *Bol Soc Med Cent Mat Infant "Maximino Avila Camacho"* 1951;2:91–9.
10. Espinosa y de los Reyes I. La labor de los Centros de Higiene Infantil dependientes del Departamento de Salubridad Pública. *Rev Mex Pueric* 1931–1932;2:5–18.
11. Avila-Cisneros I. Hitos en la evolución de la pediatría en el México independiente. *Rev Mex Pediatr* 1989;56:15–30.
12. Carrillo R. La Cuna: su pasado, su presente, su porvenir. *Gac Med Mex* (3a. serie) 1915;10:320–343.
13. Frenk S. Historia reciente de la asistencia materno-infantil en México. *Salud Publica Mex* 1983;25:513–7.
14. Toussaint-Aragón E. *Hospital Infantil de México "Dr. Federico Gómez". 1943–1983.* México: E. Toussaint Aragón, 1983;29–120.
15. Varela G, Aguirre A, Carrillo J. *Escherichia coli-Gómez,* nueva especie aislada de un caso mortal de diarrea. *Bol Med Hosp Infant Mex* 1946;3:623–7.
16. Gómez F. Desnutrición. *Bol Med Hosp Infant Mex* 1946;3:543–51.
17. Gómez F. El Hospital General de Pediatría del Instituto Mexicano del Seguro Social. *Bol Med IMSS* 1963;5:5–25.

DISCUSSION

Dr. Stern: I was pleased that the Instituto Nacional de Perinatología was mentioned. Can we hear some more about this institute?

Dr. Frenk: It was an obstetrician, Professor Isidro Espinosa y de los Reyes, who first realized the goal of integrated, preventive care of the mother and infant in the Centros de Higiene Infantil. In his honor, a maternity hospital, conceived on the same principles, was given his name. The Instituto Nacional de Perinatología was subsequently built on the same site.

In Mexico, as elsewhere, the concept of perinatology was forged in maternity hospitals. To my knowledge the first formal university course in this discipline was organized by Professor Juan Urrusti in the Hospital de Gineco-Obstetricia No. 2 of the Centro Médico Nacional (IMSS). The unique approach of the Instituto Nacional de Perinatología has made it a center of training for pediatricians and obstetricians alike.

Dr. Metcoff: I think it would be interesting to say more about Federico Gómez. I recall several things about him. One was his philosophical concept of the nature of kwashiorkor as a reversion from the alert active infant to the inactive "fetal" being. Second, I recall being impressed by his conduct of ward rounds, and particularly by the fact that one of the jobs of the house officer was to push a typewriter around and type the comments as they were made by the attending physician! I also remember his philosophical contributions to social progress. Perhaps you could comment some more on his various contributions to pediatrics.

Dr. Frenk: Federico Gómez was a totally unusual character. He was, as Dr. Metcoff has said, not only a physician but a philosopher, a very good writer, and a man of extremely deep feelings—a complete physician. When he made rounds on the nutrition ward we had to push along a little cart carrying all kinds of food—bread, bananas, and so on—that he himself fed to the small children who were struggling to recover from malnutrition. This aspect of the man was one that many people who visited us found most surprising; they were amazed that a person of such solid academic achievement and such organizing abilities, who had conceived and carried through the construction of the Hospital Infantil and who ran it so successfully, could at the same time show such humanitarian, almost nurse-like, behavior in his treatment of small children.

The Hospital Infantil was hit by the 1957 earthquake but was moved to a nearby building (a maternity hospital). Its academic and teaching role in attracting young physicians from other countries has continued. Gómez's main collaborators of the early days have retired, but his heritage is in the big network of pediatric hospitals in the metropolitan area of Mexico City and in the interior of the country. Mexico is an old country, but it has a young population (55% are less than 16 years old), and there is still an excessive morbidity rate in spite of a large reduction in infant and preschool mortality. The need for children's hospitals persists, as does the need for a more efficient maternal health education.

Dr. Waterlow: You mentioned the paper of Hinojosa on what we now call kwashiorkor, which appeared 70 years before its description by Dr. Cicely Williams. What about the one on culebrilla, which used to be quoted as one of the pioneer articles on the subject? Which one was first?

Dr. Frenk: As pointed out, the article of Hinojosa (5) preceded the one on culebrilla by Patrón-Correa (7) by 44 years. While the latter was a clinical description of the syndrome, Hinojosa performed a clever and partially correct (in present-day terms) hypothesis on its etiopathogenesis. He went right to the point. The first sentence of the article reads: "The first symptom observed in this disease is diarrhea," a fact that took about 80 more years to be universally recognized. His is a most outstanding piece of work, by a general practitioner, who was not a teacher nor an academician, but who had the solid clinical insight typical of the medicine of the past century. His paper was followed by a much longer one by Leon Coindet (remember that in those days México was occupied by the French army), which showed that the picture did not correspond to pellagra (6).

History of Pediatrics 1850–1950, edited by
B.L. Nichols, A. Ballabriga, and N. Kretchmer.
Nestlé Nutrition Workshop Series, Vol. 22. Nestec
Ltd., Vevey/Raven Press, Ltd., New York © 1991.

Infant Feeding

Samuel J. Fomon

Department of Pediatrics, College of Medicine, University of Iowa, Iowa City, Iowa 52242, USA

Changes in infant feeding practices from 1850 to 1950 were more dramatic than during any earlier period, and most of the many developments since 1950 seem trivial by comparison. I shall review infant feeding as it existed in western Europe and North America in 1850, identify the major changes that occurred between 1850 and 1950, and comment on the situation in 1950.

Infant feeding in the mid-1800s must be examined in the context of a high infant mortality in Europe and North America. Routh (1a) cites data indicating that in Brussels, Brunswick, Berlin, Hamburg, Paris, and Vienna, deaths during the first 3 months of life ranged from 1 in 3 to 1 in 11. In 1874, infant mortality in England was 18% (1b). Although I have been unable to locate similar data for American cities, infant mortality was undoubtedly high.

FEEDING PRACTICES IN 1850

From the writings of a number of authors (1–4), it is evident that, in the middle of the nineteenth century, the majority of infants in Europe and North America were breast-fed. Although the various writers do not comment on the actual percentage of infants who were breast-fed in various countries, the recommended practice for women who could not nurse their own infants (or preferred not to do so) was the employment of another lactating woman (a wet nurse). In western Europe in about 1850, most infants were breast-fed by their own mothers, some were breast-fed by other women and some, perhaps only about 10%, were "hand-reared" (also spoken of as "dry nursed").

Breast Feeding

Wet nursing, which had been widespread in western Europe in the seventeenth century, especially among the urban middle and upper classes, had begun to decline by the middle of the nineteenth century (3). In most instances, wet nurses proved to be unsatisfactory (1c,3). A woman who nursed her own infant as well as another infant often failed to provide an adequate amount of milk. Even when the woman's own infant had died or had been abandoned, the care given to the temporary foster infant was often poor. Routh (1d) reports on two communities with similar hygienic conditions in the Geronde in France: "In one the mothers suckle their own children; in the other a number of mercenary wet nurses take in children from Bordeaux in large numbers to nurse. In the first commune the mortality is 13 per cent. In the second 87 per cent." Social pressure developed to eliminate wet nursing because it was believed, with justification, that a number of women abandoned their own infants in order to obtain employment as wet nurses (5).

Although black slaves in the southern colonies were sometimes wet nurses for children of the plantation owners (6), wet nursing was much less common in North America than in Europe.

Breast feeding was frequently supplemented by thin gruels called pap or panada (1,3,4). Pap consisted of bread or flour cooked in water with or without the addition of milk (7). Panada was similar but was usually cooked in broth of meat or legumes and included a combination of cereal, butter, flour or bread. Milk, egg yolk, whole egg, beer, wine, or anise were sometimes included. These foods were generally fed from a boat-shaped vessel (pap boat), or from a pap spoon with hollow handle, permitting the speed of delivery to be controlled by pressure of the finger on a hole at the end of the handle. Pap was more liquid than the purées that are commonly fed to infants at the present time.

It was commonly recommended that weaning from the breast begin at 10 to 12 months of age, at least in vigorous, healthy infants (3,4,8). Weaning was not recommended during the months of July, August, and September, when diarrhea was prevalent.

Bottle Feeding

As the popularity of wet nursing declined during the first half of the nineteenth century, bottle feeding increased. Use of ass and goat milk decreased in favor of cow's milk. Although the mortality among bottle-fed infants was high, data are not available concerning mortality of infants who were bottle-fed in their own homes. Among bottle-fed infants in foundling institutions in France, 50% died (1e). In New York City foundling asylums in 1886, nearly all bottle-fed infants died (9).

A number of circumstances made it unlikely that bottle feeding would be successful. Sewage disposal was poor and water supplies were unsafe. Sanitary standards for dairying and for handling and storage of milk, although improving, were unsatisfactory, especially in urban areas. Cow sheds were located within cities, sometimes underground, and cows were often diseased (1f). Milk was often adulterated by the addition of water and other substances. Although glass feeding bottles had largely replaced the animal horns and other receptacles that had been used in the eighteenth century, nipples were made of cloth or leather, often stuffed with a piece of sponge. Thus, adequate cleaning of the feeding utensils was impossible. Means for safe storage of formula in the home were not available.

Knowledge of microbiology, food chemistry, and requirements for micronutrients was rudimentary. The relationship between intestinal bacteria and diarrhea was unrecognized; the need to reduce the curd tension of cow's milk was not appreciated; there were strong prejudices against heat treatment of milk because of the observation that infantile scurvy, a disease of unknown etiology, was most common in infants fed heat-treated milks.

CHANGES IN FEEDING PRACTICES, 1850–1950

Breast Feeding

During the latter part of the nineteenth century, as the popularity of formula feeding increased, breast feeding declined. Although practice of wet nursing had not disappeared (10), Bullough (11) notes that advertisements for wet nurses were no longer found in the London *Times* after about 1880.

By the end of the nineteenth century in America, breast-fed infants were frequently offered some formula feedings (12).

Knowledge of Milk Composition

In 1869, Biedert reported that the protein content of cow's milk was about twice as high as that of human milk (9). He recommended that mixtures of cow's milk, water, and lactose be used for infant feeding. By the end of the nineteenth century, information was available on the chemical composition of human milk and of various other animal milks (1,2).

General Sanitation

The widespread adulteration and contamination of the milk supply prevalent in the middle of the nineteenth century persisted to the end of the century. As cited by Cone (9), Sedgwick in 1892 wrote of the situation in Massachusetts as follows:

> Milk . . . is usually drawn from animals in stables which will not bear description in good society, from cows which often have flaking excrement all over their flanks, by milkmen who are anything but clean. It is drawn into milk pails which are seldom or never thoroughly cleansed, sent to the city, where it is still further delayed and finally delivered to the consumer in a partially decomposed condition.

In 1901 in New York City, milk delivered to customers in the summer was generally contaminated with bacteria and might contain more than 5,000,000 organisms per ml (13). It was not until 1912 that clean milk was available in New York City (13).

Chlorination of water was introduced in the United States in the 1880s and, at the same time, major improvements were made in disposal of garbage (14). Toward the end of the nineteenth century, bacilli causing dysentery were identified. Organisms of the dysentery group were suspected as the cause of bloody diarrhea in infants (9), thus stimulating efforts to improve general sanitation.

An important development toward the end of the nineteenth century was the creation of infant and child care facilities. These appeared first in Hamburg, New York, and Barcelona, and during the early 1900s became widespread in France, the United States, Germany, England, and Scotland (13a).

Processing of Milk

In 1856, Borden was granted a patent for condensing milk with heat (15). It was soon learned that the addition of sugar prevented bacterial growth and improved keeping properties, but such milk was found to be unsatisfactory for infant feeding, probably because of high energy density. Until the development of suitable methods of canning, use of "unsweetened" evaporated milk in infant feeding was not feasible because there was no satisfactory method for preventing contamination of the product after manufacture.

Pasteurization of milk was first practiced on a commercial scale in Denmark in 1890 (4) and subsequently was introduced in other countries—apparently more to improve the "life" of the milk than to reduce the number of pathogens.

In the late 1800s, it was recognized that feeding of fresh, unprocessed cow's milk resulted in formation of a tough and rubbery curd in the infant's stomach, whereas feeding of fresh human milk results in a soft, flocculent curd (16). Nevertheless, use of raw cow's milk for infant feeding was commonly practiced in the United States because of the belief of many American practitioners during the late 1800s and early 1900s that "clean" raw milk was preferable to pasteurized or other processed milk (4).

Rubber Nipples, Canning, and Ice Boxes

The rubber nipple was introduced in 1845 and a number of modifications followed (11). By the 1870s, seamless rubber nipples that could be fitted over the necks of feeding bottles were available. Thus, for the first time a satisfactory cleaning of the feeding utensils was possible. In the early 1900s, the sanitary open-top can was introduced into industry and it became feasible to market evaporated milk in cans. By 1910 safe storage of milk in the home had become possible because of the widespread availability of the kitchen ice box.

Recognition of the Importance of Vitamins

Langworthy, a leading researcher in nutrition, stated in 1898 that "Foods consist of the nutrients protein, fat, and carbohydrates, and various mineral salts (17a)." The need for vitamins was not yet appreciated. The concept of the importance of micronutrients was eloquently presented in 1906 by Hopkins (17b):

> . . . no animal can live on a mixture of proteins, carbohydrates and fats, and even when the necessary inorganic material is carefully supplied, the animal can still not flourish. The animal body is adjusted to live either on plant tissues or on other animals, and these contain countless substances other than proteins, carbohydrates and fat. Physiological evolution, I believe, has made some of these well nigh as essential as are the basal constituents of the diet . . . In diseases such as rickets, and particularly in scurvy, we have had for long years knowledge of a dietetic factor; but though we know how to benefit these conditions empirically, the real errors in the diet are to this day obscure.

In 1912 Funk suggested that beriberi, scurvy, pellagra, and possibly rickets were caused by deficiency in the diet of "special substances which are of the nature of organic bases, which we will call vitamins" (17b).

Scurvy

Scurvy was a well-recognized disease of infants in England in the 1880s. Barlow in 1883 attributed it to the widespread use of commercially prepared formulas and the reluctance of well-to-do mothers to breast-feed their infants. It was recognized that scurvy was rare in breast-fed infants and uncommon in those fed fresh cow's milk, whereas it was common in infants fed commercially prepared formulas, boiled or condensed milk (4). Infantile scurvy had been infrequently observed in North America until the 1890s (17c). Its appearance at that time seems to have been associated with the increased use of heated milks and commercially prepared formulas.

The relation between infantile and adult scurvy was slow to be recognized. As early as 1734, Bachstrom had written (18) that adult scurvy was the sole result of deficiency of fresh vegetable food in the diet. The American Pediatric Society, however, in its Collective Investigation of Infantile Scurvy in North America of 1898, had noted that the great majority of 379 identified cases of infantile scurvy occurred in infants fed sterilized, condensed, or pasteurized milk (19), but nutrient inadequacy of these products was apparently not suspected.

By 1912, Holst and Frohlich in Oslo had demonstrated that supplementation of a grain diet with fruits, fresh vegetables, or their juices prevented scurvy in guinea pigs (17c). Hess reported in 1914 that scurvy became prevalent in the Hebrew Infant Asylum in New York when orange juice was eliminated from the diet. It was largely through his efforts in the 1920s that it became customary to supplement the diets of infants with fruit or vegetable juices (17c). The prevalence of infantile scurvy then rapidly decreased.

Rickets

Rickets was well described by Glisson in England in 1650 (20), and had become common in parts of England by the eighteenth century (17d). By the middle of the nineteenth century, rickets was a major problem in European cities, reflecting the increased urban crowding, with decreased exposure of infants to sunlight. In Great Britain the disease was apparent in one-third of poor children in such cities as Manchester and London in 1870 (13b). The majority of medical writers in America stated that at least until the 1880s, rickets was rare (4). Although some authors have suggested that milder cases were not diagnosed, Meigs and Pepper stated in the fifth (1870) edition of their textbook that rickets must be much more common among the poor in London than among the same classes in large American cities (4). In 1921 McCollum is reported (13b) to have estimated that about one-half of children in cities of the United States had active or healed rickets—perhaps reflecting an unwarranted generalization from observations in Baltimore.

Schutte in Germany in 1824 recommended cod liver oil as a treatment for rickets (17d), and the Russian pediatrician, Schabad, in a series of reports published between 1908 and 1912, demonstrated that cod liver oil was effective in curing and preventing rickets (21). Because rickets was not recognized as a nutritional deficiency disease, administration of cod liver oil as a prophylactic measure must have seemed illogical.

Mellanby in 1920 (22) demonstrated that a fat-soluble substance could prevent rickets in puppies, and McCollum et al. showed that the fat-soluble substance was not vitamin A. Use of cod liver oil as a prophylactic measure against rickets became widespread in American in the 1920s.

Formula Feeding, 1875–1920

The last quarter of the nineteenth century in Europe and America was notable for the increase in knowledge of the chemical composition of foods, and improvements in formula composition. Biedert, recognizing that casein of cow's milk is less digestible than casein of human milk, recommended that formulas be made up of cream from cow's milk with the addition of water and lactose (23). Meigs in the United States made similar recommendations (4). The report of Rubner and Heubner on energy requirements of infants provided additional information for determining formula composition (23). Formulas frequently included hydrolyzed starch or cereal (1), or the milk was treated with rennet to alter the casein curd (2). Holt in 1894 (12) recommended methods of formula preparation and feeding that did not differ greatly from those that remained in wide use 50 years later.

Toward the end of the nineteenth century, Rotch (see p. 59, Fig. 3) introduced "the percentage method of infant feeding," which became so widely accepted by American pediatricians that it was referred to as the American method. It was based on the assumption that digestive capacity varied from infant to infant at the same age and from week to week in the same infant. It was supposed that minute variations in the concentration of one of the ingredients might exert a major influence on digestibility. Morbidity was less in infants fed by the Rotch method than by other methods in vogue at the time, probably because Rotch insisted on the use of clean, fresh milk, and because the method of formula preparation was so complicated that the formulas were generally prepared in commercial milk laboratories. Conditions for formula preparation were better in these laboratories than in most homes. From about 1890 through the early 1900s, many infants in the United States received formulas prepared by Rotch's method. However, Jacobi, one of the most prominent American pediatricians, did not accept the teaching of Rotch, stating that "you cannot bring up a baby by mathematics" (24).

A number of prepared formulas were patented. Liebig's food for infants, marketed in 1867, consisted of wheat flour, cow's milk, malt flour, and potassium bicarbonate (2,3). It was first marketed as a liquid and subsequently as a powder. Other formulas were introduced in rapid succession. By 1883, 27 brands of infant foods were commercially available (7). A formula developed by Gerstenberger in 1915 provided 67 kcal/dl and was made up of non-fat cow's milk, lactose, oleo oils (i.e., destearinated beef fat) and vegetable oils. The formula, called "synthetic milk adapted," was a forerunner of one of today's commercially prepared formulas.

Forsyth in 1910–1911 (3) stated that "Hand-feeding is already so well understood that beyond all dispute an infant can be reared by it with perfect safety to its health."

The Science of Coprology

In the first two decades of the twentieth century, great attention was paid to the characteristics of the infant's feces. Goldbloom (25) referred to this period of preoccupation with excreta as "the coprophilic era or era of divination by stool." Brenneman (26) discussed "the etiology and nature of hard curds in infant stools," and called attention to considerable differences of opinion among experts as to their significance.

In the early 1900s, problems in infant feeding were ascribed to excessive intakes. Biedert believed that digestive disorders were caused by excessive intakes of casein; Finkelstein and Meyer blamed sugar and salt; Czerny blamed fat (9). Protein milk was introduced by Finkelstein and Meyer in 1910 to provide a feeding low in carbohydrate, and Rotch developed his system of infant feeding primarily to decrease the harmful effects of high protein feedings.

Formula Feeding, 1920–1950

Government Regulations in the United States

The first Food and Drug Act in 1906 contained no reference to food for special dietary purposes. By 1934, however, in the second draft of the new Food and Drug

Act, specific reference to a new category of foods—foods for special dietary purposes—was included, particularly to assure the safety and quality of infant foods (27). In 1940, two years after the passage of the Act, the Food and Drug Administration declared that a food sold for use by infants should contain label declaration for moisture, energy, protein, fat, available carbohydrates, fiber, calcium, phosphorus, iron, and vitamins A, B_1, C, and D. A final order was published in 1941.

Mortality of bottle-fed infants during the early part of the twentieth century was greater than that of breast-fed infants: four to five times greater in the Hague, Netherlands, in 1908; three to six times greater in eight eastern cities in the United States in 1922; and 10 times greater in Chicago in 1924 to 1929 (10).

Once the fear of using heat-treated milks had been removed, formulas prepared with evaporated milk rapidly gained prominence. The practical advantages of evaporated milk for infant feeding were readily apparent. Not only was it free of microbial contamination but it could be stored conveniently for long periods. Impetus for its general adoption was provided by Marriott (see p. 141, Fig. 4) in 1927 when he recommended the use of evaporated milk instead of boiled whole milk in preparing the formula that he and Davison had proposed in 1923 (4). The significance of the introduction of evaporated milk may be appreciated from published comments of some of the leading pediatricians of the time (26,28). Brenneman (26) described his observations as

> . . . the most startling I have ever encountered in more than twenty-five years of hospital experience in feeding ward babies. The interns had often asked me to show them a normal stool such as I had told them all babies had in private practice and I had had great difficulty in meeting their request. At one swoop I was able to show them normal, yellow, smooth, well formed or thick pasty stools with a perfect putrefactive bouquet in practically every one of these babies.

The low incidence of gastrointestinal disturbances in infants fed evaporated milk formulas was commented upon by many observers. For the next 25 years the great majority of bottle-fed infants in the United States received formulas prepared from evaporated milk.

Beikost

By the latter part of the nineteenth century, as feeding of animal milks increased, feeding of pap decreased. Although cereals and custards were introduced by 4 months of age, other foods were introduced with great caution. During the last quarter of the nineteenth century, the recommended diet was restricted during the first 2 years of life to milk, farinaceous foods and beef tea (29). In 1887, Jacobi advised that no vegetables in any quantity be given to children before 2 years of age (4). Rotch in 1896 permitted feeding of baked potato at 17 months of age and certain vegetables at 30 months of age. Holt in 1899 recommended nothing but milk until 8 or 9 months of age. At 10 months of age beef juice and thin gruels made from various grains were permitted (4).

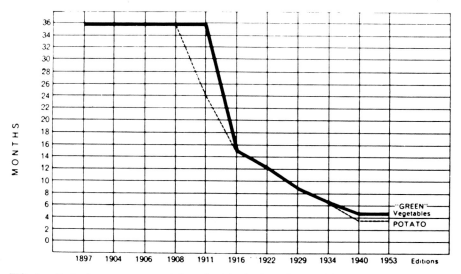

FIG. 1. Earliest age recommendations for introduction of vegetables, as indicated in 11 editions of Holt's *The Diseases of Infancy and Childhood*, published from 1897 until 1953 (5th edition missing). (From Adams, 1959, ref. 29.)

Eighteen reports published from 1900 to 1917 indicate that in the United States the feeding of sieved vegetable soup was commonly recommended at the end of the first year of life, potato at about 18 months of age, and other vegetables at 2 years of age or older (29). All vegetables were to be well cooked to increase digestibility.

The earliest ages recommended for introduction of vegetables as indicated in 11 editions of Holt's *The Diseases of Infancy and Childhood* have been summarized by Adams (29) (Fig. 1). Until 1911, green vegetables were not recommended before 36 months of age and even in 1929 they were not recommended before 9 months of age.

In 1935, Marriott (30) suggested that 6 months was the proper age for introduction of solid foods and in 1937 the AMA Council on Foods (31) stated that pediatricians favored feeding of strained fruits and vegetables at about 4 to 6 months of age.

The recommended age for introduction of beikost has fluctuated widely during the recent history of infant feeding. Between 1900 and 1950 the trend was toward earlier and earlier introduction of beikost.

INFANT FEEDING ABOUT 1950

Breast Feeding

A survey carried out in the United States in 1946–1947 indicated that at the time of discharge from the hospital (about 7 days of age), 38% of infants were solely breast-fed and 65% of infants were solely or partially bottle-fed (32). Data on the percentage of infants who continued to be breast-fed for several months are not available for 1950, but by 1958 fewer than 15% of 2-month-old infants were breast-fed (33).

By the middle of the twentieth century, knowledge of infant feeding was well advanced. Jeans and Marriott (34), in the fourth edition of their textbook *Infant Nutrition,* recommended that breast-fed infants receive a daily supplement of cod liver oil and orange juice. Supplementary formula feeding of the breast-fed infant was considered optional. The addition of soft custard was recommended at 3 to 4 months of age. Iron-fortified infant cereals and egg yolk were then to be fed, and it was considered desirable to begin weaning at 8 to 9 months of age. With the availability of good sanitation and refrigeration facilities, weaning was considered feasible even during the summer months.

In the United States, Bain (32) reported in 1948 that 65% of 8-day-old infants were wholly or partially breast-fed, but the Department of Health, Education and Welfare (10) reported that only 50.5% of first-born infants of married women were breast-fed. By contrast, in the United Kingdom, from 1951 to 1960, 61.9% of infants were breast-fed; in Brussels, from 1950 to 1958, 77.1% of infants were breast-fed (10). In Sweden, nearly 90% of 2-month-old infants in 1944 and about 75% of 2-month-old infants in 1953 were breast-fed (35).

Formula Feeding

The recommendations of Jeans and Marriott (34) for satisfactory formula feeding reflected the great advances that had occurred over the previous 50 years. They commented on the need for a sufficient intake of energy, water, protein, fat, minerals, and vitamins, the absence of harmful bacteria, and easy digestibility. They identified the more important pathogenic enteric bacteria, and explained that the size of the curd could be decreased by heat treatment, acidification, or dilution. Alternate times and temperatures for pasteurization were presented, and homogenization of milk was explained. They stated that vitamin-D-fortified fresh and evaporated milks were widely available. The quantities of various ingredients needed to make a formula from fresh milk or evaporated milk were specified.

Beikost

In the United States, beikost was introduced into the diet at earlier ages than had previously been practiced. Based on a survey of 2,000 pediatricians, Butler and Wolman reported in 1954 (36) that 66% of pediatricians recommended feeding of beikost at 6 to 8 weeks of age or earlier.

SUMMARY OF INFANT FEEDING IN 1950

By 1950, many of the infant feeding customs of the 1850s had been abandoned. The majority of infants were no longer breast-fed. The wet nurse had disappeared. Rickets and scurvy had been almost completely eliminated. Improved general sanitation, safe supplies of water and milk, better understanding of microbiology, and better understanding of nutrient requirements had led physicians and the general public to believe that formula feeding was the approximate equal of breast feeding. Almost a quarter of a century passed before there was a resurgence of enthusiasm for breast feeding.

REFERENCES

1. Routh CHF. *Infant feeding and its influence on life, or the causes and prevention of infant mortality.* 3rd ed. New York: William Wood, 1879; (a) p 33; (b) p 30; (c) p 16; (d) p 31; (e) pp 8–9; (f) p 150–153.
2. Smith E. *The wasting diseases of infants and children,* 4th ed. New York: William Wood, 1885.
3. Forsyth D. The history of infant feeding from Elizabethan times. *Proc R Soc Med* 1910–11;4:110.
4. Cone TE. *History of American pediatrics.* Boston: Little, Brown and Company, 1979.
5. Baines MA. Infant alimentation; or artificial feeding, as a substitute for breast-milk, considered in its physical and social aspects. *The Lancet* 1861; January 12:33–34.
6. Spruill JC. *Women's life and work in the southern colonies.* Chapel Hill, NC: University of North Carolina Press, 1938:55–57.
7. Bracken FJ. Infant feeding in the American colonies. *J Am Diet Assoc* 1953;29:349.
8. Duncum BM. Some notes on the history of lactation. *Br Med Bull* 1947;5/1141:253.
9. Cone TE. History of infant and child feeding: from the earliest years through the development of scientific concepts. In: Bond JT, Filer LJ, Leveille GA, Thomson AM, Weil WB, eds. *Infant and child feeding.* New York: Academic Press, 1981;4–34.
10. Reniers JR, Peeters RS, Meheus AZ. Breast feeding in the industrialized world. Review of the literature. *Rev Epidém et Santé Publ* 1983;31:375–407.
11. Bullough VL. Bottle feeding: an amplification. *Bull History Med* 1981;55:257–9.
12. Holt LE. *The care and feeding of children.* New York: D. Appleton and Co, 1894.
13. Rosen G. *A history of public health.* New York: MD Publications, 1958; (a) pp 33–5; (b) p 411.
14. Furnas JC. *The Americans. A social history of the United States, 1587–1914.* New York: Putnam, 1969.
15. Frantz JB. *Gail Borden, dairyman to a nation.* Norman, OK: University of Oklahoma Press, 1951.
16. Brenneman J. A contribution to our knowledge of the etiology and nature of hard curd in infants' stools. *Am J Dis Child* 1911;1:341.
17. McCollum EV. *A history of nutrition. The sequence of ideas in nutrition investigations.* Boston: Houghton Mifflin Company, 1957;190–1; 201–28; 252–65; 266–90.
18. Stewart CP, Guthrie P., eds. *Lind's treatise on scurvy. A reprint of the first edition of a treatise of the scurvy.* Edinburgh: Edinburgh University Press, 1953.
19. Friedenwald J, Ruhrah J. *Diet in health and disease.* 5th ed. Philadelphia: WB Saunders Company, 1915;506–7.
20. Vahlquist B. A two-century perspective of some major nutritional deficiency diseases in childhood. *Acta Paediatr Scand* 1975;64:161–71.
21. Holt LE. Letter to Editor. Let us give the Russians their due. *Pediatrics* 1963;32:462.
22. Mellanby E. Accessory food factors (vitamines) in the feeding of infants. *Lancet* 1920;1:856.
23. Davison WD. A brief history of infant feeding. *J Pediatr* 1953;43:74–87.
24. Levin S. Infant feeding as a faith. *Am J Dis Child* 1961;102:126–34.
25. Goldbloom A. The evolution of the concepts of infant feeding. *Arch Dis Child* 1954;29:385–90.
26. Brenneman J. The curd and the buffer in infant feeding. *JAMA* 1929;92:364.

27. Miller SA. Problems associated with the establishment of maximum nutrient limits infant in for-
    mula. In: *Upper Limits of Nutrients in Infant Formulas.* J Nutr 1989;119:1764–7.
28. Marriott WM, Schoenthal L. An experimental study of use of unsweetened evaporated milk for the
    preparation of infant feeding formulas. *Arch Pediatr* 1929;46:135.
29. Adams SF. Use of vegetables in infant feeding through the ages. *J Am Diet Assoc* 1959;35:362.
30. Mariott WM. *Infant nutrition,* 2nd ed. St Louis: CV Mosby Company, 1935.
31. AMA Council on Foods: Strained fruits and vegetables in the feeding of infants. *JAMA* 1937;
    108:1259.
32. Bain K. The incidence of breast feeding in hospitals in the United States. *Pediatrics* 1948;2:313–
    20.
33. Fomon SJ. *Infant nutrition,* 2nd ed. Philadelphia: WB Saunders Company, 1974;8.
34. Jeans PC, Marriott WM. *Infant nutrition.* 4th ed. St Louis: CV Mosby Company, 1947.
35. Hofvander Y, Sjölin S. Breast feeding trends and recent information activities in Sweden. *Acta Pae-
    diatr Scand [Suppl]* 1979;275:122–5.
36. Butler AM, Wolman IJ. Trends in the early feeding of supplementary foods to infants; and analysis
    and discussion based on a nationwide survey. *Q Rev Pediatr* 1954;9:63.

DISCUSSION

Dr. Barness: I have heard that it was not the icebox but the electric refrigerator, a later invention, that saved babies.

Dr. Fomon: I doubt whether either the icebox or the refrigerator should be considered
among the most important innovations. When it became possible to deliver clean pathogen-
free evaporated milk in cans to the consumer, the bacterial problem was solved. If formula
prepared from evaporated milk was not kept cold enough, it might sour, but the problem of
overgrowth with pathogens was less of a threat.

Dr. Udall: Were there any regulations about the appropriate composition of evaporated
milk when it first became available? Were there wide fluctuations in composition?

Dr. Fomon: As I understand it the patents required that whole milk be used. I believe that
the extent of the evaporation was also specified.

Dr. Suskind: Many of us grew up on 13 oz. of formula, 10 oz. of water and 2 tablespoons
of Karo syrup. What was it that stimulated the development of present day formulas?

Dr. Fomon: There were two reasons for discontinuing evaporated milk formulas. In the
first place, nearly all infants regurgitate from time to time and when an infant regurgitates formula containing large amounts of butter fat the odor is repulsive. Second, the new formulas
made with vegetable oils were aggressively marketed as being similar to human milk. These
formulas were later fortified with iron and shown to be effective at preventing iron deficiency
anemia. Evaporated milk could not be fortified in this way and still be used as a coffee whit-
ener. Thus, the evaporated milk industry eventually gave up the fight for a share of the infant
formula market.

Dr. Lockhart: Was carrot juice used in this country as a substitute for orange juice, as it
was in Europe?

Dr. Fomon: I have not come across any reference to the widespread use of carrot juice in
the United States. I was not aware that it was used in Europe as a substitute for orange juice.
I know that carrot soup was at one time widely used at least in Germany as a means of providing electrolyte replacement for infants with diarrhea. It provides a good assortment of electrolytes for that purpose, but I do not know whether it is still used.

Dr. Metcoff: The adoption of formula feeds seems to have been related mostly to incidental events. When did investigations leading to the composition of the present artificial milk formulations start?

Dr. Fomon: Although some studies of commercially prepared infant formulas were carried out in the 1940s, most sound clinical investigations began to be published in the 1950s.

Dr. Kaufmann: Schlossman was concerned about alternatives to breast feeding and actually questioned the chemical differences between cow's milk and human milk before Ehrlich. Ehrlich described immunologic differences between human and cow's milk. In the more recent past, Dr. Oscar Schloss demonstrated the passage of ingested antigens and allergens into human milk. Both Ehrlich and Schloss were concerned about the components of human and cow's milk and their possible relationship to disease in children. Schloss performed the first skin tests for foods while exploring the question of the changes in foods following ingestion. He was the first to show unaltered egg albumin in the milk of nursing mothers who had eaten eggs.

History of Pediatrics 1850–1950, edited by
B.L. Nichols, A. Ballabriga, and N. Kretchmer.
Nestlé Nutrition Workshop Series, Vol. 22. Nestec
Ltd., Vevey/Raven Press, Ltd., New York © 1991.

Breast Feeding in Fine Art

Jarmo K. Visakorpi

Department of Pediatrics, University Hospital of Tampere, 33520 Tampere, Finland

In connection with a campaign to promote breast feeding in Finland during the late 1970s, my attention was attracted to classical paintings presenting breast feeding mothers. As a layman in the history of art, I first thought that these pieces were exceptions. However, this was not the case. I found that not only was such art abundant, but also that breast feeding appears to be one of the basic motifs of art throughout the history of mankind, from the prehistoric era to the present. There is, however, considerable variation in the depiction of breast feeding over the centuries. During certain historical periods the representation of such an intimate event was even prohibited, and during other periods such "soft art" was not popular—the "hard" facts of life, such as military heroes, being more popular subjects.

THE PREHISTORIC ERA AND ANTIQUITY

In ancient Egypt, breast feeding was often depicted in papyrus-writings and in sculptural art. At that time art mainly depicted the Pharaohs and religious themes. The best known subject was the goddess Isis breast-feeding the child Horus, a well-known god (Fig. 1).

In ancient Greek and Roman art, breast feeding was rarely shown. These cultures emphasized masculine strength and feminine beauty rather than family life. However, there are several works depicting breast feeding. Perhaps the best known piece of breast-feeding art, in its own peculiar way, is the statue of the mythological founders of the city of Rome. This statue (Fig. 2) is based on an old Etruscan bronze of a wolf from 600 BC to which Romulus and Remus were added much later. This statue can be found today in the Palazzo dei Conservatori on Capitoline Hill in Rome.

The motif of breast feeding was also used in ancient cultures other than those of the Mediterranean area. This ceramic vessel from the Pre-Columbian period in Peru (Fig. 3) is a funerary object of the Mochica culture, which flourished in Peru from about the sixth to the thirteenth or fourteenth centuries.

EARLY CHRISTIAN AND MEDIEVAL ART

During the first millennium AD, breast feeding seldom appeared in art. The Catholic church was against it, insisting that the Child Jesus did not need milk at all. However, following the Synod of Ephesus in 431 AD, when this dogma was overturned, there was an increase in the portrayal of breast feeding in fine art in the form of a nursing Virgin Mary with the Child Jesus. The milk of the Virgin Mary itself became a relic, a sample of which is saved even today in many Catholic Churches.

The leading European style of art at the end of the first millennium was Romanesque. According to this style, the nursing Madonna, *virgo lactans,* was depicted in several altarpieces of small churches in southern Europe. Both the Romanesque and Gothic styles of medieval art depicted mainly religious motifs, and were usually stiff and serious (Fig. 4). The human body proportions were exaggerated and rich religious symbolism was included. This stiff medieval style still continues today in the production of icons. Breast-feeding Madonnas in icons are called *Galactotrophousa.*

THE RENAISSANCE

The Renaissance heralded a fundamental revolution in art. It was developed during the late fourteenth century in Italy and marked a return to the more natural portrayal of human beings, as in antiquity, as opposed to the symbolic representation of the first millennium. However, religious themes remained the main subjects of art. Thus the Madonna and Child were still commonly portrayed during the Renaissance, although the Virgin Mary and the Child Jesus were depicted more like ordinary human beings. However, the serious nature of religious art was still clearly visible in the early Renaissance as seen in the painting by Jan van Eyck (Fig. 5), one of the pioneers of Renaissance art north of the Alps, and in the painting of Jean Fouquet (Fig. 6), one of the great masters of the French Renaissance. A Biblical motif often depicted in the religious paintings of this time was the escape of the Holy Family to Egypt (Fig. 7).

All three great Italian Renaissance masters, Leonardo da Vinci, Michelangelo, and Raphael used this motif (Figs. 8 and 9). From Italy the Renaissance style spread over the Alps to Germany, France, and the Flemish Netherlands. The greatest German Renaissance master was Albrecht Dürer (Fig. 10). A very peculiar artist from that time was Lucas Cranach, the Elder (Fig. 11), who painted several breast-feeding pictures with his unique style during the early sixteenth century.

Although the Madonna remained the most common breast-feeding motif during the Renaissance, lactation now also began to appear in other connections. François Clouet, a well-known French Renaissance painter, produced the painting shown in Fig. 12 in 1571. The beautiful young lady is Diane de Poitiers, the mistress of King Henry II. However, she was not willing to nurse the child herself, but used instead a wet nurse, a common habit in upper-class families of the time. The painting in

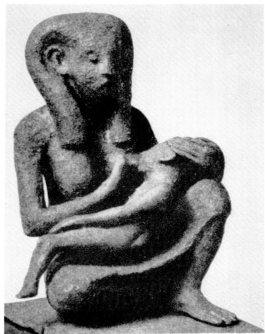

FIG. 1. The Goddess Isis nursing the Horus-child. A bronze statue from Egypt c. 1900 B.C. (Courtesy of VEB Georg Thieme, Leipzig.)

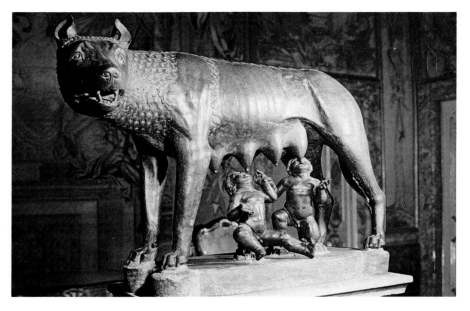

FIG. 2. Romulus and Remus. Palazzo dei Conservatori, Rome. (Courtesy of VEB Georg Thieme, Leipzig.)

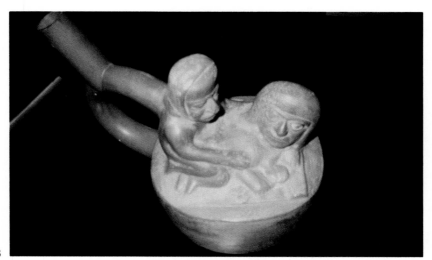

3

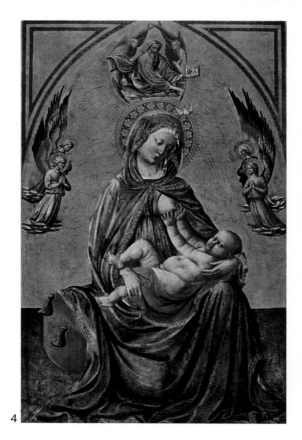

4

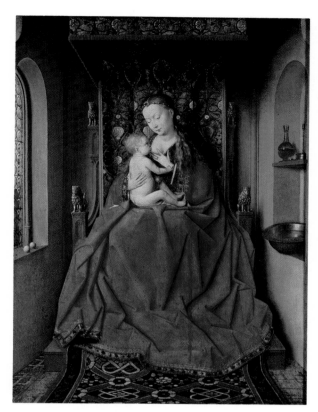

FIG. 5. "Lucca-Madonna (*Die Madonna im Gemach*)," 1436 Jan van Eyck. (Courtesy of Städelsches Kunstinstitut, Frankfurt am Main.)

FIG. 3. A Peruvian ceramic vessel from the Pre-Columbian era. The vessel depicts a breast-feeding woman with the man in a position of sodomy, which reflects the cultural taboo against vaginal intercourse during lactation period. Private collection. (Courtesy of Laurence Finberg, M.D.)

FIG. 4. Virgin Mary with the Child. Masolino da Panicale, early fifteenth century. Alte Pinakothek, Munich. (Courtesy of Bayerische Staatsgemäldesammlung, Munich.)

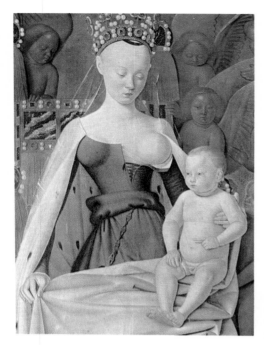

FIG. 6. Madonna and the Child, 1451. Jean Fouquet. (Courtesy of Koninklijk Museum voor Schone Kunsten, Antwerp.)

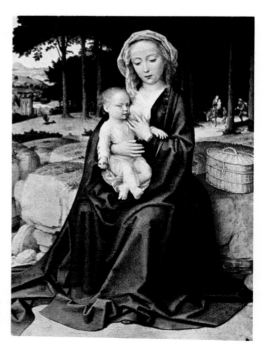

FIG. 7. The rest during the escape to Egypt depicted by Gerard David, late 15th century. (Courtesy of Museo del Prado, Madrid.)

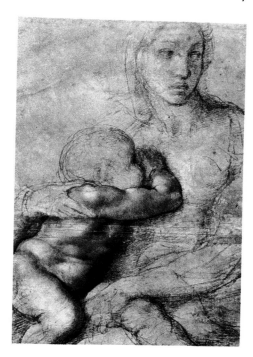

FIG. 8. "Madonna con il figlio," Virgin Mary with Child. Michelangelo, early 16th century. (Courtesy of Museo Buonarroti, Florence.)

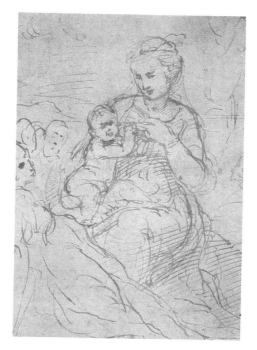

FIG. 9. "Madonna of the Balducchin." Raphael, late 15th century. (Courtesy of Graphische Sammlung Albertina, Vienna.)

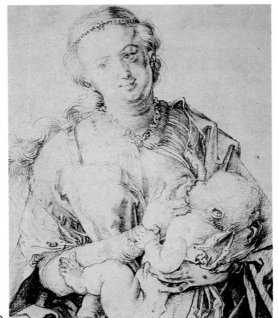

10

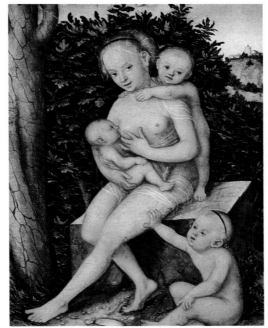

11

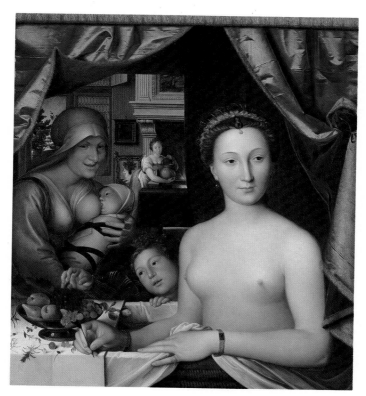

FIG. 12. The use of a wet nurse as shown in the painting "Diane de Poitiers," depicting the mistress of King Henry II. François Clouet, French Renaissance artist, c. 1571. (Courtesy of the National Gallery of Art, Washington, DC, Samuel H. Kress Collection.)

FIG. 10. The Virgin Nursing the Child. Albrecht Dürer, c. 1512. (Courtesy of Graphische Sammlung Albertina, Vienna.)

FIG. 11. Lucas Cranach de Oude (the Elder) depicted breast feeding mothers with children in several paintings during the early sixteenth century. These works bear the same name, "*Caritas*." (Courtesy of Koninklijk Museum voor Schone Kunsten, Antwerp.)

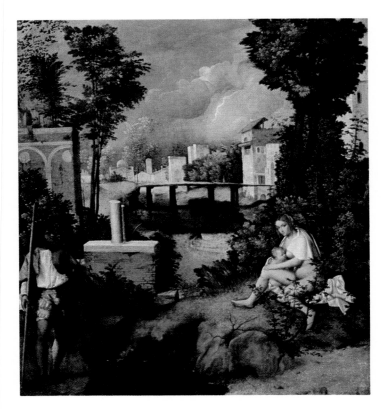

FIG. 13. "La Tempesta," Stormy Weather, 1506. Giorgione, Italian Renaissance painter. (Courtesy of Gallerie dell' Accademia, Venice.)

FIG. 14. Detail of Stormy Weather; see Fig. 13.

FIG. 15. Spanish Baroque style. El Greco. "The Holy Family with Holy Ann", 1595. (Courtesy of Museo de Tavera, Toledo.)

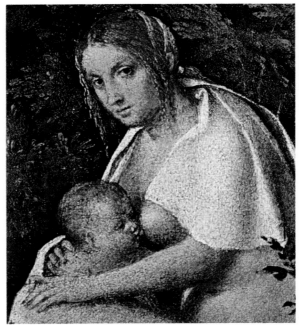

14

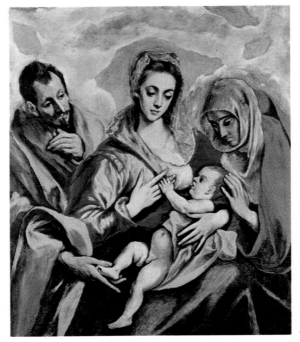

15

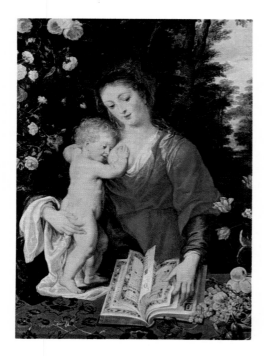

FIG. 16. "Virgin Mary with the Child." Peter Paul Rubens, late 16th century. (Courtesy of Bildarchiv Preussischer Kulturbesitz, Berlin.)

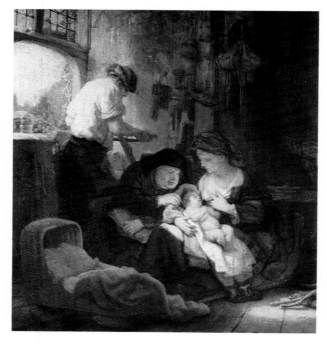

FIG. 17. "The Holy Family in the Carpenter's Workshop." Rembrandt, c. 1640. (Courtesy of Musée du Louvre, Paris.)

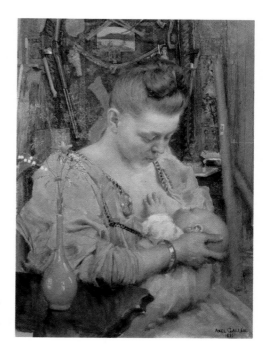

FIG. 18. "Madonna, Mary and Marjatta Gallén." Akseli Gallen-Kallela, 1891. (Courtesy of Gallen-Kallela Museum, Espoo, Finland.)

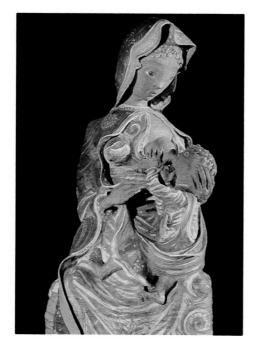

FIG. 19. Hungarian Madonna, "Szopató Madonna," in ceramic. Margit Kovács, 1948. (Courtesy of Museum of Pest County, Szentendre, Hungary.)

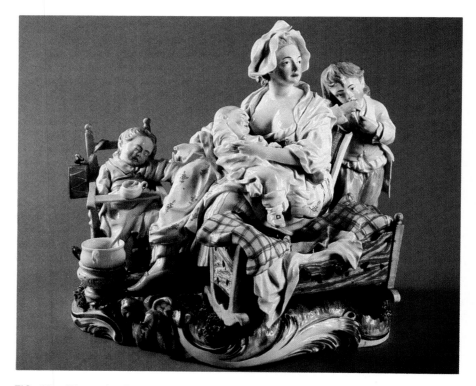

FIG. 20. "Breast-feeding mother with family," porcelain figure. Karl Gottlieb Lück, 1762. (Courtesy of Kurpfälzisches Museum der Stadt Heidelberg, Heidelberg.)

FIG. 21. "Yashoda and Krishna", a copper statue from Karnantaka, India, fourteenth century or earlier. (Courtesy of The Metropolitan Museum of Art, Purchase, Lita Annenberg Hazan Charitable Trust Gift, in honor of Cynthia Hazan and Leon Bernard Polsky, 1982.) (1982.220.8)

FIG. 22. Wooden sculpture made by an unknown Tanzanian artist. The souls of the ancestors are transferred to the child via mother's milk. (Acta Paediatrica Scandinavica 1988; vol 77:2:187, Fig. 1.)

FIG. 23. "The Charity of a Beggar at Ornans." Realism in the depiction of breast feeding. Gustave Courbet, 1868. (Courtesy of Glasgow Museum and Art Gallery, The Burrell Collection, Glasgow.)

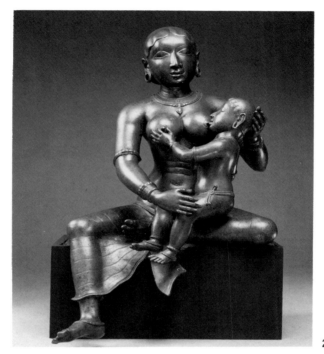

21

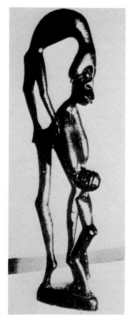

22

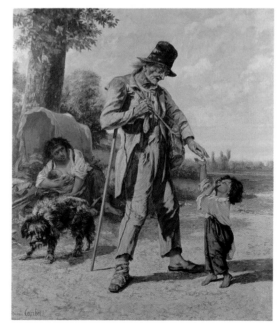

23

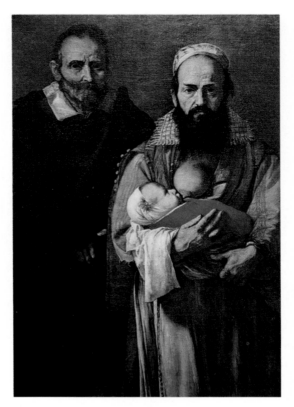

FIG. 24. Unique breast-feeding mother, "The Bearded Lady," José Ribera, 16th century. (Courtesy of Museo de Tavera, Toledo.)

FIG. 25. "The Republic," Honoré Daumier, 1848. (Courtesy of Musée d' Orsay, Paris.)

FIG. 26. "The Origin of the Milky Way." Peter Paul Rubens, early seventeenth century. (Courtesy of Musées Royaux des Beaux-Arts, Brussels.)

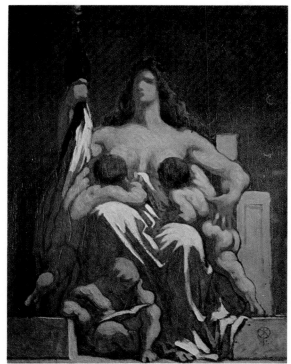

25

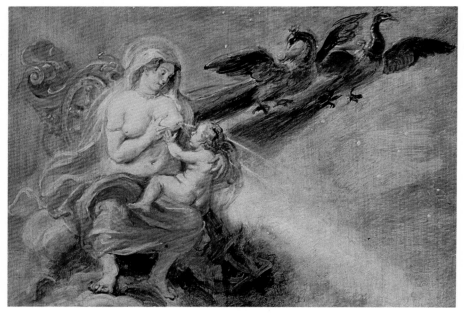

26

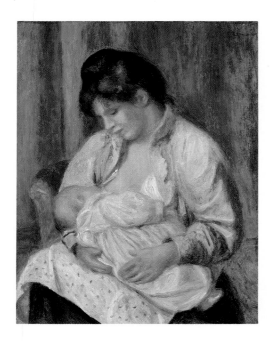

FIG. 27. "Mother with Child," Auguste Renoir, c. 1914. (Courtesy of the National Gallery of Scotland, Scottish National Portrait Gallery, Edinburg.)

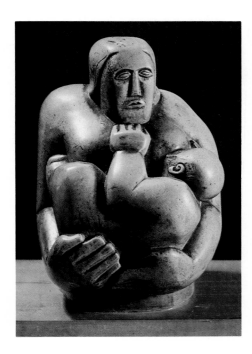

FIG. 28. "Maternity." Henry Moore, 1924–1925. (© Henry Moore Foundation, 1924–5. Reproduced by kind permission of the Henry Moore Foundation.)

Fig. 13 is another well-known work, *"La Tempesta"* (Stormy Weather), from 1502 by Giorgione. It also includes a nursing mother (Fig. 13 and Fig. 14).

THE BAROQUE STYLE IN EUROPE

The seventeenth and eighteenth centuries are often called the great centuries of art. This period was initiated by the Baroque style. The great Spanish painter El Greco was a Baroque artist, although his style is unique. His painting of the Holy Family (Fig. 15) includes Mary's mother, the Holy Ann. El Greco created two almost identical versions of this painting, one of which is today in Toledo, Spain, and the other in Budapest, Hungary. The most typical Baroque painter was Rubens, from the the famous Flemish school (Fig. 16). Another great Baroque painter, Rembrandt, also depicted the Holy Family in several paintings (Fig. 17).

NATIONAL MADONNAS FROM DIFFERENT PARTS OF THE WORLD

The representation of the Madonna and Child has been the main motif for the depiction of breast feeding in art. Over the centuries, the handling of this motif changed from a symbolic-religious to a more natural style. An example is the Madonna by the Finnish national painter Akseli Gallen-Kallela (Fig. 18).

The motif of breast feeding has also been expressed in sculptures of different materials. Margit Kovacs, a contemporary Hungarian artist, worked with ceramics (Fig. 19). Another example is a work from the eighteenth century by a German, Karl Gottlieb Lück—breast feeding is depicted in a porcelain china figurine (Fig. 20).

Most of the art reproductions I have included are from European cultures, but breast feeding has been depicted in the art of other cultures. The copper statue "Yashoda and Krishna" is from Karnantaka, India (Fig. 21), and the wooden sculpture is from Tanzania (Fig. 22).

REALISM IN ART

Most paintings show breast feeding as a warm, intimate, and almost holy interaction between the Virgin Mary and Child Jesus. There are, however, exceptions. The nineteenth century brought realism to art. The Realist master Gustave Courbet depicted breast feeding in his 1868 painting "The Charity of a Beggar at Ornans" (Fig. 23). The bearded lady, a *mujer barbuda*, in Toledo, Spain, is an exceptional example of breast feeding (Fig. 24).

SYMBOLISM IN THE DEPICTION OF BREAST FEEDING

The symbolism in breast-feeding paintings usually represents motherhood, parenthood, and Christian love. But breast feeding has also been used to symbolize other ideas. ''The Republic'' (Fig. 25) by Honoré Daumier symbolizes the love of one's neighbor. It was dedicated to the victory of the republicans in 1848 in France. Artists have been inspired by the old Greek myth of the origins of the Milky Way. This can be seen in Rubens' painting in the Royal Museum of Fine Art, Brussels, where the goddess Juno is nursing Heracles, son of Jupiter, and the strong ejection of milk gives rise to the concept of the Milky Way (Fig. 26).

IMPRESSIONISM

The Impressionists wanted to show real life as we see it through our eyes. The Impressionist master of depicting breast feeding was Auguste Renoir, who was very fond of the motif and used it in several works. His model was usually his own family (Fig. 27).

CONTEMPORARY ART

In the art of the twentieth century, and especially in contemporary art, the use of breast feeding as a motif declined in parallel with the decline in breast feeding. However, exceptions may be found, as in the work of Henry Moore. One of the main motifs for this sculptor was the mother and child, and breast feeding was included in several of his works (Fig. 28).

Deviating from the practice of most other contemporary artists, Picasso continued to depict breast feeding throughout his career and in the many styles with which he experimented. ''Maternity'' from his Blue Era in 1905, is perhaps one of his most popular nursing-mother pictures. We can also find breast feeding representing the theme of Peace in his fresco ''War and Peace'' from 1952, which is located in a small chapel in France.

ACKNOWLEDGMENTS

I wish to thank the authorities, foundations, museums, galleries, and private collectors for their kind permission to reproduce the pictures illustrated in this chapter. Fig. 3, Laurence Finberg, MD; Fig. 4, Der Bayerischen Staatsgemäldesammlungen, Munich; Fig. 5, Städelsches Kunstinstitut und Städtische Gallerie, Frankfurt am Main; Figs. 6 and 11, Koninklijk Museum voor Schone Kunsten, Antwerp; Fig. 7, Museo del Prado, Madrid; Fig. 8, Casa Buonarroti, Florence; Figs. 9 and 10, Graphische Sammlung Albertina, Vienna; Fig. 12, National Gallery of Art,

Washington, DC; Figs. 13 and 14, Ministero per i Beni Culturali e Ambientali, Venice; Figs. 15 and 24, Medinaceli, Casa de Pilatos, Seville; Fig. 16, Bildarchiv Preussischer Kulturbesitz, Berlin; Fig. 17, Musée du Louvre, Paris; Fig. 18, Gallen-Kallela Museum, Espoo; Fig. 19, Direction of the Museum of Pest County, Szentendre; Fig. 20, Kurpfälzisches Museum der Stadt Heidelberg; Fig. 21, Metropolitan Museum of Art, New York; Fig. 23, Glasgow Museums and Art Galleries, Scotland; Fig. 25, Musée d'Orsay, Paris; Fig. 26, Musées Royaux des Beaux-Arts, Brussels; Fig. 27, National Gallery of Scotland, Edinburgh; Fig. 28, The Henry Moore Foundation.

BIBLIOGRAPHY

1. Semenzato C. *Kuvataide kautta aikojen*. Helsinki: Otava, 1987;1–478.
2. Peiper A. *Chronik der Kinderheilkunde*. Leipzig: VEB Georg Thieme Verlag, 1958;1–527.
3. Koctürk T, Zetterström R. Breast feeding and its promotion. *Acta Paediat Scand* 1988;77:183–90.

DISCUSSION

Dr. Katz: In Italian Renaissance paintings both the infants and the practice of breast feeding are depicted unrealistically. The children's bodies are out of proportion—they are like small adults—and the way the mother holds the infant is unrealistic. On the other hand German Renaissance paintings depict breast feeding more realistically. Does this suggest to you that the pervading Italian cultural morés did not allow these men, who painted so beautifully, to represent this very important function realistically?

Dr. Visakorpi: I believe the church had a strong influence. Such a religious influence could already be seen in the art of ancient Egypt, where there were certain rules that had to be obeyed in depicting the Pharaohs.

Dr. Stern: I don't think these distortions were peculiar to paintings depicting breast feeding. They were typical of Italian art up to the time when Carravaggio began to paint people as they really were. Most Italian art previous to this was extremely unrealistic, whether or not it showed breast-feeding Madonnas. The figures were always out of proportion; they had a heavenly upward gaze and did not seem to be a part of ordinary earth-bound life. It wasn't until the later painters, who began to portray not only ordinary people but ordinary people doing ordinary things, that a more realistic art form emerged.

History of Pediatrics 1850–1950, edited by
B.L. Nichols, A. Ballabriga, and N. Kretchmer.
Nestlé Nutrition Workshop Series, Vol. 22. Nestec
Ltd., Vevey/Raven Press, Ltd., New York © 1991.

Pediatric Endocrinology

Andrea Prader

Department of Pediatrics, Kinderspital, CH 8032 Zürich, Switzerland

In the period covered by this workshop, pediatrics established itself as a new medical speciality and made impressive progress, mainly in the fields of nutrition and infectious diseases. However, it was only toward the end of this period that the modern pediatric subspecialities started to develop rapidly. So far as pediatric endocrinology is concerned, pediatric textbooks before 1950 contained only anecdotal descriptions of children with goitre, cretinism, dwarfism, gigantism, precocious puberty, or ambiguous genitalia. There was little understanding of endocrine pathophysiology, and there were few therapeutic possibilities.

In Cone's *History of American Pediatrics,* published in 1979, there are only 2 pages (out of 260) on endocrinology. They contain brief remarks about treatment of hypothyroidism with desiccated thyroid, treatment of diabetes mellitus with insulin, adrenal hemorrhage with fulminant septicemia, and cancer of the thyroid caused by unnecessary radiation of the thymus. There is also a short but important note stating that the first special clinics in a children's hospital in the United States were organized in 1936 by Edwards A. Park in the Harriet Lane Home at Johns Hopkins Hospital. They were for tuberculosis, psychiatry, cardiology, and endocrinology. This was an innovation introduced by a far-sighted chairman that had an immense impact on the future development of pediatrics.

The head of the endocrinology clinic was Lawson Wilkins, who may be regarded as the father of pediatric endocrinology. In 1950 he published his textbook *The Diagnosis and Treatment of Endocrine Disorders in Childhood and Adolescence.* It was the first book on pediatric endocrinology, and it had an enormous influence on the development of this field in the United States and abroad. The inclusion of adolescence as part of pediatric practice was rather new, and it had far reaching consequences on the development of pediatrics in general, such that, today, adolescent medicine is an integral part of pediatrics. Since adolescence is characterized by marked endocrine and psychological changes, this age period presents important and fascinating problems for the pediatric endocrinologist.

Lawson Wilkins (1894–1963) was a colorful personality and an enthusiastic and gifted teacher. He attracted many students who became leaders in the field. He laid the foundations of pediatric endocrinology by making full use of the knowledge available from experimental and adult endocrinology and from anthropometry. He was first a full-time pediatric practitioner, then a part-time director of the endocrine clinic. He obtained a full time academic position at the age of only 52. Fig. 1 is a picture taken in 1963, the year of his death, showing him surrounded by his former fellows.

Lawson Wilkins dedicated his book to his father, George L. Wilkins, to Edwards A. Park and to Fuller Albright, the "family physician, the pediatrician and the endocrinologist." His book dedication emphasizes the main sources of pediatric endocrinology: classical pediatrics and experimental and adult endocrinology.

Let me sketch briefly some of the milestones in the history of general endocrinology. In the last century, Claude Bernard and Brown-Séguard introduced the concept of internal secretion. They gave experimental evidence that certain glands secrete products into the circulation that control important functions of the body. Bayliss and Starling coined the word *hormones* for these secretions. In 1910, Biedl in Vienna published his famous textbook *Innere Sekretion,* which summarized all the available theoretical and practical knowledge of his time. Desiccated thyroid was the first available substance for endocrine substitution therapy and later thyroxine became the first available pure hormone. In 1922, insulin was discovered by Banting and Best, who were honored with the Nobel prize. In the 1930s, the chemical structure of the sex hormones was elucidated, and in the 1940s, cortisone and other adrenal steroids were discovered by Kendall and Reichstein and the beneficial effect of cortisone on rheumatoid arthritis was recognized by Hench. These achievements were also rewarded by Nobel Prizes. In 1949, Wilkins reported the first experience with cortisone in the treatment of congenital adrenal hyperplasia.

Wilkins' 1950 book contains most of the fundamental clinical knowledge of today, but of course most of today's laboratory endocrinology was not yet available. It was not possible to estimate the blood level of hormones. Urinary steroids could

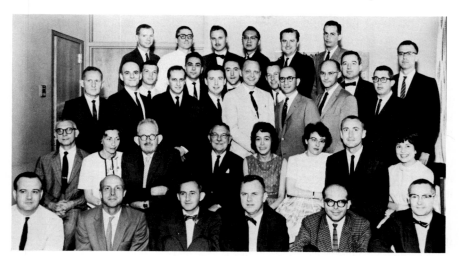

FIG. 1.   Lawson Wilkins (1894–1963), third row center, and his former fellows.

be estimated only by a few color reactions, mainly the Zimmermann reaction for 17-ketosteroids, and gonadotropins by a complicated and time-consuming bioassay in mice. The concept of bone age was rather new and did not yet take into account sex differences. The first edition of the Greulich and Pyle atlas was published only in 1951. Chromosomes could not yet be studied, and it was not yet known that Turner's syndrome and Klinefelter's syndrome were chromosomal aberrations. The main sex steroids were available for substitution therapy but their use for oral contraception had not yet been discovered. Growth hormone was not available. The variants of congenital adrenal hyperplasia were not yet known. Although the high familial incidence of this condition is mentioned, it was not thought to be hereditary and it is clear that Wilkins did not fully realize the hereditary nature of autosomal recessive disorders. This shows that scientific and clinical thinking in terms of genetics was far less developed 40 years ago than today. The tremendous progress in genetics since 1950 has played a major role in the rapid development of pediatric endocrinology and other pediatric subspecialities.

In this chapter I shall discuss some selected aspects of the history of pediatric endocrinology under the headings of hormone analysis, anabolic steroids, congenital adrenal hyperplasia, normal and abnormal sex differentiation, thyroid problems, and some aspects of growth hormone and growth factors.

HORMONE ANALYSIS

One of the most important advances in the last 40 years has been the development of analytical methods to measure hormones in blood and urine. Previously it was purely on clinical grounds, sometimes with the help of indirect laboratory tests such as cholesterol or alkaline phosphatase, that a hormone deficiency or a hormone excess was diagnosed. There were only a few methods by which urinary steroids could be determined and a few time-consuming animal tests for urinary protein hormones.

In the 1950s, the analysis of urinary steroids was improved by paper chromatography, and in the 1960s by gas chromatography, first on packed columns, then on glass capillaries, and finally assisted by mass spectrometry. Today all the urinary steroids can be measured precisely.

A major methodological breakthrough, rewarded by the Nobel prize, was the radioimmunoassay technique developed by Berson and Yallow in the 1950s. This new technique allowed us to measure the plasma concentration of insulin, growth hormone, and other protein hormones. It was rapidly adapted to plasma steroids, and it is now possible to estimate the plasma concentrations of all major hormones.

This technical progress has occurred in less than half a century and is truly impressive. However, it has its dangerous side also. It may seduce today's physicians into examining the patient only superficially, while asking for as much laboratory data as possible, and to base the diagnosis mainly or exclusively on laboratory results. This is not only unnecessarily expensive but also frequently misleading. Clinical skills and clinical judgment cannot be replaced; the wisely used laboratory helps only to confirm or refute the clinical diagnosis and to add a certain precision.

ANABOLIC STEROIDS

In the 1950s and 1960s, the so-called anabolic steroids became fashionable. The only truly anabolic natural steroid is testosterone. Its use as an anabolic hormone is limited because of its androgenic or virilizing properties. The pharmaceutical industry worked hard to develop testosterone derivatives that were supposed to have an anabolic effect without an androgenic effect. This prospect encouraged pediatric endocrinologists in the hope that they might at last have available a drug that accelerated growth in short children. Unfortunately, it was found that anabolic steroids also accelerated bone age, and thus possibly compromised future adult height. In high dosage they still had an androgenic effect and they were sometimes hepatotoxic. Anabolic steroids did not fulfill their promise and should be abandoned. They can possibly be replaced by testosterone in extremely small doses. They are better known today for their misuse by athletes than for their value in pediatric endocrinology.

CONGENITAL ADRENAL HYPERPLASIA

Congenital adrenal hyperplasia is caused by several autosomal recessive defects of the biosynthesis of cortisol. The classical form, 21-hydroxylase deficiency, is by far the most frequent. Many babies with this disorder die from salt loss if not diagnosed and treated. The 2 other forms, 3-β-dehydrogenase deficiency and 11-hydroxylase deficiency, are relatively rare.

Lifelong treatment with glucocorticoids and fluorocortisol in replacement dosage, and surgical correction of the virilized external genitalia in girls, allow normal growth and physical development without virilization, and normal fertility. Such patients look entirely normal and may produce healthy children, who are of course heterozygote carriers.

The prevalence, estimated in the 1950s to be about 1 in 70,000, is now known to be about 1 in 10,000. The discovery of a linkage between the 21-hydroxylase defect and HLA antigens revealed an impressive and not fully clarified genetic and clinical heterogeneity, with marked ethnic differences. The late-onset, or non-classical form, of 21-hydroxylase deficiency is now recognized as one of the most frequent autosomal recessive genetic disorders in humans, with a prevalence of about 1 in 1,000 in the general population and 1 in 27 in Ashkenazi Jews.

Prenatal diagnosis in a pregnant mother with a previous affected child has become possible. Prenatal treatment has even been achieved, by giving dexamethasone to the mother in order to prevent the virilization of the external genitalia of the female fetus.

SEX DIFFERENTIATION

Sex differentiation is one of the most fascinating biological processes. The first step, gonadal differentiation, is directly controlled by the chromosomes. Today it is believed that the presence of the testis-determining-factor (TDF) on the Y chromosome directs the development of the testes. In its absence ovaries will develop. Future research may reveal a more complex chromosomal regulation. The second step is the hormonal sex differentiation. The development of male genitalia is an active process induced by the hormones of the fetal testis, while the development of female genitalia is a passive non-hormonal process.

The decisive experiment that clarified hormonal sex differentiation was done by Jost in France in the late 1940s. When he gonadectomized rabbit fetuses before the gonads were differentiated, all the fetuses developed female genitalia. Jost concluded that the development of male genitalia depends on the presence of testes, whereas female development does not depend on the presence of ovaries. Wilkins immediately recognized the importance of this experimental evidence and felt that it should be possible to interpret certain inter-sex states in the light of Jost's experiment. However, this had to wait for methods to visualize and analyze the human chromosomes and for further analysis of the hormones produced by the fetal testis.

Today we know that, before 7 weeks of gestation, the gonads, the Müllerian and Wolffian ducts, and the urogenital sinus are indifferent. After this age the testes begin to secrete two hormones. One is the antimüllerian hormone, a glycoprotein secreted by the Sertoli cells causing regression of the Müllerian ducts. The other is testosterone, produced by the Leydig cells, allowing the transformation of the Wolffian ducts into vas deferens, seminal vesicle, and epididymis. Testosterone is metabolized to dihydrotestosterone in the tissues of the urogenital sinus, and this in turn causes the development of the male external genitalia and the prostate. If the gonads are ovaries, antimüllerian hormone, testosterone, and dihydrotestosterone are absent; the Müllerian ducts persist and are transformed into Fallopian tubes, uterus, and upper vagina. The Wolffian ducts regress and the urogenital sinus forms the lower vagina. This concept of hormonal sex differentiation allows us to explain the occurrence of XY individuals with female or ambiguous genitalia, also called male pseudohermaphrodites.

THYROID PROBLEMS

Thyroid problems have a long history, mainly because of the frequent occurrence of endemic goitre and endemic cretinism in certain countries. The preventive effect of iodine was already recognized in the last century. However, it was only in the 1920s and 1930s and thereafter that iodine was introduced on a large scale in countries with endemic goitre. The effect has been highly beneficial. My country, Switzerland, is an excellent example. After the introduction of iodized salt, endemic goitre and cretinism, which had previously been frequent, have completely disappeared.

The most frequent thyroid disorder in children is primary congenital hypothyroidism. In a minority of patients it is caused by hereditary defects in the biosynthesis of thyroid hormones. In the large majority, however, it is caused by dysgenesis of the thyroid gland of unknown etiology. Twelve years ago, universal neonatal screening was introduced based on increased plasma thyroid stimulating hormone (TSH) values. This revealed a prevalence as high as 1 in 4,000 and made it possible to start treatment with thyroxine in the first weeks of life, before symptoms of hypothyroidism become evident. Such early and life-long treatment allows normal physical and psycho-intellectual development. Younger pediatricians now no longer have any experience with the clinical diagnosis of congenital hypothyroidism.

GROWTH HORMONE AND GROWTH FACTORS

Diagnosis and treatment of growth hormone deficiency are based on two important advances that occurred in the 1950s. One already mentioned, was the introduction of radioimmunoassay, allowing the measurement of growth hormones. The other was the extraction of growth hormone from human pituitaries by Raben, and its successful application to the treatment of hypopituitary dwarfism, which was followed by the organized collection of human pituitaries and the extraction of growth hormone in many countries. The amounts extracted were just sufficient to treat most patients with classical hypopituitary dwarfism. The effect is highly satisfactory if treatment starts early in childhood and is continued to the end of the growth period. A few years ago a suspicion was raised that this extract could contain viral particles causing Creutzfeld-Jacob disease. Fortunately, at the same time, it became possible, by the use of new recombinant DNA techniques, to produce human growth hormone biosynthetically in unlimited amounts. Presently many studies are under way to discover whether growth hormone may help other children with short stature.

A confusion has arisen about the best way to assess the functional growth hormone status of a child. Is it best to measure plasma values before and after provocative stimuli, such as insulin or arginine, or to study the spontaneous pulsatile plasma profiles, or to measure urinary values? At the moment we do not know the best approach and we do not know which children with short stature, apart from classical hypopituitary dwarfs, will profit from treatment with growth hormone. Over the last 3 years, it has also become evident that most parents want their children to become tall, that most adolescents want to be tall, and that they are prepared to undergo expensive, uncomfortable, and still experimental therapy in the hope of achieving that goal.

Since the late 1950s, a lot of work has been done to identify growth factors in the blood. When it became apparent that the growth-promoting effect of growth hormone is mediated by such factors, they were termed *somatomedins*. At present the two best-known somatomedins are the insulin-like growth factors (IGF) 1 and 2.

They can be synthesized with recombinant DNA techniques, but have not yet been released for experimental therapy in children. We can only speculate whether they will be useful in treating short stature and other disorders. Other factors that may play a role in the regulation of growth are the carrier (binding) proteins of growth hormone and IGF.

Another new chapter in pediatric endocrinology has opened in recent years in children who had chemotherapy and cranial radiation for malignant disease. Such children frequently develop the combination of growth hormone deficiency and precocious puberty caused by hypothalamic damage. One may speculate whether this is the result of a deficiency state (of growth hormone releasing hormone) combined with a state of excess production of gonadotropin releasing hormone, or whether precocious puberty is the expression of a deficiency of a hypothetical physiological puberty supressing hypothalamic function (depression).

SOCIETIES OF PEDIATRIC ENDOCRINOLOGY

Progress in pediatric endocrinology has been greatly stimulated and accelerated by the foundation and rapid growth of two new scientific societies. In 1962, we founded the European Society of Pediatric Endocrinology in Zurich. Later, our American counterpart was founded, the Lawson Wilkins Pediatric Endocrine Society. The stimulation provided by our annual and joint meetings and by the resulting personal contacts can hardly be overestimated.

DISCUSSION

Dr. Lubin: Please comment on suggestions for protecting the utilization of some of these newer techniques from abuse.

Dr. Prader: This is a difficult question. Growth hormone and anabolic steroids can be prescribed by any physician and therefore abuse is possible.

I believe that certain treatments should be prescribed. For example, in my opinion anabolic steroids should no longer be used. Some physicians believe that in normal short stature final height can be increased by suppressing puberty with LHRH analogs and giving growth hormone simultaneously. For reasons that I cannot detail here I do not think this will be successful. Furthermore we do not know what possible complications may occur with such serious manipulation of normal growth. I am firmly of the opinion that this should not be done.

Dr. Stern: I am told that Hench discovered cortisone, or at least thought about it, because his women patients with rheumatoid arthritis improved when they became pregnant.

Dr. Prader: This is certainly true. Hench also observed that patients with rheumatoid arthritis improved when they got hepatitis—another link with cortisone metabolism.

History of Pediatrics 1850–1950, edited by
B.L. Nichols, A. Ballabriga, and N. Kretchmer.
Nestlé Nutrition Workshop Series, Vol. 22. Nestec
Ltd., Vevey/Raven Press, Ltd., New York © 1991.

Pediatric Gastroenterology

Ettore Rossi

Department of Pediatrics, University of Berne, 3010 Berne, Switzerland

A retrospective analysis of the origins of pediatric gastroenterology is difficult, since it involves a time of transition between nutrition and modern gastroenterology. In the period between 1850 and 1950, scientific pediatrics was concerned above all with pediatric nutrition and became almost synonymous with it.

In 1853, Barthez from Paris and Rilliet from Geneva published the first modern pediatric textbook, of which one fifth of the content was dedicated to problems in gastroenterology. "Catarrhal" diseases of the stomach and of the intestine are listed, differentiating simple from complicated forms, and infections from congenital malformations.

The first *Handbuch der Kinderheilkunde* (1880) appeared in 4 volumes and initiated a long series of textbooks. The problems of infection of the digestive tract already occupied an important part heralding the beginning of the golden period of research led by Pasteur and Koch. Well-recognized pediatricians thereafter made important contributions to the field and I shall continue myself to describing these pioneers.

In Germany, Otto Heubner (b. 1843) (see p. 25, Fig. 2), who graduated in Leipzig, first secured the establishment of a Children's Hospital in this town. He later moved to Berlin, where Adalbert Czerny (b. 1863) (see p. 27, Fig. 3) succeeded him and created a School of Pediatrics. He wrote a textbook on nutrition, and nutritional disorders and may be considered the first children's nutritionist. Finkelstein (b. 1865) (see p. 140, Fig. 3) was also active in Berlin and published several essays on nursling diseases and on sugar and fat as causes of intestinal disorders. His *Eiweissmilch* was accepted for many years. Shortly after this, Schlossmann, Keller, Feer, von Pfaundler, and many others in Germany were also deeply involved in nutritional problems in infants and young children.

In France, Budin (b. 1846) wrote the *Manuel pratique de l'allaitement*, and shortly after, Henri de Rothschild (b. 1872) published his work *L'allaitement artificiel*. In Italy, Fede (b. 1832) and Concetti (b. 1854) were very active in the field of alimentation.

In the United States, Rotch (b. 1849) (see p. 59, Fig. 3), who held the first chair of pediatrics in Boston, introduced the method of percentage or substitute feeding of infants. Holt (b. 1855) (see p. 52, Fig. 3), professor of diseases of children at the

New York clinic and a pediatric leader in his country, Abt (b. 1867), Howland (b. 1873) (see p. 268, Fig. 1), Marriott (b. 1885) (see p. 141, Fig. 4), Talbot (b. 1878), and many others made important contributions to nutrition in pediatrics.

This list is, of course, incomplete, but the field is covered in detail in the earlier chapters of this book.

Modern pediatric gastroenterology is still a young subspecialty because only a few, mostly non-invasive, diagnostic methods were available before the 1960s. Such investigations were limited to microscopic evaluation of the feces, Shwachman's test, the carbohydrate loading test, and the Lipiodol test. With the introduction of balance techniques and the use of endoscopic maneuvers, especially intestinal biopsies, new dimensions opened up. New diagnoses became possible, with the recognition of the anatomic features and physiologic bases of many gastrointestinal disorders and diseases of the liver and pancreas in children. It was therefore possible to establish a classification of gastrointestinal disturbances, starting in the neonatal period with predominantly surgical conditions and progressing through to the older ages.

Biopsies of the proximal small bowel produced essential information through microscopic examination and electronmicroscopy, as well as from enzyme studies and proved to be of little discomfort to the patient. Recent advances have allowed the technique to be used safely even in newborn infants. It was introduced by Shiner (1–3) and by Crosby and Kugler. The Crosby Capsule was modified for pediatric use (4).

Flexible endoscopy, ultrasonography, computerized axial tomography, radioimmunassay, H_2 blockers, radioactive scanning, manometry and nuclear magnetic resonance imaging were further important steps in diagnosing gastrointestinal diseases in childhood. These and other techniques enabled modern gastroenterology to develop in the United States between 1950 and 1960.

I shall now focus on three pediatric diseases as the first and most important fields of research in gastroenterology. Not only are they common disorders but they also show features distinct from adult pathology, and they were primarily investigated by pediatricians. These are celiac disease, cystic fibrosis, and carbohydrate intolerance. I shall mention some of the pioneers of these three diseases who made important contributions to the subject before 1960.

CELIAC DISEASE

In 1888, Samuel Jones Gee, of St. Bartholomew's Hospital in London, wrote the first accurate description of the clinical picture of celiac disease. However, Gee did not consider the disorder to be a newly recognized disease. The title *On the Coeliac Affection* reflected rather his admiration for Aretaeus, the Cappadocian, who described the celiac state a thousand years earlier. Dowd and Walker-Smith have published a very interesting study on the relationship between these two physicians.

Gee said that the "coeliac affection" was "A kind of chronic indigestion which is met in persons of all ages but especially apt to affect children between one and five years of age. Sign of the disease is the pale loose stool, more liquid and larger as natural and very stinking.''

Aretaeus spoke of celiac diathesis, or *ventriculosa passio* (belly sickness), giving a very careful description of all the clinical signs that today we consider as typical of the disease. ''The patient,'' he wrote, ''is emaciated, starved, pallid and without energy. All patients are adult.'' Gee was the first to observe the syndrome in children. He added an interesting contribution concerning the possible cause of this severe condition, which always led to death. Being an anatomist, he observed the atrophy of glandular crypts of the intestine, ''if always present I cannot tell.'' He concluded that ''error in diet may perhaps be a cause, but what error?'' Both very important questions were only answered many years later.

In the following years, the pancreas (Braunwell, 1903) or a general disturbance of intestinal function (Herter, 1908; Heubner, 1909) were held responsible for the disease. However, of the utmost importance were the studies of a group of researchers from Utrecht in Holland under the leadership of Dicke. He observed that bread or biscuits in the diet caused aggravation of the syndrome. During the International Congress of Pediatrics in New York in 1947 he reported his observations but nobody believed him. He returned disappointed but unchanged in his views. He discussed his story with several biochemists, emphasizing the fact that administration of wheat to the celiac patients resulted in an increasing amount of steatorrhea. Co-workers of Dicke, Weijers, a pediatrician, and van de Kamer, a biochemist, observed that on removal of wheat from the diet the fecal fat diminished, while reintroduction of wheat flour caused deterioration. The same phenomenon could not be observed with wheat starch. The first results of their work were presented at the International Meeting of the International Pediatric Association (IPA) in Zurich in 1950. The paper was submitted for publication to a well-known American pediatric journal but was refused, and it was only in 1953 that it was accepted, unchanged, in *Acta Paediatrica Scandinavica* (6).

At the same time, Anderson *et al.* (7) in Birmingham, England, observed that most of the fecal fat was of dietary origin and due to an absorption defect. They came to the conclusion that improvement occurred only following the strict removal of the gluten component of wheat flour. Gluten was the so-called ''wheat factor'' described by the Dutch authors.

The introduction of intestinal biopsy was a landmark in the diagnosis of celiac disease, revealing the characteristic flattening of the mucosa exposed to gluten, as described by Rubin and coworkers (1964).

CYSTIC FIBROSIS

Cystic fibrosis (CF) is not a new disease. From the mid-1600s to the early 1800s many authors described patients with steatorrhea related to pancreatic insufficiency in childhood. There is an interesting connection with Switzerland, in that the Swiss writer, Schmidt (1705), in a book of folk philosophy, described how salty-tasting children were considered bewitched, while in the mid-nineteenth century Pfyffer noted in the *Dictionary of the Swiss German Language* that children who tasted salty when kissed had a poor prognosis. Soon after, Rochholz, in his *Almanac of Children's Songs and Games from Switzerland* (1857), emphasized that salty infants soon die.

One of the first descriptions of meconium ileus with perforation and peritonitis was published by Rokitansky in 1838, and several subsequent authors described pediatric patients affected with both chronic diarrhea and bronchiectasis. But it was only in 1935 that Knauer, in a thesis, and a year later Fanconi, Uehlinger, and Knauer, in a journal publication, provided that first exact description of the typical picture of the disease that we now call cystic fibrosis, differentiating it particularly from celiac disease. The description was completed by Andersen who reported about 49 patients in 1938. Important contributions were also made by Blackfan and May (1938) and by Harper, who reported on the abnormal glucose tolerance curve and the typical generalized lesions in 10 patients.

In 1944, Farber suggested that there was a generalized disease of exocrine glands with inspissation of mucus and proposed the term *mucoviscidosis*. Glanzmann also spoke of "disporia entero-hepatica," i.e., generalized inspissated mucus secretion. The most important steps in the history of this very intriguing disease were taken in 1953 by di Sant'Agnese et al. They found a high concentration of sodium in sweat, which was more readily detected using pilocarpine iontophoresis, as proposed by Gibson and Cooke in 1959. Important contributions were made in the following years by Shwachman et al., Blanc (biliary cirrhosis), and Taussig (male fertility and infertility). Despite many theories, however, the pathophysiology remained unclear.

In the late 1960s and 1970s, Mangos et al. and Kaiser et al. contributed to the evaluation of the mechanism of sodium hypersecretion in sweat, while Spock described a serum factor responsible for the inhibition of the ciliary function. During recent years, papers on cystic fibrosis have become innumerable. Current contributions have been largely devoted to genetic evaluation, and to the precise localization of the defect on the long arm of chromosome 7.

CARBOHYDRATE INTOLERANCE AND INTESTINAL ENZYMOPATHIES

A third important chapter in modern pediatric gastroenterology is represented by the intestinal enzymopathies. Several congenital enzyme deficiencies of the small intestine have been described and many others have been identified as being secondary to other disorders.

In an historical perspective on lactose and lactase, Norman Kretchmer (8) noted that "lactose as a constituent of milk" was discovered by Bartoletus (1633) in Bologna 338 years ago, but its chemical synthesis had to wait for another 300 years. That lactose or other carbohydrates could be associated with the pathogenesis of gastrointestinal disturbances was first reported by Jacobi to the American Pediatric Society in 1901. In the same year, Plimmer studied lactase in the intestine in animals, and in 1909 Mendel confirmed that lactase was present in the intestine of infant animals and absent or diminished in adult animals. In 1921, John Howland described intestinal disorders related to abnormal responses of the intestinal tract to carbohydrates, stating that some deficit in the hydrolysis of lactose must be responsible. The first clinical description was given several years later.

Paolo Durand (1958) was the first to show the importance of the small intestinal enzymes in clinical gastroenterology, describing a child with intractable diarrhea following lactase deficiency and lactosuria. One year later, Holzel et al. (9) observed two siblings whose failure to thrive was found to be due to a selective inability to metabolize lactose. It remains uncertain whether these first two observations described the same disease. Holzel concluded that the occurrence of the same enzyme defect in two siblings suggests that the condition is hereditary. Should absence of lactase be proved, "hereditary alactasia" seemed to be an appropriate name. Later observations confirmed his thesis, but only partly, because the congenital forms are very rare and observed in only a few cases in Finland (10).

Innumerable instances of intolerance to lactose were subsequently reported. Some were verified by demonstrating inactivity of lactase in small intestinal biopsies. Numerous conditions were found to be associated with lactose intolerance and constitute a broad group of secondary lactase insufficiency. It has also been reported by Bayless (1966) and many others that approximately 70% of American blacks are lactose-intolerant, in contrast to 6%–12% of American whites. Further reports from different countries have shown that lactose malabsorption exists in many other ethnic groups. In this regard, the observations of Cook and Kajubi (1966) are of importance. They reported that the Bagandi tribe, who are non-milk-drinkers, are lactose intolerant, while the Tussi, who are milk drinkers, are tolerant. Kretchmer et al. found the same in the nomadic Fulani in Nigeria, a milk-drinking population. Eight out of 10 nomadic Fulani are lactose tolerant, in contrast to the non-milk-drinking, town-dwelling Fulani, in whom only 2 out of 10 are lactose tolerant. Fig. 1 is a map of the eastern hemisphere after Simoons, adapted by Kretchmer, showing dairying and non-dairying regions that, in general, relate to the location of peoples who can or cannot absorb lactose. It has also been very clearly shown that, in the majority of people, there is a decrease in lactase activity with age, but that this decrease occurs at different ages. This is certainly due to evolutionary adaptation. There is a small minority of the world population retaining a high titer of lactase, perhaps because of a deficiency in regression of the genetic complex.

In 1960, Weijers and coworkers reported for the first time a malabsorption state due to sucrose deficiency that was, in all instances, associated with isomaltase deficiency. In 1961, Auricchio et al. and Anderson et al. simultaneously demonstrated the combined defect in peroral intestinal biopsy specimens. It is assumed that the defect is inherited as a recessive trait.

Monosaccharide absorption defects have been reported by Lindquist and Meeu-

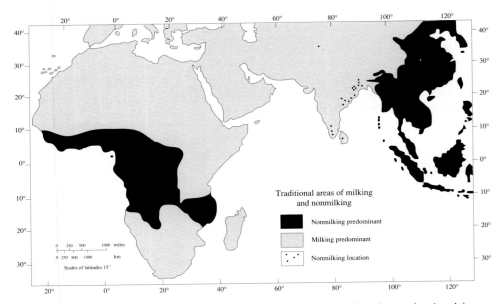

FIG. 1. Map of the eastern hemisphere after Simoons, adapted by Kretchmer, showing dairying and non-dairying regions.

wisse in Sweden (1962) and in the same year by Laplane et al. in France. Affected children tolerate neither glucose nor galactose. A formula containing fructose as the only carbohydrate decreased the diarrhea. Autoradiographic studies demonstrated that the site of the transport lesions was in the mucosal cells. Hereditary fructose intolerance was first described in 1956 by Chambers and Pratt, and 1957 by Froesch et al. They demonstrated that the administration of fructose lowered the level of serum glucose, and that there was a marked reduction of fructose-1-phosphate aldolase in the blood of the patient. The children show failure to thrive, vomiting, hypoglycemia, and convulsions.

A short overview of such a broad chapter must of course be very subjective and incomplete. I believe, nevertheless, that this summary has covered the most important developmental steps in the history of pediatric gastroenterology.

REFERENCES

1. Shiner M. Duodenal biopsy. *Lancet* 1956;i:17–19.
2. Shiner M. Jejunal biopsy tube. *Lancet* 1956;i:85.
3. Crosby WH, Kugler HW. Intraluminal biopsy of the small intestine: the intestinal biopsy capsule. *Am J Digest Dis* 1957;2:236–41.
4. McCarthy CF, Gough KR, Rodriguez M, Read AE. Peroral intestinal biopsy with a small Crosby capsule. *Brit Med J* 1964;i:1620.
5. Dowd B, Walker-Smith J, Samuel Gee, Aretaeus, and the coeliac affection. *Br Med J* 1974;ii: 45–7.

6. Dicke WK, Weijers HA, and van de Kamer JH. Coeliac disease. II. The presence in wheat of a factor having a deleterious effect in cases of coeliac disease. *Acta Paediatr Scand* 1953;42:34–42.
7. Anderson CM, Frazer AC, French JM, Gerrard JW, Sammons HG, Smellie JM. Coeliac disease:
   gastrointestinal studies and the effect of dietary wheat flour. *Lancet* 1952;i:836–42.
8. Kretchmer N. Lactose and lactase—a historical perspective. *Gastroenterology* 1971;61:805–13.
9. Holzel A, Schwarz V, Sutcliffe KW. Defective lactose absorption causing malnutrition in infancy.
   Lancet 1959;i:1126–8.
10. Savilahti E, Launiala K, Kuitunen P. Congenital lactase deficiency. A clinical study on 16 patients.
    Arch Dis Child 1983;58:246–52.

Additional Biographical Sources

Abt IA, ed. *Abt-Garrison. History of pediatrics*. Philadelphia: WB Saunders, 1965.
Anderson CM. Malabsorption—"40 years on." The Teale Lecture, 1981.
Anderson CM et al., eds. *Paediatric gastroenterology*. 2nd ed. Oxford: Blackwell, 1987.
Barthez E, Rilliet F. *Traité clinique et pratique des maladies des enfants*. 2nd edition. Paris: Germer
   Baillière, 1853.
Bohn H et al. Die Krankheiten der Verdauungsorgane. In: Gerhardt C, ed. *Handbuch der Kinderkrank-
   heiten*, vol. 4, chapter 2. Tübingen: Verlag der H Laupp'schen Buchhandlung, 1880.
Dahlqvist A et al. Rat intestinal 6-bromo-2-naphthyl glycosidase and disaccharidase activities. II. Solu-
   bilization and separation of the small-intestinal enzymes. *Arch Biochem Biophys* 1965; 109:159–67.
Davidson M. Reflections of a pediatrician on his gastroenterological roots. *Pediatr Ann* 1987;16:771–3.
Samuel Gee, 1888–1988. International Coeliac Symposium 1988. St Barth Hosp Rep. 1988;24:17.
Lebenthal E, ed. *Textbook of gastroenterology and nutrition in infancy*. 2 vols. New York: Raven Press,
   1981.
Lentze MJ. *Biogenèse des disaccharidases intestinales humaines*. In: Rambaud JC, Modigliani R, eds.
   L'Intestin grêle. Physiologie, physiopathologie et pathologie. Amsterdam: Excerpta Medica, 1988:
   63–9.
Levine MI. Pediatric gastroenterology. A pediatrician's view. *Pediatr Ann* 1982;11:109–12.
Levine MI. Colic, constipation, and diarrhea—old symptoms, new approaches (editorial). *Pediatr Ann*
   1987;16:765–7.
Moody FG. Surgical gastroenterology: problems and solutions. *Am J Surg* 1983;145:2–4.
Peiper A. *Chronik der Kinderheilkunde*. 2nd ed. Leipzig: Georg Thieme, 1955.
Peiper A. *Quellen zur Geschichte der Kinderheilkunde*. Bern und Stuttgart: Hans Huber, 1966.
Ricci FM, ed. *Dizionario biografico della storia della medicina e delle scienze naturali (liber ami-
   corum)*. Milan: FM Ricci, 1985.
Rossi E, Royer P. *Le diagnostic des syndromes de malabsorption congénitale du lactose*. Congrès Fran-
   çais de Pédiatrie. Paris, 1965.
Silverberg M, Davidson M. Pediatric gastroenterology. A review. *Gastroenterology* 1970;58:229–52.
Taussig LM. *Cystic fibrosis*. New York: Thieme-Stratton, 1984.
von Liebig J. *Suppe für Säuglinge*. 2nd ed. Braunschweig: Friedrich Vieweg, 1866.
Walker-Smith J. *Diseases of the small intestine in childhood*. 3rd ed. London: Butterworth, 1988.

DISCUSSION

Dr. Udall: Could you comment on the trend over the past 15 years for a decrease in incidence of celiac disease, at least in the British Isles?

Dr. Rossi: Professor Shmerling has observed this in Switzerland. It is difficult to understand the reasons for it. I do not think it can be entirely explained by the fact that most children are now receiving gliadin only after 6 months of age.

Dr. Visakorpi: I do not believe that celiac disease is decreasing, but rather that there is a
change in the clinical picture. In those countries where the disease is apparently decreasing
what we are seeing is a reduction in the incidence of the disease manifesting during infancy.
However, if you screen for the disease using immunological tests, you still find many cases.

There is evidence that in southern Sweden, where wheat consumption is increasing, the incidence of the disease has gone up.

Dr. Kretchmer: In celiac disease there are two genetic situations to consider, namely, the genetics of the human and the genetics of the wheat. Wheat has gone through many genetic variations and this may be a factor in the varying incidence of celiac disease. There was a great deal of celiac disease in Holland in the 1950s and now there is practically none. There is still a great deal in western Ireland. In the United States we see very little. When I was a resident we had patients with the disease in hospital, but some years later, when I was at Stanford, we saw hardly any.

Dr. Holman: We should be searching for late-onset celiac disease in cases of short stature, as described in Britain, Finland, and Italy. I trained in Canada and saw a lot of celiac disease in Saskatchewan and Manitoba. Perhaps we have a different kind of wheat in the panhandle of Texas, where I now work, since we see very little celiac disease. However, we suspect it in short-statured children with positive antigliadin antibodies. These children don't grow until taken off wheat.

Dr. Stern: Paul di Sant'Agnese discovered the sweat test of cystic fibrosis by serendipity. One hot day in New York 16 children were admitted to his ward with heat exhaustion and 12 of them turned out to be known cases of cystic fibrosis. This led him to consider that they must be losing abnormal quantities of electrolyte in the sweat, although at the time he thought it was potassium.

Dr. Rossi: No, this was not the case. Neither is it true that he diagnosed children by their salty taste. Sant'Agnese has confirmed this personally.

Dr. Farrell: Both Professors Rossi and Stern are partly correct. I completed a fellowship with Paul di Sant'Agnese in 1970 and he told me the story of the development of the sweat test. He made his initial observations before the 1948 heat wave, and in his mind he was prepared for the possibility of hyponatremic dehydration in these patients. But it was the heat wave that motivated him to pursue the research that led to the demonstration of a sweat electrolyte abnormality.

Dr. Katz: The myth of the salty kiss has pervaded our hospital, the Babies' Hospital. It may not have any historical accuracy but it certainly has historical power. Residents working with Dorothy Andersen, who was in charge of the cystic fibrosis clinic, were obliged to lick the foreheads of children suspected of having cystic fibrosis on the day of admission before the sweat test was done. We all became quite adept at it!

Dr. Prader: I should like to comment on Fanconi's thinking about cystic fibrosis. In my presentation on the history of pediatric endocrinology, I mentioned that Wilkins described congenital adrenal hypertrophy as being familial but not hereditary. Fanconi did exactly the same for cystic fibrosis. He speculated about possible causes but did not consider that it could be a genetic defect. This illustrates again how 40 or 50 years ago genetic influences were not present in our thoughts to the same extent as today.

History of Pediatrics 1850–1950, edited by
B.L. Nichols, A. Ballabriga, and N. Kretchmer.
Nestlé Nutrition Workshop Series, Vol. 22. Nestec
Ltd., Vevey/Raven Press, Ltd., New York © 1991.

Pediatric Nephrology

Malcolm E. Holliday

*Department of Pediatrics, University of California San Francisco,
San Francisco, California 94143, USA*

This chapter reviews the contributions of three individuals, two pediatricians and a physiologist, who did much to shape nephrology research in the period from 1915 to 1965. Their work had a unifying theme: it focused on the adaptive capacity of the kidney to regulate output in the face of varying input so that the volume and composition of body fluids, particularly extracellular fluid would remain stable.

The research of the two pediatricians influenced the way clinical research developed in the 1940s. The research of the physiologist helped shape the policy that emphasized basic research. These two models were complementary. In recent years an imbalance between basic and clinical research has developed that is inhibiting the capacity of either to benefit clinical practice.

The first of the three individuals, James Gamble (see p. 193, Fig. 2), a pediatrician, born in 1883, received medical training in Boston and began his research at the Harriet Lane Home around 1915. The photograph, taken by Metcoff in front of the teaching diagrams Gamble created to make basic physical chemistry intelligible to medical students of the 1940s, catches his dedication to thoughtful scholarship.

Dr. Gamble spent most of his career in his laboratory removed from patient care. However, his internship at the Boston Floating Hospital, an excursion steamer converted to a floating hospital so that infants with diarrheal dehydration would be exposed to the "healthful benefits of the sea breezes of Boston Harbor," had made him keenly aware of the problem of diarrheal dehydration. At that time, this disease had a hospital mortality rate in excess of 80%. He later commented whimsically, "We then failed to understand that *sea water* not sea breezes was what the patients needed to get well!" At the Harriet Lane Home under the guidance of John Howland (see p. 270, Fig. 6), Gamble took direction for his research from the insights of Claude Bernard, who pointed out the importance of extracellular fluid (ECF) as the true environment in which we live. To support life it must be resistant to change. Gamble studied how this environment was affected by fasting, acidosis, alkalosis, and dehydration. His first major publication (1) described observations on four children with epilepsy who were treated by fasting—then, a traditional therapy. He reported on urinary losses, composition of weight loss, and change in plasma. With this publication he introduced into clinical medicine the concepts of equivalence using "cc's of N/10 acid." By equating the losses in urine (Fig. 1) of cations to anions in accordance with basic principles in physical chemistry then unfamiliar to medical

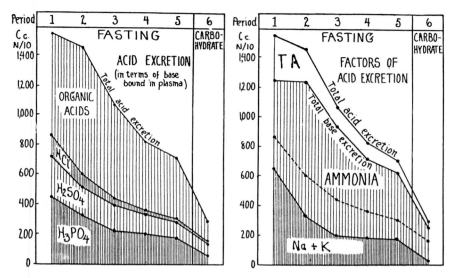

FIG. 1. Figure describing urinary excretion of anions and cations in a patient who fasted for 15 days—a conventional treatment for epilepsy in 1915. Note decrease in anion and cation excretion as fasting progressed and further decrease when carbohydrate was given. Note also that "cc N/10" were used in place of meq and that terminology of that period differed from conventions used today. The figure is a graphic representation of the formula: H^+ retention = $(Na + K) - Cl$ + retained organic acid. (Reprinted with permission from *J Biol Chem*, 1923;57.)

students and physicians, he defined renal acid excretion. These losses in urine during fasting described deficits of the cations, Na and K, and of anions, Cl and phosphate. Weight loss was due to loss of ECF, intracellular fluid (ICF), body fat, and protein. The loss of ECF was defined from the excretion of Na and Cl, the loss of ICF from the excretion of K and the loss of fat from the estimated expenditure of calories and the loss of protein from urinary nitrogen (N). Despite loss of electrolyte, retention of hydrogen ion, and loss of ECF and ICF, plasma (i.e., ECF composition) changed but little.

He drew the following conclusions from the study.

1. In fasting, renal and metabolic adaptive responses lessen the losses of Na, Cl, K, and N and the retention of hydrogen (H^+) as fasting processes.
2. Despite major losses, plasma (extracellular fluid) composition changes very little.
3. A small amount of carbohydrate further *reduces* the losses of Na, Cl, K, and N, the retention of H^+, and the changes in plasma.

This report resulted in new physiological principles and new therapeutic interventions. Over the next 11 years, each of the nine papers he read at the American Pediatric Society was cited by the historian of the Society as a highlight of that meeting. Each built on the previous work to define how the volume and composition of ECF responded to a variety of stresses. Each illustrated the role that kidney function played in maintaining ECF composition. Giving 5% glucose intravenously to provide carbohydrate (CHO) to patients had the physiological benefit of further reducing these losses.

During World War II, he joined Allan Butler in the life-raft studies conducted in normal subjects to evaluate the effect on castaways of adding carbohydrate to the water rations to be stored on life rafts (2). They found that adding 100 g of glucose to the daily ration of water reduced water, N, and electrolyte losses in urine significantly. Thus, adding glucose to the rations was warranted because less water would be required. This observation confirmed the carbohydrate effect he had described earlier and stimulated further studies on the physiological consequences of fasting.

In addition to his own contribution, Dr. Gamble helped many who spent time in his laboratory and who later became future leaders in pediatrics, medicine, and surgery. They extended the research model he developed in studying questions in body fluid physiology. Their findings had important implications for clinical practice.

The second pediatrician is Daniel C. Darrow, born in 1895 in South Dakota, trained in St. Louis and Johns Hopkins, and served on the faculty at Yale University and the University of Kansas. He is shown in Fig. 2 with his wife, who was also a pediatrician. The qualities of warmth and enthusiasm they both possessed are evident in this photograph.

Darrow made two outstanding contributions to basic physiology. Each directly affected clinical practice. The first contribution, published in 1935, was the finding that water was freely permeable across cell membranes (3). A change in the osmotic pressure of ECF caused a shift in the distribution of water between ECF and cells. With hyponatremia, cell volume increased; with hypernatremia, it decreased. This finding provided the basis for understanding the consequences of hypo- and hypernatremia and how to derive a rational treatment for each.

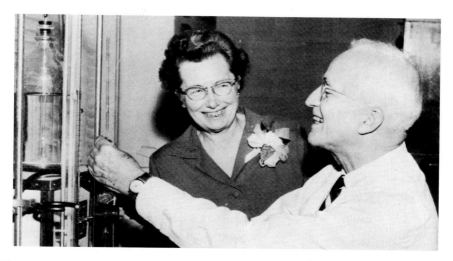

FIG. 2. Dr. and Mrs. Daniel Darrow (from *The Works of Daniel C. Darrow, M.D.* Stanley Hellertstein MD, ed., 1971). (Reprinted with permission from the editor and Sevorg Publishing, Kansas City.)

The second contribution was to describe potassium deficiency as a clinically significant problem. He reported the loss of potassium and the gain of sodium by cells in rats on a potassium-deficient diet and noted that extracellular alkalosis and hypokalemia were associated (4). He went on to show that potassium deficiency had acute effects on the electrocardiogram (5) and chronic effects on heart muscle (6), both of which had important clinical implications. He showed that giving potassium salts as part of therapy was beneficial in preventing the adverse effects of potassium deficiency (7) (Fig. 3).

Darrow was the quintessential clinician turned investigator who, in an age still dominated by teaching medical students the dogma of the past, urged that we learn basic principles and develop new approaches to therapy. In his presidential address to the American Pediatric Society in 1957, he made an uncharacteristically solemn declaration, but it was one that expressed his conviction (8) that "research is the process by which teachers and students are forced to deal with the lively facts of medical science rather than the rules of trade. . . . Ours is a learned profession in which all who enter must be prepared to deal with new ideas for the rest of their lives'' (8).

The physiologist I have chosen to describe is Homer William Smith, born in 1895 (Fig. 4). Following college and military service in World War I, he spent 3 years at Johns Hopkins with William Howell and 2 years at Harvard with Walter Cannon. During his association with these physiologists, he began his lifelong interest in comparative physiology, evolution, and philosophy.

An early project was a study of the lung fish, a primitive fish that, during the wet season, lives in the shallow estuaries of African rivers and derives oxygen through the gills. In drought, when the river dries, it buries itself in the mud flats, envelopes itself in a tough encasement and extends a tube from an air bladder through the mud in order to breathe air and get oxygen as do land-based vertebrates. When the rains come, it returns to life in fresh water and relies again on gills for oxygen. The findings from this study filled an important gap in defining the evolution of life from fresh water to land, so well described in his book *From Fish to Philosopher.* (9)

He was then drawn to the question of how vertebrates adapt to the different exter-

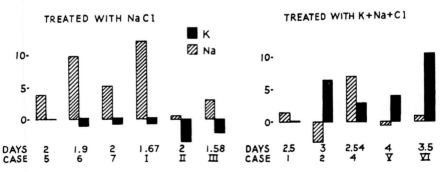

FIG. 3. Differences in retention of Na and K (in mM/kg) when therapy included K or when it did not. (Reprinted from *Pediatrics*, 1949;1:129.)

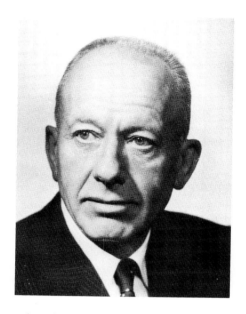

FIG. 4. Homer Smith. (Reprinted with permission from *Homer William Smith*. Chasis H, Goldring W, eds. New York University Press, 1965. Photo by Bachrach.)

nal environments in which they live, in terms of maintaining constant ECF volume and composition. Particular emphasis was placed on preserving the balance of sodium chloride (NaCl) and water by the kidney (9–11). He described the problem and the strategies used to effect a stable ECF and ICF.

He validated the method for measuring glomerular filtration rate (GFR) from the clearance of inulin and for measuring renal plasma flow from the clearance of para-amino hippurate. Using these tools he turned his attention to renal physiology in humans, especially those with hypertension. He gathered about him physiologists and physicians at Bellevue Hospital in New York who were interested in the relation of physiological mechanisms to disease.

Homer Smith's philosophy had an important influence on medical research. He served on National Committees that set the agenda for medical research in the 1940s and 1950s (12). In the immediate post-war period, he served on the Committee on Medicine, a part of an advisory group headed by Vannevar Bush to advise President Truman on what policies the government should adopt to support science. Basic research was given priority. His clinical associates at Bellevue, whom he strongly influenced, became influential leaders who gave support to this agenda within clinical departments. This policy, that basic research in biology is the best long-term investment for assuring advances in clinical care, became the predominant policy at the National Institutes of Health (NIH). While attention was to be given to clinical research, the emphasis was and is on basic research. The success of this policy is evident.

Clinical research as exemplified by Gamble and Darrow has evolved into different types:

1. Clinical observation leading to questions that stimulate research. Results are then

taken to patients for evaluation, for example, glucose (Gamble), potassium (Darrow);

2. NIH-supported clinical research projects that support research questions formally posed as hypotheses;
3. Clinical trials to answer efficacy and safety questions.

Clinical investigators continue to draw inspiration from the original Gamble-Darrow model: observe a problem at the bedside; take it to the laboratory; find an answer; bring it back to the bedside. However, in today's hospital environment, this is increasingly difficult to do.

The NIH gave support to an important offshoot of this practice in the late 1950s when they funded clinical research centers. Using resources of the centers, physicians carried out carefully designed protocols. The centers have been very useful as the body of knowledge derived from basic research increased and more sophisticated methods of clinical research were needed to exploit them.

Over the last two decades, as basic research has continued to develop, new ideas are more easily generated, but, once generated, they are less easily translated into clinical research and practice. Ward rounds are no longer leisurely; clinical decisions are made quickly. The clinical research center, designed to bridge the gap between basic and clinical practice, is today less able to do so. Results from clinical research come slowly and in a manner not well geared to abstract deadlines and grant deadlines, currencies that define success in research today.

The third type of clinical research—the controlled clinical trial—has developed to fill two needs. It may be used to test a change in therapy that is introduced informally into clinical practice or to test a therapy suggested from basic research as it reaches a stage where it is recognized as possibly useful. Its purpose is to apply the pragmatic test of whether, in the "real" world, the new therapy works and is safe. Controlled clinical trials are the means we use to answer those pragmatic questions. They are important because proposed therapies—drugs, procedures, or change in diet—have the potential for harm as well as good. The frequency of unintended consequences leading to unwanted results from promising therapies requires us to use this method of research for these purposes. Controlled trials are important in complex settings such as the intensive care unit (ICU) where new procedures or modifications of old ones can have unforeseen and unwanted consequences, just as new drug therapies can in the ward or outpatient setting. The disasters of blindness that followed the uninhibited use of oxygen in premature infants, and of fetal anomalies that followed the use of thalidomide and diethylstilbestrol (DES) by pregnant women are but three examples that compel caution in the application of research. Today, no new drug can be put on the market without passing the rigorous test of proving safety and efficacy for the condition it is designed to treat. This is a responsibility of pharmaceutical companies. Current costs limit them to testing drugs that have market potential to warrant the cost. There are few incentives for evaluating approved drugs for new treatments. The current system in academic institutions for testing new treatments and procedures to evaluate this efficacy-safety issue is not adequate to the task. Use of public research funds for clinical trials is hampered by a number of questions that are not readily addressed by the research establishment.

1. Who decides a clinical trial is needed in relation to the public and patient interest?
2. Who develops the protocol and patient population?
3. Who reviews and evaluates the study, design, and budget?
4. Where does the money come from?

Fig. 5 shows a diagram that illustrates my perception of the growth of basic and clinical research over three different periods. In the first two, there was parallel growth. For the period from 1965 to the present, basic research has continued its growth but clinical research, by contrast, appears to have declined. This seems to be true whether we consider clinical research from the perspective of the Gamble-Darrow model, or its derivative, the NIH-supported clinical research centers, or the support available for controlled clinical trials. This is not the place to analyze reasons, consider consequences, and propose remedies for this development. I have chosen to use the historical perspective to highlight the problem, in keeping with the goals set forth in the announcement of this workshop. It is a long-term problem for those doing basic research, whose support depends on the public awareness that basic research improves clinical practice. It is a more urgent problem to sustain and enlarge the capability for clinical research, which, in my view, is at risk. Given this imperative, I trust that means will be found to strengthen the clinical research on which future progress depends.

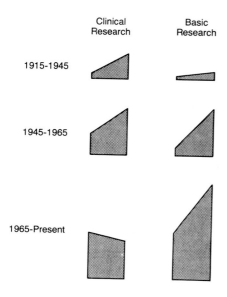

FIG. 5. Diagrammatic representation of the growth of clinical research and basic research in three different periods.

REFERENCES

1. Gamble JL, Ross GS, Tisdall FF. The metabolism of fixed base during fasting. *J Biol Chem* 1923;57:633.
2. Gamble JL. *Physiological information from studies on the life raft ration.* Harvey Lecture Ser 42, 1946;247.
3. Darrow DC, Yannet H. The changes in the distribution of body water accompanying increase and decrease in extracellular electrolyte. *J Clin Invest* 1935;14:266.
4. Darrow DC, Schwartz R, Iannucci JF, Coville F. The relation of serum bicarbonate concentration to muscle composition. *J Clin Invest* 1948;27:198–208.
5. Darrow DC. Body fluid physiology: The role of potassium on clinical disturbances of body water and electrolyte. *N Eng J Med* 1950;242:978–1014.
6. Darrow DC. Miller HC. The production of cardiac lesions by repeated injections of desoxycorticosterone acetate. *J Clin Invest* 1942;21:601–11.
7. Darrow DC, Pratt EL, Flett J, Gamble AH, Wiese HF. Disturbances of water and electrolytes in infantile diarrhea. *Pediatrics* 1949;1:129.
8. Darrow DC, Presidential Address—American Pediatric Society. *Am J Dis Child* 1957;94:359–66.
9. Smith HW. *From fish to philosopher—The lungfish.* Boston: Litttle, Brown and Company, 1953;75.
10. Smith HW. *The kidney structure and function in health and disease.* New York: Oxford University Press, 1951.
11. Chasis H, Goldring W. *Homer William Smith ScD.* New York: New York University Press, 1965; 262.
12. Ibid. 270.

DISCUSSION

Dr. Barness: Researchers in the eighteenth and nineteenth centuries and in the early twentieth century considered that they were doing basic research—for example, the development of calorimetry and the understanding of nitrogen metabolism were basic research undertakings.

Dr. Holliday: I meant to indicate that there had been important basic research before 1915 and the research you describe is certainly included under this heading. What I am saying is that today there is inadequate support for clinical research compared with the level of support given to basic research. In particular there are inadequate resources for translating basic research findings into safe and effective clinical products that have been through the process of clinical research.

Dr. Ballabriga: Some of the basic knowledge that is the foundation of modern physicochemical research stems from the work of nineteenth century investigators such as the Dutchman, Van't Hoff and the Swede, Arrhenius, and from Ostwald's book *Lehrbuch der Allgemeinen Chemie* published in 1891, which served as a basis for modern knowledge of the metabolism of water, electrolytes and hydrogen ions, and of stereochemistry.

Dr. Holliday: That is what Gamble and Darrow built on. It is interesting to see how they hesitatingly introduced the now accepted principles of physical chemistry into their papers, which described both basic and clinical research. Gamble made some basic clinical observations that could be directly translated into improved clinical care. It is much harder today for a single investigator to do this. A bridge needs to exist between the basic researcher and the clinical investigator to reproduce the Gamble-Darrow paradigm.

Dr. Harrison: You have overlooked an important point. Gamble worked with Henderson, a physiologist, and learned his physiology and chemistry from him. He was recruited by John

Howland because he was a physiologist, not because he was a clinician. He was able to make his clinical contributions because he was a good physiologist and had a basic training in physical chemistry. Marriott was also recruited by Howland, because he wanted a department that was devoted primarily to the application of chemistry to clinical medicine. I think that as long as we have department chairmen of Howland's perspicacity there will be no problem in clinical research.

Dr. Holliday: The gap between basic and clinical research is harder to close and there is usually a much longer trip from a basic research finding to a change in clinical practice.

Dr. Ballabriga: Progress in research constitutes a non-stop continuum and much of present day knowledge, for example in the field of physiology, stems from the studies of Müller in the period of transition after the *Naturphilosophie*, and from those of Ludwig, from whose School of Physiology in Leipzig more than 200 eminent disciples emerged. Some of the principles that were studied at that time could not be applied practically until 40 or 50 years later and others have remained basic concepts to this day.

Dr. Holliday: I do not disagree with what you say. However there are several tools that are needed for good clinical research today, and only when they are provided can it happen. They are epidemiology and biostatistics.

Dr. Grunberg: I think that some kinds of research are missed in the dualistic approach of ''basic'' and ''clinical'' research. Research on appropriate health technology has a tremendous impact on the future of medicine. Health technology includes all forms of knowledge that can be used in solving or reducing health problems, including drugs, devices, and procedures used in medical care and the organizational and support systems that allow the provision of care. ''Appropriate technology for health'' is defined as the capability of the technology to achieve a defined practical purpose for the prevailing conditions. To be appropriate, health technology must be scientifically sound, acceptable by the population, and affordable.

History of Pediatrics 1850–1950, edited by
B.L. Nichols, A. Ballabriga, and N. Kretchmer.
Nestlé Nutrition Workshop Series, Vol. 22. Nestec
Ltd., Vevey/Raven Press, Ltd., New York 1991.

Pediatric Allergy and Immunology

Joseph A. Bellanti and *Sheldon G. Cohen

*Departments of Pediatrics and Microbiology, and the International Center for
Interdisciplinary Studies of Immunology, Georgetown University School of Medicine,
Washington, DC 20007; and *The National Institute of Allergy and Infectious Diseases,
National Institutes of Health, Bethesda, Maryland 20892, USA*

Pediatric allergy and immunology emerged during the period from 1850 to 1950 as part of the development of three main disciplines: microbiology and infectious disease, hypersensitivity and clinical allergy, and immunobiology and immunologic disorders (1). Although knowledge in these fields did not develop concurrently, as information emerged from one area it contributed to the growth of the other two.

Pediatric allergy and immunology did not exist in 1850, for a knowledge base from which to take root had not yet evolved. Seminal observations had appeared by 1850, although the rapid ascendancy of this subspecialty lay many years ahead (2).

The evolution of pediatric allergy and immunology differs from other pediatric specialties that by 1850 had found identity in well-defined organ systems. In many of these, anatomic and physiologic bases could be traced to the medical writings of antiquity. Allergy and immunology did not have comparable origins or foundations.

The historical development of pediatric allergy and immunology can be viewed from three aspects: (1) milestones in microbiology and infection, hypersensitivity, and immunobiology; (2) the interrelationships of these areas; and (3) the resultant clinical applications of this knowledge to pediatrics. In this review, we shall discuss the relevance of immune phenomena to health and disease in infancy and childhood as well as the special contributions that pediatricians have made to the field.

MICROBIOLOGY AND INFECTIOUS DISEASES

The contributions of microbiology and infectious diseases to pediatric allergy and immunology are shown in Table 1 (3–6). With the exception of Jenner's pioneering work on smallpox vaccination, little was known in 1850 about the causative agents of infectious diseases. It was appreciated that individuals who contracted communicable diseases rarely developed the same illness again and were protected, but this host resistance was poorly understood.

The pioneering work in this area was particularly relevant to the prevalent infectious diseases of childhood. A variety of factors—poor sanitation, lack of public health measures, overcrowding, poor nutrition, and disadvantaged economic set-

tings—all contributed to the high incidence of diseases such as smallpox, tuberculosis, streptococcal pharyngitis and scarlet fever, diphtheria, tetanus, rabies, and
typhoid fever.

Eighty years lapsed after Jenner's work in 1798 before another significant advance in microbiology and infectious diseases took place. This was the work of
Louis Pasteur who was the first to establish the germ theory of disease (Table 1). Although his research led to the discovery of the causative agents of many infectious
diseases in animals, it also provided insights for studies of human diseases. The first
of these was Pasteur's introduction of vaccination against rabies in humans. As in
Jenner's earlier introduction of smallpox vaccination, children served as subjects for
Pasteur's first clinical trials of rabies vaccine.

TABLE 1. *Milestones in pediatric immunology and allergy, 1850–1950:*
microbiology and infectious diseases

Individual	Date	Contribution
Pasteur	1880–1885	Developed methodology for killed and attenu-ated vaccines
Koch	1891	Described delayed hypersensitivity to tubercu-losis bacillus
Klebs and Koeffler	1883–1884	Discovered diphtheria bacillus
Metchnikoff	1884–1908	Described role of phagocytosis in antimicro-bial defense
Roux and Yersin	1885	Described bacterial toxins (diphtheria toxin)
von Behring and Kitasato	1890	Described antitoxins
Bordet	1895	Elucidated action of complement and antibody
Widal	1896	Described serum agglutinin test for diagnosis of typhoid fever
Mantoux	1908	Described an intradermal test for diagnosis of tuberculosis
Schick	1913	Introduced a skin test for determination of sus-ceptibility to diphtheria
Dick	1915	Introduced a skin test for determination of sus-ceptibility to scarlet fever
von Pirquet	1915	Introduced intracutaneous (scratch) tuberculin test as a diagnostic aid in tuberculosis
Calmette and Guérin	1921	Developed an attenuated vaccine (BCG) for prevention of tuberculosis
Ramon	1923	Demonstrated that formalin-treated toxin, ana-toxin (toxoid), possessed advantages as an immunizing agent
Fothergill	1933	Described the striking relationship between age and incidence of *H. influenzae* type B (HIB) meningitis
Enders, Robbins and Weller	1949	Cultivated poliomyelitis viruses in tissue culture
Salk	1950	Conducted clinical trials with killed poliovirus vaccine
Sabin	1936–1962	Developed live attenuated oral poliovirus vaccine

The contributions of Pasteur in the field of microbiology and infectious diseases provided the basis for future development and design of vaccines for the prevention of other infectious diseases. In addition to initiating a whole new field of protective immunotherapy, this experimental procedure introduced an entirely new problem— that of unforeseen adverse reactions to vaccination. Thus autoimmune processes were added to the future fields of allergy and immunology.

In 1891, a contemporary of Louis Pasteur, the German physician-scientist, Robert Koch, discovered the causative agent of tuberculosis. While attempting to develop a vaccine against this disease, his observation of an associated skin reaction led to identification of delayed hypersensitivity, or cell-mediated, immunity. Koch's culture extract, which came to be known as tuberculin, was unsuccessful as a specific therapeutic agent for tuberculosis, but it was to provide one of the first applications of an immune reaction to the diagnosis of an infectious disease.

Among Koch's foreign students in 1885 was William Welch, who brought to America the evidence for bacterial etiology of disease. The contributions of Welch, Flexner, and Longcope, furthered the development of bacteriology. Their investigations on a disease familiar to pediatricians, glomerulonephritis, would provide a model for understanding immune system disorders.

The presence of organisms, however, was only part of the understanding infectivity and host responses. One year after isolation of the diphtheria bacillus by Klebs and Koeffler in 1883–1884, Roux and Yersin demonstrated the existence of a chemical toxin elaborated by this organism. Von Behring and Kitasato then used diphtheria toxin to raise a neutralizing serum factor in laboratory animals that they termed *antitoxin*. These investigators performed the first trial of serum therapy on a child with diphtheria on Christmas night, 1891. This innovative and successful study was rewarded with the first Nobel prize in 1901.

As a result, the concept of serum therapy was added to bacteriology and the discipline of immunology was born. For many years, passive immunization played a role in the conquest of diphtheria and tetanus.

At the forefront of the application of this new knowledge on induced immunity, Wright established a laboratory and clinical unit at the turn of the nineteenth century, the Inoculation Department of St. Mary's Hospital in London. Wright's visionary concept of the developing field was best represented in his widely publicized statement "the physician of the future may yet become an immunisator."

Another pioneer was Metchnikoff. His studies on host defenses revealed that immune capability did not entirely reside in humoral antibody but was also mediated through cellular and phagocytic functions of leukocytes. Metchnikoff shared the 1908 Nobel prize with Ehrlich. In later years, investigators building on Metchnikoff's observations would demonstrate granulocytic dysfunction in some immunodeficiency diseases and the chronic granulomatous disease of childhood.

It was subsequently shown by Bordet in 1895 that there was also a substance in serum distinct from antibody, called *complement*. He demonstrated that complement possessed the biologic activity necessary for the destruction of bacteria. Bordet's findings also led to investigations that made immunologically related diagnostic contributions. One of the prominent applications was the complement fixation serologic test for syphilis (Wasserman, Kahn, Kolmer, and Kline modifications). Its use in obstetric practice enabled the prevention of the disastrous consequences of congenital syphilis in the newborn. Later studies identified inherited absence of serum complement components in a number of childhood deficiency syndromes.

Although typhoid fever was a prevalent disease of all age groups, contaminated sources of water posed a special risk to infants and children. Public health control to eliminate adulteration of milk was often lacking. In 1896, Widal demonstrated the ability of sera from previously infected individuals to agglutinate typhoid baccilli in vitro. Thus, a year later, Wright showed that mass immunization with killed typhoid vaccine was at least partially effective.

Extending Koch's discovery of tuberculin, Mantoux in 1908 described its use in an intradermal technique for the diagnosis of tuberculosis. Seven years later in 1915, von Pirquet, who would be especially remembered for his later contributions to allergy, introduced the scratch test modification. Although the immune reactants of cell-free bacterial toxins and circulating antitoxins in diphtheria and scarlet fever differed in character from those responsible for positive tuberculin tests, there was nevertheless a common denominator. Thus the principle was successfully adapted to provide in vivo cutaneous tests for diphtheria (Schick test, 1913) and for scarlet fever (Dick test, 1915). The Schultz-Carlton cutaneous reaction, described in 1918 as an aid to the diagnosis of scarlet fever, used the immune capability of streptococcal antitoxin to neutralize streptococcal toxin and produce localized blanching of the hypersensitivity-related eruption at a skin test site.

In the continued war against tuberculosis, Calmette and Guérin in 1921 developed an attenuated vaccine, the bacille Calmette-Guérin (BCG). This vaccine, used worldwide, has been effective in reducing the incidence of tuberculosis in infancy.

Meanwhile, passive immunization using antitoxins recovered from the blood sera of actively immunized horses was proving to be a mixed blessing. While effective against diphtheria and tetanus if given early enough and in sufficiently large doses, the complicating side effects of serum therapy, i.e., serum sickness, were often distressing and life threatening. Actively induced immunization was demonstrated by Ramon in 1923 when he found that formalin-treated diphtheria or tetanus toxins, termed *anatoxins* (i.e., toxoid), could serve as safe vaccines.

The unique structural and biochemical characteristics of specific types of microorganisms gave further impetus to pediatric immunology. In 1933, Fothergill described a relationship between age and incidence of meningitis caused by *H. influenzae* type B. His work formed the basis for subsequent effective vaccines for the prevention of other infectious diseases due to encapsulated polysaccharide microorganisms (e.g., pneumococcal pneumonia).

In 1950, poliomyelitis remained high on the list of communicable diseases of high epidemicity, mortality, and morbidity. The work of Enders, Robbins, and Weller in 1949, showing that poliomyelitis virus could be cultivated in tissue culture, was a milestone that merited the award of a Nobel prize in 1954. This laboratory endeavor led to the development of poliovirus vaccines by Salk and Sabin, and to the development of other tissue-culture-grown vaccines against mumps, rubeola, and rubella. Rubella vaccine has done much to reduce one infectious source of birth defects.

HYPERSENSITIVITY

Early pioneers in microbiology and infectious diseases laid the groundwork for later investigations of hypersensitivity and allergic and autoimmune disorders. These contributions to pediatric allergy and immunology are shown in Table 2 (7–10).

TABLE 2. *Milestones in pediatric immunology and allergy, 1850–1950: hypersensitivity*

Individual	Date	Contribution
Wyman	1872	First described familial pre-disposition to hay fever and pollen as the specific causative agent
Richet and Portier	1902	Described anaphylaxis
von Pirquet	1903	Developed broad theory that both host and foreign substance contribute to disease. Coined the term *allergy*
von Pirquet and Schick	1905	Described serum sickness
Noon and Freeman	1911–1914	Introduced concept and procedure of immunotherapy for allergy
Schloss	1912	Developed intracutaneous (scratch) test in food allergic child
Talbot	1914	Described relationship of asthma to egg "poisoning"
Cooke and Vander Veer	1916	Described factor of inheritance of allergic disease
Rackemann	1918	Differentiated classes of asthma (intrinsic *vs* extrinsic) and their age associations; established that not all cases of asthma were of allergic origin
Park	1920	Described first case report of hypersensitivity to cow's milk in infancy on first exposure
Prausnitz and Kustner	1921	Demonstrated skin sensitizing antibody by passive transfer
Coca	1923	Described concept of atopy
Ratner	1927	Described *in* utero sensitization to milk proteins in guinea pig
Donnally	1930	Demonstrated passage of dietary antigens into breast milk
Stuart	1934	With Hill, developed nutritionally balanced palatable soybean formula; developed first standardized growth charts for children
Cooke and Loveless	1937	Described induction and character of "blocking antibody"
Guy	1938	Introduced feeding program of soybean "milk" for infants in China where genetically related high prevalence of lactase deficiency existed

In 1850, there was only Jenner's observation on the inflammatory nature of accelerated immune (''non-take'') reactions to vaccinia in previously inoculated individuals to point to the existence of delayed hypersensitivity reactions. The potential of this phenomenon for the development of serious iatrogenic disorders would not be realized until the twentieth century. In 1949, instances of encephalitis, myelitis, and neuritis appeared when large-scale immunization was undertaken during a smallpox scare in New York City. The first contribution to pediatric infectious disease immunology in the 1850–1950 period also simultaneously provided another example on a theme. Thus some of those who were successfully protected against the development of rabies by Pasteur's vaccine escaped the infectious disease only to develop encephalomyelitis. It was later shown that this was due to an autoimmune process occurring as a reactive response to the rabbit neural tissue in the vaccine.

In 1902, Richet and Portier tried to develop a protective antiserum for Prince Albert of Monaco, who was adversely affected by the toxin of stinging sea anemones. During the course of immunization of experimental animals, they found that dogs repeatedly injected with anemone toxin developed shock with respiratory and circulatory collapse; thus anaphylaxis was discovered. Smith's observations associated with attempts to standardize toxin-antitoxin reagents by in vivo techniques (1902–1904) and Rosenau and Anderson's studies on hypersensitivity (1906) demonstrated the guinea pig's exquisite susceptibility to anaphylactic reactivity. This proved to be an especially suitable model for studies in allergy.

In 1903, von Pirquet, who had been introduced to immunology through his work on tuberculin skin tests and, henceforth, would be considered the father of allergy, developed the theory that both host and foreign substances could contribute to disease. From this concept he coined the term *allergy* (*allergie*). Intending to define the phenomenon of altered reactivity, he differentiated those responses that were protective from those that led to adverse or allergic reactions. Following the introduction of passive immunization by von Behring and Kitasato, von Pirquet, together with Schick, pursued studies on one type of human allergic response that frequently followed the administration of animal sera antitoxins. Their observations described the nature of the clinical entity, serum sickness.

In the field of natural allergic disease, the observations of Wyman in 1872 were noteworthy. His was the first description of familial predisposition to seasonal hay fever (allergic rhinitis), recording that pollen of Roman wormwood was the specific causative agent of autumnal catarrh and responsible for its early appearance in childhood.

From 1911 to 1914, Noon and Freeman attempted the treatment of allergic disease by immunotherapy—a concept based upon the erroneous belief that pollens liberated toxin and that repeated injections of pollen extract might generate neutralizing antitoxin. Nonetheless, they introduced a tool for allergy practice.

In 1937, Cooke and Loveless, seeking to explain the mechanism of desensitization in hay fever, discovered a type of antibody that arose during the course of injection treatments with pollen extracts. Because of this ability to neutralize atopic reagins, this humoral factor was given the name, *blocking antibody*.

In 1912, Schloss' development of the scratch test enabled specific diagnoses in allergy. Utilizing extracts from suspected food allergens, this technique was based on von Pirquet's earlier test for tuberculosis. Schloss' contribution offered a practical diagnostic test for the identification of many allergens responsible for allergic respiratory and skin disorders. All of Schloss' studies were performed in children. In 1914, the pediatrician, Talbot, using the scratch test, showed the relationship of asthma to egg "poisoning". His work, evolved from an interest in infant and child nutrition and metabolism, formed the basis for subsequent studies of food allergy.

In 1915, Cooke modified Schloss' approach and introduced intracutaneous allergen testing, based upon the original Mantoux tuberculin technique. Cooke, a dominant figure in allergy research in the United States, made several pioneering contributions to the field. In 1916, he and Vander Veer were the first to examine and report on the factor of inheritance in allergic disease. Then in 1923, Coca, an early collaborator of Cooke, described the concept of *atopy* or "strange disease". This important contribution formed the basis for later insights into the constitutional nature of familial allergy and the propensity to develop IgE.

Rackemann in 1918, showed that the majority of instances of extrinsic asthma presented in children, whereas most cases of intrinsic asthma occurred in adults. He helped to dispel the previously held belief that all asthma was allergic in origin. Although an internist, Rackemann did much through these studies to point pediatricians to potentially productive and appropriate avenues of research on asthma.

In 1920, Park reported the first detailed description of hypersensitivity in an infant upon first exposure to cow's milk. Park's research was derived from his interest in nutrition. His own son was believed to be the infant reported in the case study.

Ruth Guy, a student of Coca and later an associate of Park, is recognized as the first female allergist. She and Schloss were the only two pediatricians taken into Cooke's original small and selective study group. She later went to China to accept a faculty position at the Peking Union Medical College, which was supported by the Rockefeller Foundation, where she introduced a soybean milk feeding program for Chinese infants.

In 1921, Prausnitz and Küstner made their discovery that specific skin sensitizing antibody could be passively transferred by serum (P-K test). The ability of donor serum from Küstner, who was allergic to fish, to provide a positive skin test to fish on transfer to Prausnitz, a pollen-sensitive patient, had important applications in pediatric allergy. The P-K test allowed normal volunteer recipients to provide undamaged skins for testing the allergic reactivity in blood serum from infants and children with atopic dermatitis; in this disorder eczematous skin precluded the direct diagnostic procedure.

Many of the early investigations of pediatric allergy were by investigators of infant and child nutrition, as exemplified in the reports of Talbot and Park. Studies on guinea pig anaphylaxis by Rosenau and Anderson in 1906 provided evidence that experimental sensitization could be induced by the gastrointestinal route, and in 1927 Ratner described in utero sensitization to milk proteins in the guinea pig. Donnally in 1930 demonstrated the transmission of maternal dietary antigens into human milk. This early observation formed the basis for measures that are commonly used today in pediatric allergy: lactating mothers are given guidelines about their intake of cow's milk and other highly allergenic foods.

In 1934, Stuart and Hill developed the first nutritionally balanced soybean infant formula. During the course of Stuart's studies in allergic children, he noted an absence of standards of growth and development with which to compare allergic and normal children. This motivated him to develop the first standardized pediatric growth charts in the United States which continue in common use today.

It was not long before problems of soybean allergy were encountered in infants fed on soybean formulas. With the need to find another milk substitute, Glaser in 1944 introduced an infant formula utilizing strained meat as a source of protein.

IMMUNOBIOLOGY AND IMMUNOLOGIC DISORDERS

Contributions to the knowledge of immune function and its relevance to pediatric immunology and allergy had their sources in studies of infection, host defense, hypersensitivity, and clinical allergy (Table 3 [6, 9, 11]).

From 1897 to 1908, Ehrlich's studies led to many contributions to immunology. Among these were the standardization of immunochemical techniques, their theoretical foundations, and the description of tolerance. He suggested that a breakdown in tolerance occurred as a rare event (*horror autotoxicus*). This phenomenon came to be known as autoimmunity.

In 1900, Landsteiner discovered the ABO blood groups. In addition to placing blood transfusions on a rational and feasible basis, this system also provided an immunologic method for paternity identification. Another contribution to clinical pediatrics was the identification of the Rh blood group system by Levine and Stetson in the early 1940s. This discovery led to the understanding of the role of isoimmunization in the pathogenesis of erythroblastosis fetalis.

Another of Landsteiner's contributions was the concept of *haptens*, or low molecular weight antigens, that become immunogenic when coupled to carrier proteins. His studies formed the basis for the understanding of hypersensitivity reactions, transplantation reactions, and immune reactions to low molecular weight chemicals and drugs. The work represented the first step in the development of immunogenetics and was an important precursor of the description of the histocompatibility system.

That microorganisms could cause antigen-antibody reactions was suggested by studies in Welch's pathology laboratories, where Longcope demonstrated the role of streptococci in glomerulonephritis. Later epidemiologic and microbiologic investigations would also implicate streptococcal infection with rheumatic fever.

In 1928, Witebsky and Steinfeld showed that injections of brain suspensions could elicit antibody responses. This work was among the first to show that autoimmune reactions were possible. It had relevance to allergic encephalitis as well as to other autoimmune diseases. Extended studies on autoimmune systems, however,

TABLE 3. *Milestones in pediatrics immunology and allergy, 1850–1950: immunobiology and immunologic disorders*

Individual	Date	Contribution
Ehrlich	1897–1908	Introduced standardization of immunochemical techniques and their theoretical foundations; described the body's vigilance in maintaining tolerance to its own molecular constituents (*horror autotoxicus*)
Metchnikoff	1884–1908	Introduced concepts that laid foundation for cellular basis of immunology
Landsteiner	1900	Described ABO blood groups; described concept of *haptens* and carrier proteins
Witebsky and Steinfeld	1928	Demonstrated that brain suspension could elicit antibody when injected into a foreign species
Heidelberger	1930	Described quantitative relationship of antigen and antibody
Tiselius and Kabat	1939	Developed technique of electrophoresis and demonstrated that antibodies are γ globulins
Freund	1942	Developed immunizing adjuvant that provided new approaches for study of autoimmunity
Medawar and Burnet	1944	Established that rejection of grafts is an immunologic phenomenon; described tolerance in "self" *vs* "non-self" phenomena
Levine and Stetson	1941–1947	Discovered Rh blood system; described role of isoimmunization in pathogenesis of erythroblastosis fetalis
Bruton	1946–1952	Described agammaglobulinemia, a clinical discovery that ushered in modern clinical and molecular immunology
Good	1950	Translated experiments of nature and basic immunologic phenomenon
Witebsky	1950 +	Developed "postulates" for autoimmune diseases; described classic model of autoimmune thyroiditis in rabbit

could not be undertaken without the modification of host proteins made possible by the subsequent introduction of Freund's adjuvant in 1942. In the 1950s, Witebsky developed ''postulates'' for autoimmune diseases and described autoimmune thyroiditis in rabbits. These studies provided the basis for future investigations that would help to explain immunopathologic mechanisms for a spectrum of autoimmune diseases in childhood: juvenile diabetes, rheumatoid arthritis, systemic lupus erythematosus, and thyroiditis.

Heidelberger, in 1930, examining the chemical structure of pneumococcal polysaccharide and the relationship with antibody, discovered quantitative precipitin reactions. His studies have formed the basis for modern immunochemical microtechniques.

In 1939, Tiselius and Kabat developed the technique of electrophoresis. They were the first to observe that antibodies in serum were γ globulins, and they paved the way for identification of IgA formed at the surface of secretory membranes. IgA has been shown to be the protective factor transmitted from mother to nursing infant in colostrum and human milk and the defense against respiratory and gastrointestinal tract infections.

Medawar and Burnet, in 1944, established that rejection of organ and tissue grafts is an immunologic phenomenon. Burnet described the concept of tolerance and the clonal selection theory. Their studies and observations during this era provided the incentive for extended studies by future investigators that translated transplantation biology from laboratory experimentation to applications in clinical medicine and surgery. What began as a search for ways to promote skin graft survival in war injuries led to the knowledge that made possible the use of fetal thymus grafts and bone marrow transplants in the treatment of certain immunodeficiency syndromes and leukemia, and donor organ replacement in destructive kidney, liver, and heart diseases of childhood.

At the end of the era, 1850–1950, Bruton's description of agammaglobulinemia in an 8-year-old boy ushered in modern cellular and molecular immunology. The work of Good was responsible for the translation of such experiments of nature into applications of clinical relevance.

DEVELOPMENT OF THE SPECIALTY OF PEDIATRIC ALLERGY AND IMMUNOLOGY

The development of specialists in pediatric allergy and immunology in the United States occurred in the latter 30 years of the 1850–1950 period. In addition to Schloss, Talbot, and Stuart, there were several other outstanding figures in the history of academic pediatrics who contributed to pediatric allergy and immunology in the United States, e.g., Park, Blackfan, and Rubin.

Growth of the allergy field was, however, heavily influenced by specialists in internal medicine who believed the specialty to be under their purview. Schloss and Guy were the only two pediatric representatives of the 13 founding members of the first professional organization in 1924, the (Eastern) Society for the Study of Asthma and Allied Conditions under the leadership of Cooke. Later, Donnally, a former student of Cooke, was the only other pediatrician taken into the selective group. He became in 1928 the first and only pediatrician to serve as president of the Eastern Society.

In 1942, a clinically oriented professional society was founded under the name, the American College of Allergists. Prominent in the initial organization, development, and leadership of this group were two highly regarded and respected pediatric allergists, Ratner and Glaser, who, through academic affiliations, publications, and investigative endeavors, had already contributed much to the new field. A subspecialty Board in allergy and immunology, the Conjoint American Board of Allergy and Immunology (ABAI), was established in 1972 under the American Board of Internal Medicine (ABIM) and the American Board of Pediatrics (ABP). From 1972 through 1988, the Board certified 3,183 candidates, of whom 44% were pediatricians. It is thus clear that pediatric allergy and immunology have come of age.

REFERENCES

1. Bellanti JA, ed. *Immunology*, vol. 3. Philadelphia: WB Saunders Co, 1985;1–7.
2. Cohen SG. The American Academy of Allergy. An historical review, *J Allergy Clin Immunol* 1979;64:332–474.
3. Kolmer JA, Tuft L. *Clinical immunology, biotherapy and chemotherapy*. Philadelphia: WB Saunders, 1943.
4. Dubos RJ, ed. *Bacterial and mycotic infections of man*. Philadelphia: Lippincott, 1948.
5. Clark PF. *Pioneer microbiologists of America*. Madison: University of Wisconsin Press, 1961; 91–102.
6. Bibel JB. *Milestones in immunology. A historical exploration*. Madison: Science Tech, 1988.
7. Ratner B. *Allergy, anaphylaxis and immunotherapy. Basic principles and practice*. Baltimore: Williams and Wilkins, 1943.
8. Glaser J. *Allergy in childhood*. Springfield: Charles C Thomas, 1956.
9. Samter M, ed. *Excerpts from classics in allergy*. Columbus: Ross Laboratories, 1969.
10. Cohen SG. *Firsts in allergy, Boston remembered. N Engl Reg Allergy Proc* 1983;1:309–34; 1984;2:48–64.
11. Longcope WT. The susceptibility of man to foreign protein. *Am J Med Sci* 1916;152:625–50.

DISCUSSION

Dr. Katz: The reason for the development of soybean milk in China was not the prevalence of lactase deficiency, although that is a common problem. The reason was the lack of cattle husbandry in China. There is insufficient cow's milk so the production of soy milk is necessitated by a lack of weaning foods.

Dr. Bellanti: However, lactase deficiency is significant in the Far East, as Dr. Rossi pointed out in his presentation, and it is prevalent in a major part of China. The Chinese simply don't drink milk. The use of soybean products actually originates from the Far East and the idea was imported into the United States. The studies of Ruth Guy, who introduced a palatable soybean formula, are important in this regard.

Dr. Kaufman: I want to point out the importance of clinical research in the allergy field. It was economics, not basic science, that took Richet to Monte Carlo. The prince was losing money because vacationers wouldn't come to swim on his beach, being deterred by sea anemone stings. Richet was brought down on the royal yacht and they conducted experiments on board in search of a treatment for the anemone sting. It was this that led to the coining of the term ''anaphylaxis'' and to later work on allergy in the pediatric sphere, culminating in the publication of the book, *Alimentary Anaphylaxis*, a textbook on food allergy.

In the 1960s, I visited the Wright-Flemming Institute at St Mary's hospital in London to try to find out about the early immunotherapy injections of Noon and Freeman. The present Director had been there when they gave their very first injections of antigen. Although this is not generally known, a large number of patients died from anaphylaxis before a safe and effective method of antigen injection was developed. It was not an easy beginning.

History of Pediatrics 1850–1950, edited by
B.L. Nichols, A. Ballabriga, and N. Kretchmer.
Nestlé Nutrition Workshop Series, Vol. 22. Nestec
Ltd., Vevey/Raven Press, Ltd., New York © 1991.

Developmental Biology

Norman Kretchmer

*Department of Nutritional Sciences, University of California,
Berkeley, California 94720, USA*

As a biologic phenomenon, human development has been recognized since ancient times by literate man. In his *Generation of Animals*, Aristotle states, "He who sees things grow from their beginning will have the finest view of them" (1). Many other philosophers were also concerned with development and growth, but the exposition of the phenomenon had to await the stepwise, interdependent advance of many sciences. The years 1850–1950 are particularly pertinent since they encompass a time from the first explosion of scientific thought to the advent of the remarkable change in biological perspective that is molecular biology. Those hundred years encompassed social and intellectual upheavals that affected the entire development of medical science and education.

To some, developmental biology is a composite of methodologies used to solve problems, specifically in embryology (2). To others, the term is all-encompassing and includes studies that are behavioral, anatomic, physiologic, or molecular (3). In this essay on the history of developmental biology in pediatrics (1850–1950), I shall limit myself to consideration of the external scientific influences on non-behavioral pediatrics, as well as the intellectual progression within pediatrics that has resulted in the outburst of research activity after 1950. Studies in developmental biology must incorporate this philosophy of gradual unfolding ontogeny. To simplify matters, I shall discuss only those steps that yielded information contributing to the advance of biochemical and cellular development.

Prior to 1875, the physician who attended children was concerned only with disease and a variety of personalized forms of treatment. Scientific activity in pediatrics was minimal. In the text published in 1776 by von Rosenstein, consideration of diseases and their problems had no scientific basis. This approach to diseases of children and to medicine in general persisted until the middle of the nineteenth century.

Embryology and cellular biology were the first important influences on a scientific approach to pediatrics. The volume by K.E. von Baehr, *Ueber Entwicklungsgeschichte der Thiere, Königsberg, 1828–34*, was one of the most important contributions to embryological thought and is still cited in any text concerned with development. Karl Ernst von Baehr (1792–1876) was educated in Riga, Latvia, a city of great beauty. It was a time when many still believed that the formation of the embryo was initiated from a homunculus (Fig. 1). Development was thought to

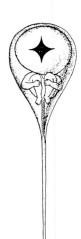

FIG. 1. Homunculus. (Reprinted by permission. Curtis H. *Biology*, 5th ed., New York: Worth Publishers, 1989, p. 237.)

evolve only by an increase in size of the primitive organism. Gavin de Beer (4) pointed out that the foundations of knowledge of the ontogenetic stages during development were initially promulgated by von Baehr in 1828. Von Baehr believed that during development from the ovum (which he described), general characteristics appeared first and were followed by specialized characteristics. This statement has subsequent biochemical implications for enzymatic development. He wrote that the early stages of development in animals resembled one another and these stages deviated as embryogenesis continued. Although von Baehr described the primordial germ-layers, he did not identify the cell as the primary morphologic unit. That revelation had to await the microscopic description of the plant cell by Matthias Joseph Schleiden (1804–1881) and the animal cell by Theodor Schwann (1810–1882).

Schwann thought "There is one universal principle of development for the elementary parts of organisms, however different, and that principle is the formation of the cells." Robert Remak (1815–1865) modified the postulates of von Baehr on germ-layers and disagreed with Schleiden and Schwann. He demonstrated that the growth of tissues resulted from cellular division. Schleiden and Schwann had had a more vitalistic philosophy than did Remak. These four scholars provided the basis for all future developmental thought. In the book published by Needham in 1964 (5), there is a definition of development and growth. Needham states that development involves growth, a quantitative aspect, coupled with differentiation, the appearance of qualitative characteristics.

The epoch from 1850–1900 was replete with scientific advances. The outstanding contributions of Rudolf Virchow (1821–1902) (Fig. 2), Charles Darwin (1809–1882), Ernst Haeckel (1834–1879), Justus von Liebig (1803–1873), and Claude Bernard (1813–1878) appeared during the first decades of these years. They were

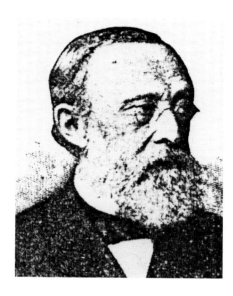

FIG. 2. Rudolph Virchow (1821–1902).

giants of science whose work affected the trend of all medicine. Osler described Virchow on the occasion of his 70th birthday in 1891 saying,

> The influence of his work has been deep and far-reaching, and in one way or another has been felt by each one of us. It is well to acknowledge the debt which we every-day practitioners owe to the great leaders and workers in the scientific branches of our art. . . . The lesson which should sink deepest into our hearts is the answer which a life, such as Virchow's, gives to those who to-day as in past generations see only pills and potions in the profession of medicine, and who utilizing the gains of science fail to appreciate the dignity and the worth of the methods by which they are attained (6).

Virchow wrote *Cellular Pathology* (7), a book that is still exciting to read. This father of pathology was also a brigand who fought Bismarck and his regime with intensity. Although he was a political revolutionary and a socialist, he was a reactionary in science and opposed the hypotheses and works of Koch and Darwin.

The man of this era who exerted the greatest influence on physiology and experimental medicine was Claude Bernard in Paris. A romantic, he wrote frivolous plays as a youth but was advised to enter medicine since that was a more practical and lucrative career. His discoveries were revolutionary. They include studies of carbohydrate metabolism, pancreatic juice, and neural physiology. His book, *An Introduction to Experimental Medicine* is still available in modern paper-back.

Liebig was the founder of physiological chemistry, with studies of purines, fats, urea, and fermentation. According to Garrison (8), he was the first to introduce the term *metabolism (stoffwechsel)*, although some claim that it was Schwann who coined the phrase "metabolic-phenomena." Haeckel and Darwin both promulgated hypotheses relating ontogeny to phylogeny and evolutionary processes. These five scientists provided the foundation of scientific medicine.

In 1852, Charles West (1816–1898) (see p. 32, Fig. 1) established the Children's Hospital in Great Ormond Street, London. There was a burst of activity to establish pediatrics as a field separate from general medicine. An interest in developmental maturation and the effect of maturation on health and disease was the unique aspect that underlay the emergence of pediatrics as a separate medical specialty.

During the latter half of the eighteenth century, pediatrics was thriving in Germany, the Austro-Hungarian Empire, and the United Kingdom. France suffered because the medical profession was late in utilizing the work of Virchow in their educational system. The United States was politically torn by the issue of slavery. Then the ravaging Civil War erupted and the political aspects of reconstruction took their toll. Young Americans traveled abroad to become educated in modern medicine and science. When they returned, the only real opportunities were in the practice of medicine. William Camerer (1842–1910), Adolf B. Baginsky (1843–1919), and Arthur Schlossman (1867–1932) in Germany, and Theodor Escherich (1857–1911) in Austria, were some of the European pediatricians who supervised scientific services that were popular with Americans. In general, their reseach was dedicated to metabolic problems. The interest in European training continued until after World War I and had a recrudescence following World War II. But science was moving much faster than pediatrics. Genetics evolved as a major addition to the scientific influences on pediatrics following the work of Gregor Mendel (1822–1884) that was to become the foundation of the laws of heredity. Sir Archibald Garrod (1857–1936) sometime later (1908) utilized these laws to explain his discovery of inborn errors of metabolism. Garrod practiced pediatrics and general medicine at St. Bartholomews Hospital until he succeeded Osler as Regis Professor of Medicine at Oxford.

Camerer, Baginsky, Escherich, and Schlossman accomplished research concerning the nutrition and metabolism of the infant and child. Camerer extended his work to include longitudinal studies of growth and development, work subsequently carried on by his son. Development as a province for the pediatrician was an important part of the first presidential speech to the American Pediatric Society by Abraham Jacobi (1830–1919).

[Pediatrics] does not deal with a special organ, but with the entire organism at the very period which presents the most interesting features to the student of biology and medicine. Infancy and childhood are the links between conception and death, between foetus and the adult. The latter has attained a certain degree of invariability. His physiological labor is reproduction; that of the young is both reproduction and growth. . . . the most interesting time, and the one most difficult to understand, is that in which persistent development, increase, solidification, and improvement are taking place (9). . . .

The history of the embryo and foetus finds its legitimate termination in that of the infant and child. Thus embryology, teratology, and pedology, with pediatrics, are but chapters of the same book. The scientific consideration of any one of them is impossible without that of the others. The theories of heredity and consanguinity refer equally to all. The most important changes and diseases met with in the young human being cannot be studied without the knowledge of its previous history, and the intelligent appreciation of embryology cannot be attained without the exact knowledge of its final outcome. Excessive or defective growth, arrest of development, and foetal inflammation are the heads under which a large number of anomalies of the infant can be subsumed (10).

Development as a pediatric responsibility was identified by Thomas Morgan Rotch of Boston (1849–1914) (see p. 39, Fig. 3) in the third presidential address to the American Pediatric Society.

Wise iconoclasm and patient originality must be the weapons by which we shall fight our way to the front and place the standard of pediatrics where it ought to be, —place it side by side with the already perfected anatomical and physiological investigations which have become the true basis for the enlightened clinical study of human beings.

To intelligently understand the fully developed man in health and disease, it seems self-evident that . . . the various stages of development, from embryo to infant and infant to child and child to adult, should successively be dealt with. This in the past, however, has been but little done. On the contrary, the very opposite method has been adopted (11).

Rotch applied his ideas and was one of the first to develop the principles of bone-age using x-rays.

These ideas were forcibly stated again by W. S. Christopher of Cincinnati (1895–1905) when he spoke in 1902. The title of his address was, "Development, the Keynote of Pediatrics." (12)

The one feature which characterizes pediatrics and is its framework is development . . . Inasmuch as development is primarily determined by heredity, it is necessary to know first the course of natural development, and next the pathological conditions resulting from deviations from that course, together with the causes of these deviations. Finally, the environmental factors must be classified, and their influence in maintaining normal development and in permitting and causing deviations therefrom, determined. These aspects have been studied conjointly, and while not so much is known as is desirable, yet there exists a body of knowledge sufficient to make an efficient, constructive pediatrics. . . .

Functional development has not been subjected to so searching an inquiry, except in the case of the nervous system, which presents rare opportunities for quantitative investigation, of which advantage has been taken by the physiologists whose results we would do well to make our own. The functions of the kidneys have been fairly well studied, and through the urine, some attempts, although very inadequate ones, have been made to study developmental metabolism. Of remaining organs, a knowledge of whose functional development would be most serviceable, the most important are the liver and the ductless glands. However, in view of the insufficiency and uncertainty of present information regarding the specific functions of these organs, it seems too much to hope that the near future will afford any adequate insight into the natural history of the development of these functions. While we are waiting for the physiologists to supply us with this natural history . . . much can be accomplished by clinical methods of observation.

Rotch in 1903 was at Harvard and was appointed the first professor and head of a department of pediatrics in the United States. It is interesting to note that pediatrics was part of the Department of Medicine at the Massachusetts General Hospital until the late 1960s.

As the new century dawned, there was an atmosphere of excitement in the belief that a potential existed for great advances in medicine. The pediatrician was still fully occupied by clinical and social matters concerning children. The shanty towns and the unclean milk in New York were well documented by Job Lewis Smith (1827–1897) (13) as were the problems associated with summer diarrhea, a disorder that caused massive mortality in children. Basic science had not penetrated into pediatrics, in part due to the preoccupation of the clinician with overpowering clinical problems. Biochemistry was established in the United States by Lafayette B. Mendel (1872– 1935) at Yale. He published a series of papers on the biochemistry of development (14). He worked with T.B. Osborne (1859–1929) and made major contributions in nutrition that were later utilized by pediatricians. Laboratory methods that could be used by clinicians were made available from the evolving biochemical work.

The Flexner report (15) stimulated major revisions in medical education in the United States, making it possible for faculty to conduct research and have time to think. Harold K. Faber (1884–1979) and Rustin McIntosh (1894–1986) described the next period of pediatrics in the title of a chapter (16): "Period 3, 1914–1926. Pediatric Biochemistry Flowers." The title was based on the outpouring of papers related to physiological chemistry and nutrition. Time was now becoming available to the academic pediatrician to consider these problems.

Following World War I, Germany, Austria, and Europe were in descent. There was a shift of industry, science, and medicine to the United States. The United States was now becoming an industrial giant. Major research centers were established, the foremost being the Rockefeller Institute. Pediatricians sought training in these centers, but many still went to Europe for training. The prime clinics for biochemical and nutritional training in Europe were those of Heinrich Finkelstein (1865–1942) (Fig. 3) and Adalbert Czerny (1863–1941) (see p. 27, Fig. 3), but they were beginning to have severe competition from the American cadre of clinician-scientists.

Dr. Luther Emmett Holt (1855–1924) (see p. 52, Fig. 3) is pre-eminent in American Pediatrics in his contributions to the science of pediatrics. He replaced Abraham

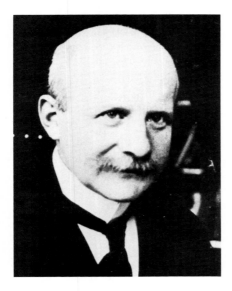

FIG. 3. Heinrich Finkelstein (1865–1942).

Jacobi as Professor at the College of Physicians and Surgeons of Columbia University. His work was primarily on infant metabolism. He published with the great biochemists, P.A. Levene (1869–1940) and D.D. Van Slyke (1883–1971). In a paper published in the *Transactions of the American Pediatric Society* (17) entitled "The Food Requirements of Children II: Protein Requirement" he discussed in great detail the differences between proteins of high quality and poor quality. He presented a number of charts relating protein intake and requirements to age, from birth to maturity. An amazing aspect of this paper is the paucity of references. However, this was a beginning in developmental biochemical studies in pediatrics.

After John Howland (1873–1926) (see p. 268, Fig. 1) worked with Czerny in Germany and with Holt in New York, he was appointed full-time head of pediatrics at Johns Hopkins Hospital in 1912. Howland established pediatric biochemistry in pediatrics. He had a remarkable series of associates—Edwards Park (1877–1969), Benjamin Kramer (1882–1972), Grover Powers (1887–1968) (see p. 61, Fig. 4), Kenneth Blackfan (1883–1944), McKim Marriott (1885–1936), and James Gamble (1883–1959) (see p. 193, Fig. 2). These scientists (see p. 270, Fig. 6) were all interested in biochemistry and development—Park and Kramer in bone, Gamble in electrolytes, Powers (eventually) in child development, Blackfan and Howland in diarrhea. Although their focus for the most part was not developmental biology, their studies provided the physiologic and biochemical background upon which future developmental studies were based. The career of Marriott (Fig. 4) was most interesting. He was trained as a biochemist and casually received his MD from Cornell in 1910. He then went to Washington University in St. Louis where, after a sojourn in biochemistry, he worked with Howland in St. Louis and joined the Department of Pediatrics at Johns Hopkins. Their scientific contributions in explaining

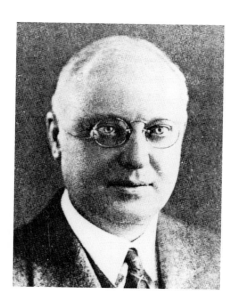

FIG. 4. McKim Marriott (1885–1936). (Reprinted by permission. *Semi-centennial volume of the American Pediatric Society 1938–1988*, p. 370. Menasha, WI: George Banta Publishing Co., © 1938.)

acidosis resulting from diarrhea and low calcium in tetany gained them fame throughout the world. In 1917, Marriott was appointed full-time head of the Department of Pediatrics at Washington University. He became Dean of the Medical School at Washington University in 1923, and in 1936 he became Dean and Professor of Research Medicine at the University of California, San Francisco. The disappointing aspect of the outstanding work of Marriott was that it lacked a developmental philosophy. On the other hand, the biochemical studies that he accomplished were impressive. Another hereditary academic line was that fostered by Oscar Schloss (1882–1952) and exemplified by Samuel Z. Levine (1895–1971) (Fig. 5) and Harry H. Gordon (1906–1988). Schloss utilized Van Slyke's methods to study acidosis and impairment of renal function. Levine carried the work further to metabolic studies of the young infant. Harry Gordon was the true believer in developmental studies with a focus on the infant. He was effective politically in the establishment of the National Institute of Child Health and Human Development. After that Institute was formed, he created the Rose F. Kennedy Center at the Albert Einstein College of Medicine. These laboratories were dedicated to developmental studies with a particular emphasis on mental retardation.

The rise of enzymology and metabolism characterized the mid-period of the twentieth century. Many Nobel prizes were awarded for dissecting and reconstructing metabolic pathways. These studies answered the central questions of how these pathways are regulated and what are their controls. This burst of knowledge stimulated interest in development in the pediatric community. Many studies were undertaken to respond to the original adage of Jacobi, ". . . that a child is not a small adult."

Research on physical growth and development was initiated by Camerer and Camerer, followed by Rotch, and much later by Harold C. Stuart (1891–1977). The

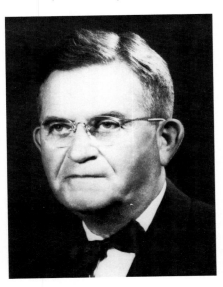

FIG. 5. Samuel Z. Levine (1895–1971).

work in this area has been summarized by Tanner (18). Alfred H. Washburn (1895–1988), who was an active investigator in this field, delivered an address to the American Pediatric Society in 1955, entitled "Human Growth, Development, and Adaptation." Placing great emphasis on longitudinal studies, Washburn was an important worker in the field of auxology. In this period, the physiological development of various organs was investigated by a number of pediatricians. The kidney, an organ that had been subjected to exhaustive scrutiny by Homer Smith (1895–1962) (see p. 117, Fig. 4) and Jean R. Oliver (1889–1976), was studied carefully by pediatricians. Their extensive work on developmental renal physiology showed unequivocally that an infant is vastly different from a small adult. Developmental endocrinology was fostered by Lawson Wilkins (1894–1936) who trained a whole school of pediatric endocrinologists, some of whom dealt primarily with disease and others whose interests were in developmental regulatory phenomena. Work in neonatal physiology was implied in the writings of Ballentyne and then investigated by Barcroft (1872–1947) and carried on by John Lind (1909–1983) who was Professor of Pediatrics at the Karolinska Institute in Stockholm. Many Americans trained in his laboratory and brought the techniques for studying neonatal physiology back to the United States. Studies of the development of the gastrointestinal tract were influenced by I. P. Pavlov (1849–1936), a Nobel Prize winner in 1904, who worked in Leningrad, and by Lafayette B. Mendel in New Haven. The work of Claude Bernard greatly influenced the pursuit by the French of problems related to the development of the liver.

The 1950s heralded the initiation of the new biology. The work of Avery (19) and Pauling (20) initiated the field of molecular biology and genetic control. These seminal works were closely followed by the paper of Watson and Crick (21,22) in 1953. The model of DNA as a double helix demanded an immense amount of previous work. DNA was synthesized in 1960 (23) and the most important work relating to developmental biology was published in 1961 by Jacob and Monod (24), less than two decades after the initial report by Avery.

In this essay, I have tried to give an insight into the flow of events concerning all of developmental biology in pediatrics. It required time away from the clinic for the overworked clinician to participate in these efforts. Biology and medicine do not proceed without many seemingly extraneous influences. I have tried to outline these influences on the pediatrician. I have attempted to relate a story, albeit incomplete—a story with my scientific prejudice for biochemistry and with my national prejudice for the United States. I believe that if I had come from another country, I might have woven the story with a different set of threads and actors. The story here clearly gives an insight into those investigators who influenced me and into those people close to me, philosophically. I have assiduously adhered to restricting my review to the years, 1850–1950, and in addition, I have avoided the mention of any living pediatrician.

I have not discussed behaviorial and social development, a critical and major field in pediatrics. This movement of child development is well documented by Milton Senn (25).

Pediatrics is now well established as a specialty. Academic departments have grown immensely, thus giving more time to the faculty for investigation. In fact, some departments of pediatrics house units of basic and developmental science much more extensive than an entire department of basic science in the recent past. The methods of molecular biology, molecular immunology, and molecular genetics have penetrated scientific pediatrics. All of these methodologies are utilized for unraveling the mysteries of development.

I am still sufficiently old fashioned to believe that, regardless of these dramatic advances in scientific thought and method, the pertinent research questions in pediatrics will emanate from direct confrontation with the developing organism.

ACKNOWLEDGMENT

This work was supported in part by NIH grant No. 5P30 HD2224.

REFERENCES

1. Aristotle. *Generation of animals*. Cambridge, Mass: Harvard University Press, 1943.
2. Brown DB. How embryologists became developmental biologists and other matters. *Persp Biol Med* 1986;29:S149–53.
3. Kretchmer N. On the homology between human development and pediatrics. *Pediatr Res* 1968;2:283–6.
4. de Beer G. *Embryos and ancestors*. London: Oxford University Press, 1958;1–13.
5. Needham AE. *The growth process in animals*. London: Pitman Press, 1964.
6. Cushing H. *The life of Sir William Osler*, vol 1. Oxford: Oxford University Press, 1926;355.
7. Virchow R. *Cellular pathology*, translated from 2nd ed. Philadelphia: JB Lippincott, 1863.
8. Garrison FH. *An introduction to the history of medicine*, 4th ed. Philadelphia: WB Saunders Company, 1929.
9. Jacobi A. The relations of pediatrics to general medicine. *Trans Am Pediatr Soc* 1890;1:6–7.
10. Idem. 13–4.
11. Rotch TM. Iconoclasm and original thought in the study of pediatrics. *Trans Am Pediatr Soc* 1892;3:6–11.
12. Christopher WS. Development, the keynote of pediatrics. *Trans Am Pediatr Soc* 1902;14:10.
13. Cone TE. *History of American pediatrics*. Boston: Little, Brown and Company, 1979.
14. Mendel LB, Mitchell PH. Chemical studies on growth. I. The inverting enzymes of the alimentary tract, especially in the embryo. *Am J Physiol* 1907;20:81.
15. Flexner A. Medical education in the United States and Canada. New York, 1910. *Medical education in Europe*, New York: Carnegie Foundation for the Advancement of Teaching, 1912.
16. Faber HK, McIntosh R. *History of the American Pediatric Society, 1887–1965*. New York: McGraw-Hill Book Company, 1966.
17. Holt LE, Fales HL. The food requirements of children. II. Protein requirement. *Trans Am Pediatr Soc* 1921;33:142–51.
18. Tanner JM. *A history of the study of human growth*. Cambridge: Cambridge University Press, 1981;269–81.
19. Avery OT, MacLeod CM, McCarty M. Studies on the chemical nature of the substance inducing transformation of pneumococcal types. Induction of transformation by a deoxyribonucleic acid fraction isolated from pneumococcus type III. *J Exp Med* 1944;79:137–58.
20. Pauling L, Itano HA, Singer SJ, Wells IC. Sickle cell anemia: a molecular disease. *Science* 1949;110:543–8.
21. Watson JD, Crick FHC. Molecular structure of nucleic acid. A structure for deoxyribose nucleic acid. *Nature* 1953;171:737–8.

22. Watson JD, Crick FHC. Genetic implications of the structure of deoxyribonucleic acid. *Nature* 1953;171:964–7.
23. Kornberg A. Biologic synthesis of deoxyribonucleic acid. *Science* 1960;131:1503–8.
24. Jacob F, Monod J. Genetic regulatory mechanisms in the synthesis of proteins. *J Mol Biol* 1961;3:318–56.
25. Senn MJE. Insights on the child development movement in the United States. *Monographs Soc Res Child Devel* 1975;40:1–107.

Additional Bibliographic Sources

American Pediatric Society. *Semi-centennial volume of the American Pediatric Society 1888–1938.* Menasha, WI: George Banta Publishing Company, 1938.

Barcroft J. *Researches on pre-natal life.* Oxford: Blackwell Scientific Publications, 1946.

Castiglioni A. *A history of medicine.* New York: Alfred A Knopf, 1941.

Halpern SA. *American pediatrics: the social dynamics of professionalism, 1880–1980.* Berkeley: University of California Press, 1988.

Levinson A. *Pioneers of pediatrics.* New York: Froben Press, 1943.

Meyer AW. *Human generation: conclusions of Burdach, Dollinger and von Baehr.* Stanford: Stanford University Press, 1956.

Pearson HA, Brown AK. *The centennial history of the American Pediatric Society 1888–1988.* New Haven: Yale University Printing Service, 1988.

Ruhrah J. *Pediatric biographies.* Chicago: American Medical Association, 1932.

Stryer L. *Biochemistry.* 2nd ed. San Francisco: WH Freeman and Company, 1981.

Stuart HC. Standards of reference for physical development: suggestions for presentation and use in clinical appraisement. *Trans Am Pediatr Soc* 1934;46:36.

Veeder BS, ed. *Pediatric profiles.* St. Louis: The CV Mosby Company,1957.

Waddington CH. *Principles of development and differentiation*, New York: Macmillan, 1967.

DISCUSSION

Dr. Ballabriga: I was with John Lind in 1947 at the Children's Hospital, Stockholm, then directed by Wallgren. Lind was dedicated to pediatric cardiology, particularly neonatal cardiology, and his studies were oriented towards the fetal circulation.

The pediatric clinic at Stockholm was an important European center in the field of research, which was mainly devoted to the application of biochemistry in pediatrics. At the end of the Second World War, European pediatrics flourished in Sweden and Switzerland, the countries that had remained neutral. Progress was made at that time in social aspects of pediatrics and in clinical pediatric biochemistry. This was the start of a new stage in the evolution of medicine, the stage of enzymatic-biochemical study of the cell.

History of Pediatrics 1850–1950, edited by
B.L. Nichols, A. Ballabriga, and N. Kretchmer.
Nestlé Nutrition Workshop Series, Vol. 22. Nestec
Ltd., Vevey/Raven Press, Ltd., New York © 1991.

Auxology

James M. Tanner

*School of Public Health, University of Texas at Houston, and Institute of Child Health,
University of London, London WCIN IEH, United Kingdom*

Three strands can be discerned in the history of auxology, the study of growth and development (1). We may call them the social, the medical (or perhaps clinical), and the intellectual (or scientific). In the strict context of clinical pediatrics, we have less to do with the third strand, auxology as a branch of human biology, than with the other two.

That undernutrition caused stunted growth must have been apparent since time immemorial, but the earliest clear description known to me is in the seventeenth century—*Touchstone of Complexions* (1633), an English translation of a book written in the previous century by the Dutch physician, Levinus Lemnius (1505–1568).

"Comely tallnesse and length of personage," said Lemnius, "cometh and is caused of the abundance of heat and moisture, where the spirit is thoroughly and fully perfused" (p. 42). "Schoolmasters and others that take the chance upon them to teach and boord young boyes . . . pinch their poore Pupils and Boorders by the belly, and allow them meate neither sufficient nor yet wholesome . . . whereby it cometh to passe, that in growth they seldome come to any personable stature, to the use of their full powers, to perfect strength and firmity of their members, or to any handsome feature or composition of bodily proportion: and the cause is for that in their tender and growing age, being kept under by famine and skanted of common meate and drinke, their natural moisture which requireth continuall cherishing and maintenance, was skanted and bebarred of his due nourishment and competent allowance" (p. 43).

At much the same date Hippolyt Guarinoni (1571–1654), physician in the town of Hall, near Innsbruck, and the forerunner of public health medicine in Germany, suggested another cause of growth failure: emotional stress in school. "Many children do not grow properly despite good food," he wrote, "because coming home from school they feel still the pain of rough blows (i.e., received there) and anticipate their renewal with anxiety and fear, so that they are never happy nor lighthearted" (*Die Greuwel*, 1610:p. 246).

Johann Augustin Stöller, the German who in 1729 wrote what is the first textbook on human growth (which, incidentally predated the first textbook on pediatrics by some 40 years), shared a general opinion derived from humoral pathology. "Amongst the things which hinder growth I think that an artificially soft treatment and regimen is the greatest. The more luxurious is the living and upbringing in youth, the more is the sickness and the smaller the growth" (*Wachstum*, 1729; p. 59).

Stöller gave the first clear description of catch-up growth.

"Lastly," he writes, "I note that people grow really visibly, and chiefly in length, when they have fully overcome a severe illness, provided they behaved appropriately during it, and the course of the illness was not disturbed by false treatment. Frequently illnesses stop people growing. . . . But if a feverish or not very long-standing malady is properly overcome then people grow very much; so as a rule those persons shoot up in height, who particularly in their childhood have been held in check by hot or cold fevers. This is the basis of the well-known proverb: 'Illness laid him low and stretched him out.' "

A hundred years later, at the beginning of the nineteenth century, little had changed. Growth was a product of nutrition, and nutrition of a particular sort. Virey (1775–1846), writing the article on growth in the French *Dictionary of Medical Sciences* (1816), remained firmly in the humoral era:

"Nourish a man or an animal parsimoniously, with dry and hard foods, smoked, salted, spiced or sharp and stringent; permit him to drink only a little and then a sharp and sour wine such as tartarous vin rouge, give him primarily acid and bitter things which harden and contract the fibres; it is very obvious that such a person will become thin, short, compact in all his organs. In contrast, stuff a child with soggy foods, get him used to taking milk and gruel and dough, to slimy drinks like beer, mead, whey and oily-chocolate, to warm and dilute liquids; cram him with all the foods apt to distend and enlarge him, in the way one fattens geese and pigs; then he is able to become colossal and gigantic in stature compared with a person nourished in the opposite way" (p. 553).

VILLERMÉ, CHADWICK AND AUXOLOGICAL EPIDEMIOLOGY

As Virey was writing his piece for the *Dictionary*, what I have called *auxological epidemiology* was being born. This is defined as "the use of growth data to search out and later to define suboptimal conditions of health" (1). Its two *accoucheurs* were Louis-Réné Villermé (1782–1863) in France and Edwin Chadwick (1800–1890) in England. Returning from the horrors of the Napoleonic war in the Spanish Peninsula, Villermé dedicated his life to ameliorating the conditions of the poor— *les miserables*. In 1829, he published in the *Annales D'Hygiene Publique*, a journal he himself had founded, a classic paper on the relation of the height of French conscripts to the conditions of their lives as children. In Paris, he showed that conscripts coming from *arrondisements* (districts or wards) where few persons owned their own houses were considerably less tall than those from *arrondisements* where more persons were house-owners. Surveying the whole of France, Villermé concluded that poverty was much more important than climate (a current opinion) in influencing growth. He summed up his findings in words that have never been bettered: "Human height," he said, "becomes greater and growth takes place more rapidly, other things being equal, in proportion as the country is richer, comfort more general, houses, clothes and nourishment better and labor, fatigue and privation during infancy and youth less; in other words, the circumstances which accompany poverty delay the age at which complete stature is reached and stunt adult height'' (1829, p. 385).

This view was at once challenged: Boudin (1806–1867), a distinguished Army surgeon and colleague of Villermé on the editorial board of the *Annals*, said the view that, between populations, differences in heights were due to differences in nutrition was quite mistaken: altitude, climate, and race were the important factors. And Paul Broca (1824–1880), the leading physical anthropologist in France, was admirably explicit on the point. ''I have recognized, '' he wrote, ''that the height of Frenchmen, considered generally, depends not on altitude, nor latitude, nor poverty or riches, neither on the nature of the soil nor on nutrition, nor on any of the other environmental conditions that can be invoked. After these have all been successively eliminated, I have been brought to consider only one general influence, that of ethnic heredity'' (Dally, 1879; p. 348). Broca and the anthropologists recognized that poverty and poor nutrition slowed down growth and postponed the age at which mature height was reached; but they denied that in France, at any rate, mature height itself, like the cranial index, was other than hereditarily determined.

Villermé himself never measured any children, although his younger and more brilliant friend, the Belgian, Adolph Quetelet (1797–1874), did so, in 1830–32. But Quetelet was primarily interested in the intellectual, not the public health problem. He wished to establish the form of the curve of human growth rather than to identify the disadvantaged or reform the conditions of life. (He was after all a mathematician and astronomer.) But Quetelet played a large part in establishing the Statistical Society of London (later the Royal Statistical Society) and in that connection undoubtedly met Edwin Chadwick, the civil servant, who was the founder of public health in Britain. In 1833, Chadwick initiated the first study of growth designed to use growth failure as a measure of conditions of life. At this time children aged 8 and upward worked 10 to 14 hours a day in factories under conditions we should be astonished to find nowadays even in the industrial slums of the Third World. For his *Report on the Conditions of Children in Factories* (1833) Chadwick had commissioners measure a sample of factory children in the Manchester area. The children's heights were below the modern third centile (and thus below those of most contemporary children in the slums of the Third World). In addition, as Villermé had said, their tempo of growth was slow; they reached their point of maximum velocity in the pubertal spurt a year or more later than children nowadays.

In the 1833 study, there was a control group of ''non-factory'' children, but these were clearly also of the manual laboring classes. In the 1870s Galton initiated the measurement of middle-class children attending the famous English boarding schools, (the so called Public Schools) as well as working-class children. The results are shown in Fig. 1. There is a wide discrepancy between the manual and nonmanual children, both in tempo (see the bottom section of the graph) and in final height.

From the 1870s to the present time, there has been an uninterrupted history of child growth surveys. Henry Bowditch (1840–1911), first Professor of Physiology and Dean of Harvard Medical School, made the first extensive American survey in

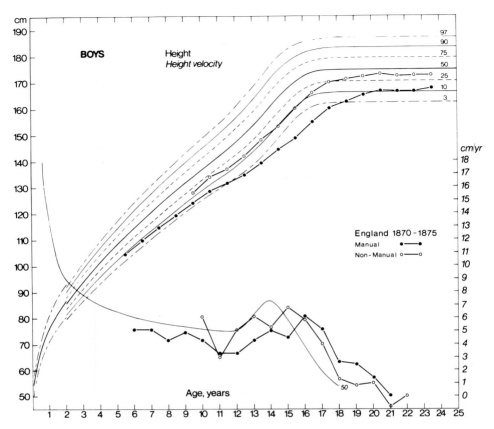

FIG. 1. Heights of boys of manual workers and of the non-manual, mainly professional, class in England in about 1870 (1).

1875, and Luigi Pagliani (1847–1932), Professor of Hygiene the University of Turin, the first large-scale survey on the European continent. Soon school committees everywhere demanded surveys to see if the conditions of their schools were such as to encourage healthy growth. A journal, the *Zeitschrift für Schulgesundheitspflege*, was founded in 1888. Agonizing discussions took place as to whether the "overpressure" of work in schools—particularly secondary schools with their factory-like hours and conditions—affected the growth and health of the pupils (especially, in America, the girl pupils, whose pubertal development was said to be irreparably compromised by all this brain work). A second important American contribution came from St. Louis, where William Porter (1862–1949), like Bowditch one of the founding fathers of American physiology, showed that pupils who achieved above-average grades were taller than pupils of identical age who received below average grades. He thus started a series of investigations on social mobility, social class, height, and achievement that continues to the present day.

POPULATION SURVEYS, SECULAR TRENDS
AND SOCIAL CLASS DIFFERENCES

Repeated surveys showed that, in industrialized countries, there was a trend toward greater height and a faster tempo of growth. An example is given in Fig. 2, from Sweden (2), where a series of comprehensive surveys of school children have taken place, beginning with that of Axel Key in 1882. More detail is revealed in the data of the Oslo school system (3), where in 1920 Schiötz established annual measurements of all pupils (Fig. 3). The drop during the Nazi occupation can be seen, the continued increase thereafter, and the more recent leveling out of the trend. The trend in height is a good guide to the existence of pockets of relative growth failure in a population. As conditions improve, the trend slows down. The greatest recorded trend has been recently in Japan, but it has now ceased. Conversely, when conditions deteriorate, the trend, as we see in the figure, may reverse.

Comprehensive surveys of a country's whole population of children, or even of defined parts of it, are of rather recent origin. They have been made to define regional differences, differences between socioeconomic classes, and differences between races in multiracial societies. A major problem has been to obtain representative samples of children below and above school-going ages. In Great Britain, the National Survey of Health Development (1946) pin-pointed all children born in the first week of March, 1946, and followed up a sample at ages 2, 7, 11, and 15 years. A second national sample was recruited during a week of March, 1958, (the National Child Development Study) and this time as many of the entire sample of 17,000 as could be located were followed at 7, 11, 15, and 21 years. Such geographically widespread surveys have problems with accuracy of measurement, but yield exceptional information on the factors enumerated above.

Other countries have conducted periodical cross-sectional surveys: Holland in 1955, 1965, and 1980; Czechoslovakia in 1951, 1961, 1971, and 1981; the United States National Center for Health Statistics intermittently from the 1960s (HES II, 1963–65) to the present. The most comprehensive such national survey was made in Cuba in 1972–73, conducted jointly by the Cubans and a team from the Institute of Child Health of London University, supported by the World Health Organization (WHO) (4). Here, some 50,000 subjects aged 0–20 years were measured, a sampling fraction of 1.3% of the population.

Finally, instead of periodic surveys, there is continuous *surveillance*, which, at least in theory, should yield quicker results on which public health and political action can be based. Such a system was set up in Britain in 1972 following the outcry aroused by a government decision to discontinue the issue of free milk in schools that had hitherto been a feature of the British welfare system. The surveillance was divided into two parts, that for pre-school children (Pre-school Child Growth Survey), which was based on a relatively small sample of areas of the country, with household-based sampling within these areas, and a school survey of pupils 5–11 years old (National Study of Health and Growth), based on a wide sample of schools. As the years went by, changes in sampling were introduced so that groups most disadvantaged and deemed to be at risk of growth failure were up-weighted.

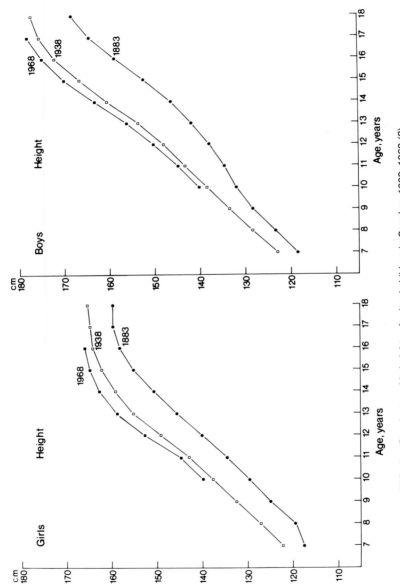

FIG. 2. Secular trend in heights of school children in Sweden, 1882–1968 (2).

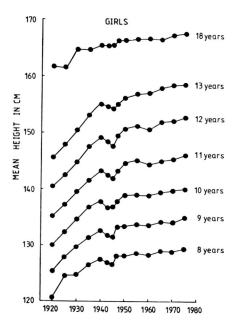

FIG. 3. Secular trend in growth of girls in Oslo schools, 1920–1975 (3).

An important event in the investigation of the epidemiology of growth failure occurred in connection with the International Biological Program of 1967–1972, organized by the International Council of Scientific Unions (ICSU). This wide-reaching program included a section called "Human Adaptability," and within this Phyllis Eveleth and I collected comprehensive and often unpublished statistics on growth and maturation around the world. The result was published in 1976 as *World-Wide Variation in Human Growth* (5). A new edition, incorporating the enormous amount of new data accumulated since that time, was published in 1990.

In all this survey activity, then, growth is regarded as a proxy for health, and growth failure of one group relative to another as an indication of a failure of health delivery systems, public health activity, or political will, all of which should be aimed at eliminating those subpopulation differences that are not due to genetic distinction. In Sweden and Norway, indeed, these actions have in the last 20 years succeeded in eliminating differences in height between social classes; elsewhere, as in the United Kingdom and the United States such differences remain.

CLINICAL STUDIES AND GROWTH STANDARDS

The medical, or clinical, motivation to the study of growth is the reverse side of the same coin. Just as cross-sectional studies of populations aim to monitor growth failure in populations, so longitudinal studies of individuals aim to monitor provision, or lack of it, *within* the population, in the individual family. Here the German pediatricians of the 1870s and the German school doctors led the way.

Measurements of birth length, weight, and head circumference started, of course, much earlier, but they were made in pursuit of reduced perinatal mortality rather than to diagnose growth failure (1). In the 1850s, Guillot (1852) advocated regular weighing of infants as a guide to the amount of human milk being provided, but it was Cnopf (1872) in Nuremberg, Fleischmann (1877) in Vienna, and Russow (1880–1) in St. Petersburg who first systematically weighed infants beyond the perinatal period. Russow, in particular, thought artificial feeding injurious and compared the lengths and weights of infants who were breast-fed with those fed by bottle. Between 1873 and 1878, he and one nurse carried out, he says, 5000 weighings. The children he measured suffered from nothing worse than coughs and colds. He wished to establish standards—the first ones—for well, breast-fed infants. He gives mean lengths and weights each month from birth to 1 year and each year from age 1.0 to 8.0 for a total of 900 children. Although his comparison of breast-fed and bottle-fed infants is largely vitiated by lack of control of social class, birthweight, and other factors, he was a pioneer of growth standards and of the idea that growth is a guide to well-being in infancy.

A few years later (1893), Wilhelm Camerer, Sr. (1842–1909), a dominant figure in German pediatrics, published a paper on infant growth that was the foundation for his son's (Wilhelm, Jr.) very influential chapter on growth of children in Pfaundler and Schlossman's textbook of pediatrics published in 1906, and in English translation in 1908.

Camerer, Sr., was one of the few pediatricians to discuss with clarity and understanding the differences between the longitudinal (''individualizing'') and cross-sectional (''generalizing'') methods of studying growth—a distinction upon which modern standards for diagnosing growth failure are founded.

The foundation of infant welfare clinics from 1892 onward, with their supplies of sterilized milk, gave an added impulse to the monitoring of growth. The first growth standard used in England was introduced in 1906; it was a copy of that made in Leon Dufour's *Goutte de Lait*, a pioneer milk center established at Fécamp in northern France. The history of the study of individual growth failure is largely a history of the creation of standards, for it is only in relation to standards of normality that individual growth failure has any meaning (which is in contrast to population failure, assessed in relation to other populations, not a standard).

Standards of a sort were published by a Munich pediatrician, von Lange, in 1903 (Fig. 4). The sources of his tables were Hermann Vierordt's *Daten und Tabellen* of 1893. He draws channels for tall and short children, apparently by projecting backward for each 10 cm of adult height. Vierordt's tables provide no basis for such projections and Lange evidently knew nothing of the percentiles that Francis Galton had invented in 1875. Henry Bowditch was aware of these and used the 5th, 10th, 20th, 80th, and 95th centiles in formulating standards of height for Massachusetts school children in 1891. Sargent, the physical educationist at Harvard, used them in 1889, and Porter in his charts of 1922. In Europe, however, the divide between clinicians and auxologists was wide indeed. Camerer, Jr.'s chapter on children's growth in height and weight, though sound enough, ignores entirely the classical

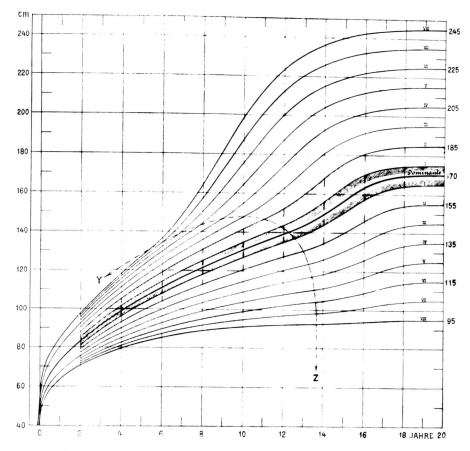

FIG. 4. Lange's chart of height growth ((1) reproduced from Lange, 1903).

work of the anthropologist, Franz Boas, and the successors to Galton. It gives means for growth, but no variances. When Camerer died, the chapter on growth was dropped from Pfaundler's textbook entirely. American textbooks of the same period endeavor to deal with the issue, but it was not until the publication of Harold Stuart and Howard Meredith's chapter in the 1946 edition of Nelson that real standards of growth over the whole age range first became available.

The many longitudinal growth studies that were done in the United States between about 1925 and 1955 were set up in the context of child development seen from the educational and psychological points of view, and their influence on pediatrics was slight. Two, however, were directed by pediatricians: The Harvard School of Public Health Study under Harold Stuart, which recruited children from 1930 to 1939, studied them until maturity, and continues seeing them at intervals to this day; and the Denver Child Research Council study under Alfred Washburn, which recruited in exactly the same years. The studies of the anthropologist W.M.

Krogman in Philadelphia Children's Hospital from the 1940s onward had perhaps a greater influence, partly because of the study's location in a hospital faced with practical problems, and partly because Krogman trained a whole generation of physical anthropologists in the techniques of auxology. His students and grand-students have dominated the field of American auxology for the last 30 years.

In Europe there was also a period of intense longitudinal growth study activity, with children recruited in five capital cities in the early 1950s. These studies which were directed mostly by pediatricians, although they included an equal number of psychologists, were much more oriented toward the clinic than were the American studies. They had a correspondingly greater effect on the creation of growth standards and the general level of knowledge of auxology. Prominent in this transfer of knowledge was Andrea Prader, Professor of Pediatrics in Zurich and also the director of the Zurich longitudinal growth study.

The growth standards produced by Stuart and Meredith made no allowance for whether a child was an early or late developer. Thus they ignored the difference between individual clinical and population standards known to auxologists for nearly 100 years. It was a psychologist, Nancy Bayley, who in 1956 first provided standards that today are what we call tempo-conditional (6). She was before her time, and it took a further 10 years before Whitehouse, Takaishi and I (7) successfully introduced them, with the help of the editor of *Archives for Disease in Childhood* (who had in 1952 already published what seems to have been the first relatively clear statement of the models underlying the construction of clinical standards (8)).

The rest is recent history. There have been many mathematical advances both in the construction of standards and in their use to diagnose growth failure as early as possible (e.g., (9)). There has been debate as to the relative importance of nutrition and infection in causing growth failure. The measurement of growth over periods of weeks or even days has been introduced, and the modern model of this interaction clarified: in infection, food intake falls below requirement; after infection, catch-up restores the situation—but only if a high level of nutrition is available to fuel the burst of growth. Methods are now available for monitoring growth both in individuals and communities, and for correcting incipient failure, but, in so many countries, the political will is lacking. Where it is present, as in the Scandinavian countries, growth failure of the sort we have been discussing has been banished as surely as the disease of smallpox. It can be done. So let us pay homage to the pioneers, who, with all their quaintness, their mistakes, and their myopias, laid the foundations of modern auxology.

REFERENCES

1. Tanner JM. *A history of the study of human growth*. Cambridge, England: University Press, 1981.
2. Ljung B, Bersten-Brucefors A, Lindgren G. The secular trend in physical growth in Sweden. *Ann Hum Biol* 1974;1:245–56.
3. Bruntland GH, Liestøl K, Walløe L. Height, weight and menarcheal age of Oslo school children during the last 60 years. *Ann hum Biol* 1980;7:307–22.
4. Jordan JR, Ruben M, Hernandez J, Bebelagua A, Tanner JM, Goldstein H. *The 1972 Cuban national*

child growth study as an example of population health monitoring: design and methods. Ann Hum Biol 1975;2:153–71.
5. Eveleth PB and Tanner JM. *World-wide variation in human growth.* Cambridge England University Press, 1976. Second ed., 1990.
6. Bayley N. Growth curves of height and weight by age for boys and girls, scaled according to physical maturity. *J Pediatr* 1956;48:187–94.
7. Tanner JM, Whitehouse RH, Takaishi M. Standards from birth to maturity for height, weight, height velocity and weight velocity: British children, 1965. *Arch Dis Child* 1966;41:454–71,613–35.
8. Tanner JM. The assessment of growth and development in children. Arch Dis Child 1952;27:10–33.
9. Healy MRH, Wang M, Tanner JM, Zumrawi FY. The use of short-term increments in length to monitor growth in infancy. In: Waterlow JC. ed. *Linear Growth Retardation in Less Developed Countries* New York: Raven Press 1988;41–55.

DISCUSSION

Dr. Kretchmer: Al Washburn, who died last year, was president of the American Pediatric Society in 1955. He was the preeminent US pediatrician in the study of longitudinal growth curves and his presidential address was on this very subject.

Dr. Tanner: It is sad that the Denver group, which was an extremely good group and produced excellent data, was never able to put their data to use. I do not think that Washburn knew what to do with the growth data, apart from using them to teach medical students.

Dr. Hansen: You brought up the question of growth performance under conditions of unemployment, but I'd like to point out how useful and successful it has been to have charts for following children's growth available in under-developed countries. In South Africa, 20 years ago, about half the children were below the third percentile. This number has now dropped to about 13%. It has been politically useful to be able to show data in this way.

Dr. Tanner: I feel badly that I have confined my remarks to the developed world, but everything I have said applies to a greater extent to the Third World. Growth monitoring is practical and useful in developing countries.

History of Pediatrics 1850–1950, edited by
B.L. Nichols, A. Ballabriga, and N. Kretchmer.
Nestlé Nutrition Workshop Series, Vol. 22. Nestec
Ltd., Vevey/Raven Press, Ltd., New York © 1991.

Rickets

Harold E. Harrison

Johns Hopkins University School of Medicine, Baltimore, Maryland 21205 USA

Rickets was possibly the first environmental disease to be recognized. Long before anything was known of its biochemistry and physiology, rickets was recognized by virtue of the visible deformities it caused to the skeleton, and the resulting functional disturbances. The early decay of the teeth was so striking that it could not be overlooked. Rickets was known in England and continental Europe in the seventeenth century. The name probably derives from the Middle English word *wrikken*, to twist, and was the common name in use in England. In 1650, an English physician published the first important monograph describing this disease (1), *De Rachitide sive Morbo Puerili qui vulgo The Rickets dicitur. Tractatus*. Since he wrote in Latin, Glisson had to find a more classical name than the common term *rickets,* and derived the term *rachitis* from the Greek *rhakis*, the spine. The similarity to the common name was convenient. We now use the common term as the noun and Glisson's derived name *rachitic* as the adjective. There had been previous descriptions of rickets in medical writings, but Glisson's treatise provided the most comprehensive description of the physical findings. In 1645, another English physician, Daniel Whistler, had presented a discussion of rickets as his thesis for the MD degree at Leyden (2), but this was little noted until Glisson's monograph was published. Arnoldus Bootuis in 1649 wrote that rickets was common in Ireland as well as in England. Rickets was also present on the continent of Europe but, because of the preponderance of authoritative writings by English physicians, it was known as the "English Disease" (Die Englische Krankheit).

It is uncertain whether rickets was recognized as a disease of infants before the seventeenth century. In 1609, Guillemeau, a French surgeon, published a treatise on the nursing of children in which he described deformities that he ascribed to swathing of children with tight binding of their limbs. The descriptions of the chest deformities and those of the lower limbs suggest that he was dealing with rickets. An American pediatrician, John A. Foote (3) examined paintings of artists of the fifteenth century in which naked children were portrayed. Foote believed that some of these children showed deformities of rickets such as Harrison's groove. I cannot convince myself that I see these deformities in the reproductions of the paintings in Foote's paper (Fig. 1).

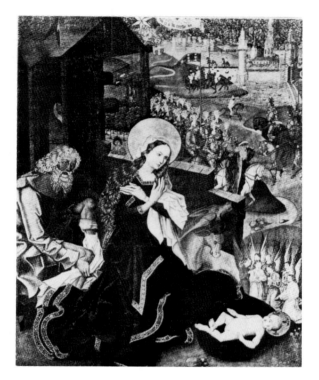

FIG. 1. "Adoration of Christ" 1460—purporting to show Harrison's groove as evidence of rickets, from Foote, p. 447 (3). (Reprinted with permission. Copyright © 1927, American Medical Association.)

An explosive increase in the incidence of rickets in England and other European countries occurred with the Industrial Revolution. The etiology remained a mystery, however. A nutritional cause was apparently ruled out because "rickets appears at a time when the child is independent of the general table. The percentage of breast-fed babies among the poorer classes is very high . . . and yet in certain areas of all large industrial towns, practically all the children show signs of rickets of a more or less severe form" (4).

Although the bone deformities of rickets were severe, the disease was not fatal per se, but children with severe chest deformities might be more susceptible to pneumonia, which did have a high mortality. In addition, rickets appeared to be an important predisposing factor for convulsive seizures associated with laryngeal spasm and tetany that could be fatal. Despite the fact that the disease appeared to be self-limited, the extraordinarily high incidence in infants living in crowded slum districts in England and the Continent prompted intensive interest in its pathogenesis and possible methods of treatment.

An important deformity caused by rickets is that of the pelvis, which results in a contracted pelvis in the adult. In the female, this was associated with serious problems in childbirth, and mortality and morbidity due to prolonged difficult deliveries should be properly charged against rickets. It is possible that rickets was an important factor in the emergence of medical obstetrics in the eighteenth and nineteenth centuries due to the need for instrumental intervention in women with contracted pelvises.

The possibility of an infectious basis for rickets was considered by many physicians and there was confusion in the differential diagnosis of rickets and congenital syphilis, both of which affect long bones and the enamel of the permanent teeth. It is therefore not surprising that eminent authorities considered that syphilis was an important factor in the causation of rickets. The French pediatrician, Parrot, insisted that congenital syphilis was the most common cause of rickets. The founder of American pediatrics, Abraham Jacobi, also considered syphilis as a cause of rickets. He wrote in 1896, "Thus there are a great many cases of early rhachitis which are due to the influence of mitigated syphilis in the parents" (5). His colleague, Job Lewis Smith, concurred with this at first but later changed his mind and argued for a dietetic cause. The basis for Smith's conversion to the dietetic theory will be discussed later.

Inevitably, the question of hereditary factors and prenatal influences in the pathogenesis of rickets was raised. In view of the geographic distribution of the disease and its high incidence in the crowded slum areas of the industrial cities of Europe and the United States, a genetic etiology seemed highly improbable. However, the German physician, Siegert, believed, on the basis of family studies, that heredity was an important factor. The concept of diathesis, i.e., a predisposition to a disease, was a favored one in the nineteenth century and rickets was thought by some to be due to a "scrofulous diathesis."

The most widely held theory of the etiology of rickets was that it was an environmental disease caused by pollution in the home. This has been most thoroughly discussed by Dick in his book entitled *Rickets* (4). He wrote: "What, then, is the nature of the environment which produces rickets? It is that associated with the overcrowding of immense populations into slum areas. . . . It implies several factors: (i) absence of sunlight; (ii) deprivation of fresh air and of the means of proper oxygenation of the blood and removal of carbonic acid required for the metabolism of the healthy infant; (iii) deprivation of the means of exercise which is so essential a stimulus to the proper regulation of the process of growth; (iv) the breathing of an atmosphere polluted by overcrowding in confined and badly ventilated rooms; (v) the want of the opportunity for proper cleanliness. . . ."Whether in England, or Europe or America, the greatest prevalence of rickets is associated with the greatest density of population."

Although Dick included the absence of sunlight in his list of causative factors, most emphasis by medical authorities was placed on the injurious effects of the internal environment; the breathing of impure air and the restricted activity of the infant confined in a close, stuffy room and exposed to vitiated air. This was thought to be consistent with the observation that children suffered from rickets primarily during the first 2 or 3 years of life. Although the deformities persisted, the progression of the disease ceased once the child could walk and run and was no longer confined to the house.

In the absence of a proven theory of the pathogenesis of rickets, there was no effective method of prevention or treatment. Since the disease developed in infants fed on either human or cow's milk, an insufficiency of calcium intake could not be the cause. As is usually the case, physicians, when confronted with a disease of unknown etiology, try a variety of treatments and, on occasion, claim beneficial effects that cannot later be confirmed. In Europe, elemental phosphorus was recommended as a curative agent. This was given in minute amounts dissolved in oil and, interestingly enough, cod-liver oil was often used as the solvent. Either because not enough cod-liver oil was given or because the antirachitic potency of cod-liver oil was variable, most pediatricians considered this treatment of no value. It also seemed unlikely that the minute amounts of elemental phosphorus (0.5 mg per dose) could be effective in children on milk feedings that were known to contain considerable amounts of phosphate. Elemental phosphorus feeding did produce an interesting change in bone demonstrable by x-ray—a line of increased density at the metaphysis. (Fig. 2 shows an x-ray from an unpublished study by Dr. Edwards A. Park and me using this technique to investigate the rate of growth of bone. The two lines represent periods of phosphorus administration separated by a known time interval allowing the rate of bone growth during that interval to be determined.) Hygienic measures and what we now call physiotherapy were of course, recommended.

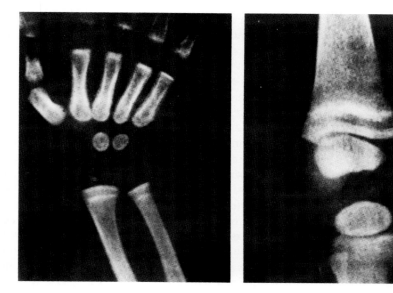

FIG. 2. X-ray of tibia and hand showing 2 phosphorus lines as method of measuring rate of linear growth of bone.

Stimulation of the skin by baths was thought to be helpful not only for cleanliness but for "toning up the system in the debility of rickets."

The major fundamental investigations on rickets in the nineteenth and early twentieth centuries were studies that correlated its pathology with the mineral content of bone. The eminent pathologist, Rudolf Virchow (see p. 137, Fig. 2), published an important treatise in 1853 on the histology of bone and cartilage in infants with rickets (6). He reported histological evidence of rickets in infants who had died in the second month of life. The most definitive study of the pathology was that of Schmorl in 1909 who examined the bones of infants who had died between the ages of 2 months and 4 years (7). Infants in Dresden showed a startling incidence of rickets—345 infants out of a total number of 386, i.e., 89.4% had evidence of rickets.

Clues to the etiology of rickets were consistently disregarded by the medical establishment. The evidence from Schmorl's data that rickets tends to heal during the summer months did not persuade the English pediatrician, Findlay, that exposure to sunshine might be the curative factor. This was even more surprising in view of the evidence published in 1890 by Palm (8), an English missionary physician in Japan, who was struck by the absence of rickets in that country. Through correspondence with other medical missionaries, he determined that, despite the high incidence of other diseases such as tuberculosis, and the poor sanitation in the homes, rickets was unknown in China, India, Ceylon, and Morocco, confirming his own experience in Japan. The common factor in all these vast communities was the open-air life and the brilliant sunshine.

The other clue that was disregarded was the experience of the London Zoo. The veterinarians at this famous zoo were unable to raise lion cubs because they developed bone changes resembling rickets and became immobile and died. Bland-Sutton (9) tried feeding them a diet including crushed bones and cod-liver oil that succeeded in preventing the skeletal abnormalities and made it possible to raise the animals to maturity. Bland-Sutton used cod-liver oil because it had been a folk remedy for rheumatism and other skeletal disorders used by fishermen along the northern coast of Europe. In Holland, it evidently had been used for the treatment of rickets in the early nineteenth century and there were reports from Germany and France of the therapeutic value of cod-liver oil in infantile rickets (10). Nevertheless, it was not generally accepted by physicians, probably because of the lack of objective evidence of healing. Determinations of calcium and phosphate concentrations in serum were unknown and the x-ray had not yet been discovered. In the 1893 meeting of the American Pediatric Society, Job Lewis Smith (11) presented a paper on rickets in which he cited the experiences with rickets in animals at the London Zoo and concluded that the successful prevention of rickets by addition of cod-liver oil and crushed bones indicated that rickets was a deficiency disease. Despite his eminent position in American pediatrics, little attention was given to this paper. The following year, Irving Snow (12) of Buffalo discussed the high incidence of rickets in black and Italian children in that city and cited Palm's observations on the role of sunshine, but the audience was not impressed.

In 1908, the British pediatrician Findlay (13) published studies on experimental rickets in puppies. He was able to produce deformities resembling human rickets in puppies kept in cages, whereas animals given the same diet but allowed fresh air and freedom of movement remained healthy. His conclusion was that exercise was the important factor, neglecting the influence of sunlight. However, these studies provided the basis for the important investigation of experimental rickets by Mellanby (14) (Fig. 3). He kept the puppies confined in accordance with Findlay's concept but also tested the effect of various dietary changes, particularly the effect of fat. He used histologic changes in the bones and, for the first time, x-rays as evidence of the the degree of rickets and the progression of healing. The basal diet was bread and skimmed milk, with yeast and orange juice added to provide water soluble vitamins that had already been discovered. One of the fats added was cod-liver oil, since Mellanby knew about Bland-Sutton's experience at the London Zoo. He found that rachitic puppies in confinement could be cured by the addition to the diet of cod-liver oil, whole milk, or egg yolk. Mellanby knew that cod-liver oil was a rich source of vitamin A, which had already been discovered by E. V. McCollum. He concluded, therefore, that vitamin A was the active, fat-soluble factor that prevented or healed rickets. Vitamin A, however, is readily destroyed by oxidation and although Mellanby heated cod-liver oil to 120°C for 4 hours while bubbling oxygen through it and found no loss of antirachitic effect, he contended that the vitamin A

Special Report Series, No. 61.

Pribụ Council

MEDICAL RESEARCH
COUNCIL

———

EXPERIMENTAL RICKETS

BY

EDWARD MELLANBY, M.A., M.D.

LONDON
PUBLISHED BY HIS MAJESTY'S STATIONERY OFFICE
1921
Price 4s. net.

FIG. 3. Cover of Dr. Howland's copy of Mellanby's *Medical Research Council Report on Experimental Rickets*, 1921.

content of oil was so great that enough was left despite oxidation to be effective in the healing of rickets.

In addition to his definite proof of the antirachitic action of cod-liver oil, and to a lesser extent, of butter fat and egg yolk, Mellanby also stirred the Johns Hopkins group to action. E.V. McCollum, who had discovered vitamin A while at Wisconsin, was now at the Johns Hopkins School of Hygiene and Public Health. McCollum's studies of vitamin A had involved the albino rat. He was convinced that his vitamin-A-deficient rats showed no evidence of rickets and felt compelled to see whether he could produce rickets in rats and determine the nature of the antirachitic factor. He developed diets that produced bone deformities that he thought were rickets, but being unfamiliar with the disease, he sought help in 1918 from John Howland (see p. 268, Fig. 1), Pediatrician-in-Chief at Johns Hopkins. Dr. Howland, who had long been interested in the biochemistry of rickets, cabled Edwards A. Park, an expert in rickets histology then working with the Red Cross in France, to return to Baltimore so that he could collaborate with McCollum. By 1922, McCollum, with the assistance of the pediatricians, Park and Shipley, and his technician Miss Simmonds, had shown that production of rickets in the albino rat was in part dependent on a diet with an unusual ratio of calcium to phosphorus, and confirmed the presence of an antirachitic factor in cod-liver oil and to a much lesser extent, in butter fat (15). Lard, olive oil, and many other fats tested were deficient in this substance. Oxidation of cod-liver oil or butter fat destroyed the vitamin A content, but the antirachitic property was unaffected. Hence they concluded that the rickets preventive factor was distinct from vitamin A, and it was named vitamin D.

Park and his colleagues immediately set to work to transfer these findings to human rickets. Benjamin Kramer (Fig. 4), in Howland's department, had developed a

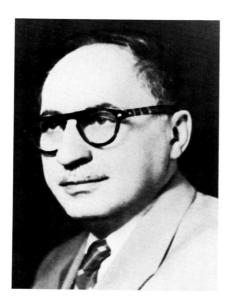

FIG. 4. Benjamin Kramer. (Courtesy of The United States National Library of Medicine.)

semi-micro method for serum calcium determination in children, and Howland and Kramer (16) (see p. 270, Fig. 6) had been among the first to measure the concentration of calcium in the serum of children with rickets. They had also made the important observation of the lowered serum phosphate concentration in rickets. Armed with the capacity to determine serum calcium and phosphate as well as the ability to detect evidence of rickets and healing rickets by x-ray, Park and colleagues (17) quickly showed the efficacy of cod-liver oil in the treatment and prevention of rickets in infants. A group of English physicians also verified the value of cod-liver oil in the treatment of rickets in a study conducted in post-war Vienna, where rickets was severe (18). Meanwhile, however, there had been another important contribution to the understanding of the pathogenesis of rickets.

Heliotherapy, i.e., artificial sunlight using a quartz lamp, which emitted ultraviolet light, had become a popular therapeutic agent in Germany, particularly for the treatment of bone tuberculosis. In 1916, a booklet on heliotherapy (19) contained the statement ''sunlight exercises as marked an action on the local and systemic condition of the rachitic child as on patients suffering from bone tuberculosis.'' No notice was taken of this until 1919, when Huldschinsky (20), a Berlin pediatrician, described treatment of four children with advanced rickets by exposure to a mercury vapor quartz lamp. He obtained cures, demonstrated by x-ray. Alfred F. Hess, a New York pediatrician, confirmed Huldschinsky's findings. At the 1921 meeting of the American Pediatric Society (11), Park and colleagues reported on the antirachitic factor in cod-liver oil and Hess and Unger reported on the antirachitic effects of ultraviolet light, explaining the seasonal variations in rickets and the extremely high incidence in black infants in New York, since ''the pigmentation of their skins . . . prevents the penetration of the short actinic rays.'' Hess irradiated excised human skin and found that it developed antirachitic activity. He also had the idea of inducing antirachitic activity into foods devoid of this activity by exposing them to ultraviolet radiation. Cottonseed oil, linseed oil, dried milk, and many vegetables could be activated by ultraviolet radiation (21). Steenbock, a biochemist at the University of Wisconsin, also had the idea of exposing food stuffs to ultraviolet light to induce antirachitic activity (22). It was at first thought that cholesterol was the component of the non-saponifiable fraction of fats that was activated, but it was soon discovered by organic chemists in England (23), Germany (24) and the United States, that pure cholesterol could not be activated, and in 1927 Windaus and Hess (25) identified the provitamin as ergosterol, a plant sterol. Later, intensive research by a number of organic chemists, stimulated by the research of Waddell (26), led to the identification of the provitamin in skin, 7-dehydrocholesterol. Although Steenbock patented the process of production of vitamin D by ultraviolet irradiation of provitamins, Hess must be given much credit for initiating the concept, and perhaps for encouraging Windhaus in his work on the structural changes in the provitamins that produce the antirachitic factor, for which he received the Nobel prize in chemistry in 1928.

The story has not ended. Cod-liver oil was effective in preventing and curing rickets but there were major drawbacks to its use in infants and children. It had to be given in teaspoonful amounts. Because of its bad taste and smell, children hated to take it and mothers were reluctant to force it upon them. Aspiration with consequent lipid pneumonia was reported in infants due to cod-liver oil administration. A more potent fish liver oil was discovered, percomorph liver oil, but the answer was developed by Steenbock's process of irradiating ergosterol or 7-dehydrocholesterol. Concentrated preparations of vitamin D could be produced by this method and vitamin preparations became available in which only a few drops could contain prophylactic quantities of vitamin D. The real answer, however, was provided by Philip C. Jeans (27) (Fig. 5), Professor of Pediatrics at the University of Iowa. He was invited by the Committee on Foods of the American Medical Association to report on the possible fortification of milk with vitamin D. He persuaded the Committee in 1936 to recommend fortification of milk with vitamin D produced by the irradiation of provitamin D. This could be done at little cost because of the efficiency of the process, and without affecting the flavor of the milk. Jeans recommended such fortification at the concentration of 400 units per quart of whole milk or equivalent quart in the case of concentrated or dried milk products. This dose was based on studies of calcium and phosphate balances in infants by Jeans and Stearns (28). Although 90–100 units of vitamin D daily might be sufficient to protect infants from clinical rickets, maximum mineral balances were achieved with the 400-unit daily dose. There was, at first, opposition from public health officials against any kind of adulteration of milk. Initially, evaporated milk was fortified and, subsequently, fluid milk, homogenized and fortified with vitamin D according to Jeans' recommendation, became the standard product in the United States. All infant feeding preparations developed as a substitute for breast feeding were also fortified. Rickets was thus transformed from the most common chronic disease of infancy and early childhood to a rare disease.

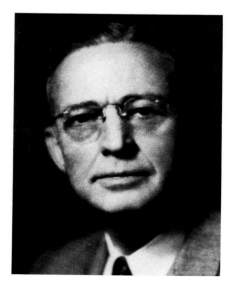

FIG. 5. Philip C. Jeans. (Courtesy of CNRC Archives; gift of L.J. Filer.)

Interest in the biochemistry and physiological action of vitamin D continued. Balance studies in infants and experimental studies in animals using intestinal preparations indicated that a major action of vitamin D was to increase the absorption of calcium and phosphate. This effect in in vitro preparations of intestine could be obtained only by administration of vitamin D to the intact animal, and there was a latent period of many hours before the effect could be shown. An explanation for this latent period was found by Hector DeLuca (29), one of Steenbock's students. When tritium-labeled vitamin D was injected intravenously into vitamin-D-deficient rats, chromatography of tissue extracts showed that a more polar metabolite of vitamin D was present. This was identified as 25-OH vitamin D and was a physiologically active metabolite. Later, the English investigator, Kodicek (30), identified a further metabolite, 1,25 (OH)$_2$ vitamin D, which was much more potent than 25-OH vitamin D. It is now recognized that vitamin D is physiologically inactive until metabolized by successive hydroxylations. The 25-OH derivative is the product of liver metabolism and is then the substrate for a renal tubule cell oxidase system to form 1,25 (OH)$_2$ vitamin D. The rickets resulting from severe hepatic disease and the disorders of calcium metabolism in renal insufficiency can now be explained. There are genetically determined disorders of 1,25 (OH)$_2$ vitamin D formation or function, so that the role of heredity in rickets was not entirely without foundation. In addition, disorders of renal tubular transport of phosphate can result in hypophosphatemia and rickets not responsive to ordinary vitamin D treatment. Rickets, therefore, has not disappeared, but it is now one of the uncommon genetic disorders of which the pediatrician must be aware.

REFERENCES

1. Glisson F. *De Rachitide Sive Morbo Puerile qui vulgo The Rickets dicitur, Tractatus.* Londinensum, Little Britain, 1650; cited by Dick JL in: *Rickets.* New York: EB Treat, 1922.
2. Whistler D. Disputatio medica innauguralis do morbo puerili anglorum quem patrio idomate vocant the rickets. Leyden, 1645; cited by Dick, JL ibid.
3. Foote JA. Evidence of rickets prior to 1650. *Am J Dis Child* 1927;34:443–52.
4. Dick JL. *Rickets.* New York: EB Treat, 1922.
5. Jacobi A. *Therapeutics of infancy and childhood.* Philadelphia: JB Lippincott Co, 1896. Cited by Cone TE in: *200 Years of feeding infants in America.* Ross Laboratories, 1976.
6. Virchow R. Das normale Knochenwachstein und die rachitische Stoerung desselben. *Virchow's Archiv* 1853;5:409–507.
7. Schmorl G. Die pathologische Anatomie der rachitischen Knochenerkrankung mit besonderer Berücksichtung ihrer Histologie und Pathogenese. *Ergeb Inn Med Kinderheilkd* 1909;4:40–48.
8. Palm TA. The geographic distribution and aetiology of rickets. *The Practitioner* 1890;45:270–9.
9. Bland-Sutton J. Rickets in monkeys, lions, bears and birds. *J Comp Med Surg* 1889;10:1.
10. Guy RA. History of cod-liver oil as a remedy. *Am J Dis Child* 1923;26:112–6.
11. Faber HR, McIntosh R. *History of the American Pediatric Society, 1887–1965.* New York: McGraw-Hill, 1966;32.
12. Ibid, p 35.
13. Findlay L. The aetiology of rickets. *Br Med J* 1908;ii:13.
14. Mellanby E. *Experimental rickets.* Medical Research Council Special Report no. 61, 1921.
15. Shipley PG, Park EA, McCollum EV, Simmonds N, Parsons HT. The effect of cod-liver oil administered to rats with experimental rickets. *J Biol Chem* 1921;45:343–8.
16. Howland J, Kramer B. Calcium and phosphorus in the serum in relation to rickets. *Am J Dis Child* 1921;22:105–19.

17. Park EA, Howland J. The radiographic evidence of the influence of cod-liver oil in rickets. *Bull Johns Hopkins Hosp* 1921;32:341–4.
18. Chick H. Study of rickets in Vienna, 1919–1922. *Med Hist* 1976;20:41–51.
19. Rollier A. Cited by Hess AF in: *Rickets including osteomalacia and tetany.* Philadelphia: Lea and Febiger, 1929.
20. Huldschinsky K. Heilung von Rachitis durch Künstliche Hohensonne. *Deutsch Med Wochenschr* 1919;45:712–3.
21. Hess AF, Weinstock M. Antirachitic properties imparted to most fluids and to green vegetables by ultraviolet irradiation. *J Biol Chem* 1924;62:301–13.
22. Steenbock H, Black A. The induction of growth-promoting and calcifying properties in fats and their unsaponifiable constituents by exposure to light. *J Biol Chem* 1925;64:263–98.
23. Rosenheim O, Webster TA. The relation of cholesterol to vitamin D. *Biochem J* 1927;21:127–9.
24. Pohl R, cited by Bills CE in: Physiology of the sterols including vitamin D. *Physiol Rev* 1935;15:1–97.
25. Hess AF, Windaus A. The development of marked activity in ergosterol following ultra-violet irradiation. *Proc Soc Exp Biol Med* 1927;24:369–70.
26. Waddell J. The provitamin D of cholesterol. I. The antirachitic efficacy of irradiated cholesterol. *J Biol Chem* 1934;105:711–39.
27. Jeans PC, Vitamin D milk. *JAMA* 1936;106:2066–9,2150.
28. Jeans PC, Stearns G. Growth and retentions of calcium, phosphorus and nitrogen of infants fed evaporated milk. *Am J Dis Child* 1933;46:69–89.
29. Blunt JW, DeLuca HF, Schnoes HK. 25-Hydroxycholecalciferol, biologically active metabolite of vitamin D_3. *Biochemistry* 1968;7:3317–22.
30. Kodicek E. The story of vitamin D. From vitamin to hormone. *Lancet* 1974;i:325–9.

DISCUSSION

Dr. Frenk: Children with rickets appear in many old paintings, most of them depicting Madonna and Child. Foot's classical paper (1) omits the most beautiful pictorial description of a child with ''florid'' rickets, namely the little Cupid, painted in 1603 by Caravaggio, which may be admired in the Uffizzi gallery in Florence.

Dr. Metcoff: Over the doorway of the lovely fifteenth century orphanage of Brezotrofio in Florence there still stands a ceramic medallion by Andrea del Sarto that is now the symbol of the American Academy of Pediatrics. It shows an infant with legs bound in the way that was usual at the time, when it was generally thought that this would prevent bowing of the limbs. Just after the Second World War, I had the opportunity to visit the orphanage and noted that every day the nurses took the children and placed them in the outdoor arcade, religiously ensuring that they remained in the shadow cast by the pillars. It was thought that if they were in the sun they would have seizures and die.

Dr. Harrison: The notion that sunshine is harmful to infants is still prevalent in many societies. After the Second World War, I was told by one of my colleagues who was working in Ethiopia in the field of public health that rickets was extremely common in Addis Ababa, where there is plenty of sunshine. Infants and young children were not allowed in the sun because it was felt that it was injurious. There is also now a considerable problem of rickets in Saudi Arabia, where mothers are not permitted outdoors unless they are completely covered from head to foot. This means that the infants never get out in the daytime either. They are breast-fed and do not receive vitamin supplements because it is felt that human milk must provide all the necessary nutrients.

Dr Kretchmer: The trend now of course is to say that the sun is harmful!

Dr. Benkappa: In India, although there is plenty of sunshine, rickets still exists in certain communities where infants are not exposed to sunlight. This is particularly the case in Muslim households where the purdah system dictates that the mother stays at home with the children. Rickets is seen in breast-fed infants because formulas are now fortified with vitamin D. It is not commonly seen in protein-energy malnutrition because there is so little growth in the malnourished state. It is important to give vitamin D during recovery from malnutrition however.

Dr. Snyderman: We are now seeing rickets again in New York City among members of the black Muslim group. The mothers are vegetarians and have no source of vitamin D. They breast-feed their babies for a long time without any supplements and the babies develop rickets.

Dr. Harrison: We are seeing the same thing in Baltimore among the black Muslims, and also among other black children who have been breast-fed. It has been confirmed that melanin in the skin shields provitamin D in the basal layers from ultraviolet radiation. Heavily pigmented babies therefore require more sunlight or exogenous vitamin D. Human milk does not contain adequate amounts of vitamin D so breast-fed babies need sunshine. This is heretical because vitamin D is regarded as a nutrient and human milk must in theory contain every nutrient that the baby requires! However vitamin D is not a nutrient—it is a hormone. Rickets is an environmental disease resulting from the lack of an energizing factor, ultraviolet radiation.

REFERENCE

1. Foote JA. Evidence of rickets prior to 1650. *Am J Dis Child* 1927;34:443.

History of Pediatrics 1850–1950, edited by
B.L. Nichols, A. Ballabriga, and N. Kretchmer.
Nestlé Nutrition Workshop Series, Vol. 22. Nestec
Ltd., Vevey/Raven Press, Ltd., New York © 1991.

Vitamin Deficiencies

Lewis A. Barness

*Department of Pediatrics, University of Wisconsin Hospital and Clinics, Madison,
Wisconsin 53792, USA*

Up to the end of the nineteenth century, the significance of the macronutrients and their sources was still not completely clear. Energy requirements had been estimated in general by 1890. The nutritional characteristics of protein, carbohydrate, and fat were recognized by 1890, and amino acids and specific dynamic action by 1900. This was the era of the contributions of Atwater, Voit, Liebig, Pettenkofer, Rubner, Lusk, and others. Fletcher had indicated the adverse effects of obesity and recommended prolonged mastication of food and a vegetarian diet.

As chemists were able to determine the composition of foods, experiments began with purified mixtures. Some animals did not grow and some died. Artificial milks made with casein, sugar, and water had been fed to infants during the siege of Paris in 1871 and children died. Dumas suggested that something essential was lacking from the macronutrients.

With the the use of purified experimental diets, effects of minor substances were sought. In retrospect, the recognition that trace elements of any kind could be important to human nutrition occupied many centuries of observation, first in animals and later in humans. As McCollum summarized: "The experience of mankind with good and bad foods through many centuries led reflective men to conclude that the diet had much to do with health" (1).

By the first decade of the twentieth century, rickets, scurvy, beriberi, pellagra, and other diseases were recognized as probably due to nutritional factors. Funk in 1912 theorized that these diseases were caused by deficiency or lack in the diet of special organic bases that he called *vitamines*. As late as 1916, however, McCollum and Kennedy suggested "the desirability of discontinuing the use of the term vitamins, and the substitution of the term fat-soluble A and water soluble B for the two classes of unknown substances concerned in inducing growth" (2).

In recounting the history of the discovery of the presently accepted vitamins, the names of many significant investigators are necessarily omitted, chemical syntheses are not discussed, and biochemical effects are mentioned only when absolutely pertinent. The order of presentation is arbitrary.

VITAMIN A

Night blindness had been recognized for many centuries and was treated with raw liver, usually with good results. Other eye diseases were also felt to be due to dietary factors. Mori, in 1904 (3), used cod-liver oil to treat conjunctivitis. Others showed that rats on a fat-free diet developed xerophthalmia (4). Because of the conjunctivitis and other infections, vitamin A was thought to be an anti-infectious factor until 1928 when Wolbach and Howe (5) showed that the defect in vitamin-A deficiency was due to the replacement of various epithelia by stratified squamous keratinizing epithelium. This epithelium then had lowered resistance to infection.

In 1913, McCollum and Davis (6) found that rats did not grow well when fed cereal grains. They started systematically studying different combinations of nutrients and found that a substance in butter fat or egg yolk improved growth. About the same time, Osborne and Mendel (7) had described a form of "infectious" eye disease that was rapidly alleviated by the addition of butter fat to the rat diet. McCollum and Davis then used a system that they called the *biological method of analysis*, in which they fed an incomplete food with the addition of single or multiple supplements. They deduced that the minimum diet for rats must contain fat-soluble A and water-soluble B. The latter was a substance that prevented beriberi.

Though cod-liver oil had been used for some time for treatment of infectious conjunctivitis and rickets, it was not until 1925 that vitamin A was separated from vitamin D. Its structure was determined by Karrer in 1931. Moore showed that β carotene, a yellow substance that colors butter and certain vegetables, was converted biologically to vitamin A. β Carotene was also synthesized by Karrer (8).

Since night blindness was simultaneously corrected, studies by Wald (9) and others determined that a biochemical effect of vitamin A, distinct from its effect on epithelial cells, was occurring in the eyes. It was found that retinol binds with opsin to form rhodopsin in the rods of the retina. Energy from light reverses the binding with release of energy, providing vision in decreased light. Functions of vitamin A are now also known to involve stability of membranes, visual purple, growth, and reproduction.

THIAMIN

Beriberi was recognized in China 12 centuries ago and in Europe, three centuries ago. Beriberi means "sheep" because people with beriberi walk like sheep. It became widespread with the development of the steam-powered rice mill in the nineteenth century. In 1897 Eijkman (10) noted that chickens developed a paralytic condition similar to the polyneuritis of beriberi, and that this was curable with rice polishings. Grijns (11) concluded that both diseases were caused by the lack of a dietary factor in rice bran, concentrated by Funk in 1911 (12) and purified by Jansen and Donath 15 years later (13). Shortly afterward the significance of thiamin pyrophosphate in the respiratory cycle was determined by Peters and others (14), and explained the heart disease in beriberi. The effects in the brain are less clear (15).

In 1932, Anhagen studied effects of crude preparation of rice bran extracts and noted carboxylase activity. Two years later, Williams determined its structure, and in 1937 Lohmann described its cocarboxylase activity. The oxidative decarboxylation of α-keto acids plays a critical role in attaining cellular energy through the Krebs cycle. Depending on additional factors, beriberi can be fatal in infants and presents as wet or dry beriberi in older children and adults.

RIBOFLAVIN

In the study of rice polishings, two factors were recognized. One affected polyneuropathy. The other was apparently a growth factor. In 1932, Warburg and Christian isolated a yellow enzyme from yeast involved in oxidation reduction (16). Shortly thereafter, Kuhn and Gyorgy (17) isolated and characterized a similar substance from eggs and milk that they called ovoflavin or lactoflavin. When, over the next 3 years, it was realized that all of these substances were identical, the name *riboflavin* was adopted. In 1935, Karrer and Kuhn synthesized riboflavin and in 1938 Warburg and Christian published their monograph on the coenzymic role of riboflavin.

Riboflavin deficiency in humans causes cheilosis, keratitis, glossitis, and seborrheic dermatitis. The coenzymes, flavin mononucleotide and flavin adenine dinucleotide, are essential for electron transport.

NIACIN

Pellagra was unrecognized as a disease until maize was introduced into Europe. Casal called it pellagra, meaning ''rough skin.'' It was considered an infectious disease or due to a toxin until Goldberger (18) and his co-workers showed that it was not transmissable but was endemic in maize-eating areas. They isolated a pellagra-preventing factor from protein-free yeast extracts.

Hopkins and Cole had isolated tryptophan in 1900 and had found that animals fed zein extracted from maize did not grow but, when tryptophan was added to the diet, growth improved. The significance of this to human nutrition was not recognized until it was realized that tryptophan was a precursor of niacin. High-protein diets had been shown to ameliorate pellagra and for a time, tryptophan was considered the anti-pellagra substance. However, in the late 1930s, Spies and coworkers (19) and Elvehjem (20) showed that nicotinamide was identical to Goldberger's factor and cured blacktongue in dogs. Goldsmith (21) determined much later that tryptophan was a precursor of niacin.

Niacin is essential for oxidation in cells as part of the coenzymes nicotinamide adenine dinucleotide and nicotinamide adenine dinucleotide phosphate.

PYRIDOXINE

In 1934, Gyorgy (22) noted the presence of a growth factor for rats that was distinct from the yellow substance later termed *riboflavin*. This factor prevented acrodynia in rats, characterized by a dermatitis. He called this vitamin B_6. It was later isolated and the chemical structure determined by six different groups. It was synthesized by Harris and Folkers in 1938. The difference in activity of pyridoxal and pyridoxamine was discovered by Snell and coworkers in 1939 (23). Because of its structural relationship to pyridine, Gyorgy and Eckhart (24) proposed its presently accepted name *pyridoxine*. It functions in the synthesis and catabolism of amino acids, as in transamination. Deficiency results in seizures, anemia, or in xanthurenic acidemia. Neuritis and seizures may occur in those receiving the anti-tuberculosis drug isonicotinic acid hydrazide. In contrast to other vitamins of the B group, requirement is related to dietary protein.

PANTOTHENIC ACID

Dermatitis in chicks was noted as early as 1930. Pantothenic acid was recognized as a growth factor for yeast by Williams in 1933 (25). It was also found to be a growth factor for chicks. Elvehjem, Jukes, and coworkers showed that this factor could be found in a yeast filtrate, and Williams finally isolated it.

A syndrome of burning feet was described in prisoners of war in 1945. This is said to have been relieved by pantothenate. No other human disease has been attributed to its deficiency. Pantothenate, however, is a constituent of coenzyme A, discovered by Lipmann in 1945 (26). As such, it occupies a central role in carbohydrate metabolism. Its wide distribution in foods partially explains the rareness of deficiency signs. Even in volunteers, deficiency produces only vague symptoms such as fatigue, sleep disturbances, and numbness of hands and feet.

BIOTIN

In 1901, Wildiers described growth- and life-promoting effects in yeast that he termed *bios*. Much later, Gyorgy (27) and his coworkers studied a factor in yeast and liver that was protective against the toxic effects of high concentrations of egg white in rats. They called this factor *vitamin H*. Kogl and Tonnis (28) in 1936 isolated a crystalline substance from egg yolk that they called *biotin* because of its relationship to bios, the yeast growth factors. Gyorgy and his coworkers established that biotin, vitamin H, and another factor, Allison's coenzyme R, essential for the growth of a nitrogen-fixing organism, were identical. Within 3 years Du Vigneaud (29) established the structure of biotin and Harris (30) synthesized it.

Biotin is bound to avidin, a glycoprotein in raw egg white. It is required in carboxylation reactions such as conversion of pyruvate to oxaloacetate in mitochondria. Deficiency in man is rare.

FOLIC ACID

In 1931, Wills (31) studied megaloblastic anemia in pregnant women in Bombay. She produced the disease in monkeys and was able to cure the anemia with autolysed yeast, *Marmite*, that she had found ineffective in the treatment of pernicious anemia. Mitchell et al. (32) in 1941 studied a growth factor for *Lactobacillus casei* from spinach that they called *folic acid*, because it came from foliage. Stokstad crystallized pteroylglutamic acid in 1943 and Shorb, about 5 years later, showed that certain Lactobacilli require it for growth. This became the basis for a test for folate. In 1945, Spies found folic acid effective in the treatment of macrocytic anemia of pregnancy and tropical sprue.

Folic acid as tetrahydrofolate is essential in purine and pyrimidine synthesis. Herbert (33) determined that folate deficiency could be induced in a relatively normal person, himself, after 133 days.

VITAMIN B_{12}

In 1849, Thomas Addison described an anemia that led to death in 2 to 5 years. Austin Flint, in 1860, noted that this specific anemia was related to stomach disorders. This disease was invariably fatal until, in 1926, Minot and Murphy produced remission with raw liver. At about the same time Castle (34) determined that patients with pernicious anemia had reduced gastric secretion of an unidentified protein. The factor in liver was termed the extrinsic factor and the gastric secretion, intrinsic factor. The extrinsic factor became known as vitamin B_{12}, isolated and identified in 1948 (35,36), and was the first compound discovered with a bond between a metallic ion and an organic ligand.

Vitamin B_{12} is the coenzyme for methyltransferase and methylmalonyl CoA mutase. The latter is responsible for excess methylmalonate (37) in patients with pernicious anemia.

Deficiency of the vitamin occurs in vegetarians, while defective absorption occurs in those who lack intrinsic factor or carrier proteins, the transcobalamins. Deficiency affects the brain and nervous system as well as the blood.

VITAMIN C

Controversy over who discovered vitamin C—and when—stirred the scientific community for two decades, and caused much confusion over the true nature of the vitamin. Controversy continues to rage concerning its function and proper dosage (38–40).

The clinical description of scurvy is contained in the Ebers Papyrus of about 1500 BC. Hippocrates also is said to have recognized this as a common disease. It was widespread until the introduction of the potato from the new world. Indians treated Cartier's troops with spruce needles in 1536.

Though various people recognized the importance of fresh fruits and vegetables in the prevention of this disease, Lind in 1757 first reported that fresh orange or lime juice was the most effective cure. The next advance in the study of the disease was accidental. Holst and Frolich (41) were attempting to induce beriberi in guinea pigs. Instead they developed scurvy. From that time, guinea pigs have remained the animal of choice for studying this disease they being one of a small number of animals that cannot synthesize ascorbic acid.

In 1928, Szent-Györgyi (42) isolated hexuronic acid from lemon juice, adrenal glands, and cabbage. In 1932, Waugh and King (43) isolated the antiscorbutic factor from lemon juice and showed that it was identical to hexuronic acid. It was synthesized by Rechstein in 1933, and re-named ascorbic acid.

Ascorbate is recognized as a non-specific water-soluble reducing agent. As such, it increases absorption of, and is involved in, the metabolism of iron and folate. It is involved in collagen metabolism and is important in wound healing. Stress of any kind, as well as smoking, increases its requirements. Although no enzyme requirement has been established for its activity in tyrosine metabolism, when infants consume high protein diets, excretion of urinary phenolic compounds is decreased after addition of ascorbate.

Though scurvy and blatant vitamin-C deficiency are now uncommon except in those on limited diets, the place of vitamin C in stress and prevention of disease continues to foster clinical and biochemical investigation.

VITAMIN D

The history of the discovery of vitamin D and its use in the treatment of rickets is given in chapter 16.

VITAMIN E

Evans and Bishop in 1922 (44) fed a diet consisting of purified protein, fat, carbohydrate, salt mixture, and adequate doses of fat-soluble A and water-soluble B and noted fetal resorption and infertility in rats, correctable by adding vegetable or butter fats. The factor was isolated and termed *vitamin E*.

The effects of deficiency in animals are multiple and include sterility, myopathy, liver disease, and encephalomalacia. The vitamin was finally isolated and synthesized by Karrer in 1938. It is recognized as an important fat-soluble antioxidant. Deficiency in premature infants consuming large amounts of polyunsaturated fatty acids results in a normocytic normochromic hemolytic anemia (45). Chronic deficiency, as occurs in persons with severe fat malabsorption, results in severe peripheral neuropathy (46). In abetalipoproteinemia, central nervous system degeneration may occur.

Although the claims for vitamin E in human nutrition are multiple, the widespread consumption of the vitamin is not justifiable on the basis of clinically proved information.

VITAMIN K

In 1929 Dam (47) noted that chicks fed a fat-extracted diet developed hemorrhagic disease due to a defect in blood clotting. He determined that the hemorrhagic disease was distinct from scurvy and that it was due to a new fat-soluble vitamin, vitamin K. McFarland noted especially severe disease when chicks were fed dried fish meal. Others then concentrated the fat soluble material and in 1939 Dam, Karrer, and associates (48) and Doisy and associates isolated it (49).

Because for many years synthesis was difficult, an artificial vitamin K was developed, which though favorably affecting prothrombin formation, also caused hemolysis. The natural compound is now available and does not cause hemolysis. Vitamin K also regulates factors VII, IX, and X in the coagulation cascade and transfers CO_2 to glutamate to form one of the factors in osteocalcin (50). Semantic argument continues since intestinal bacteria produce vitamin K. However, until suitable flora are established, external sources are required.

CONCLUSION

The history of vitamins belongs to the ages. Diseases were recognized in the early history of man, usually ascribed to what we now consider as bizarre events. Only in the present century, after the recognition of the importance of food for the development and well-being of humans, were techniques invented that permitted the study of trace substances such as vitamins that cannot be synthesized in human biochemical pathways.

Recognition of vitamin deficiencies, like many of our present concepts about nutrition, arose from problems identified in animal husbandry. As human investigation became more sophisticated, both human and non-human animals were used for experimentation. Of the former, some of the investigators were their own experimental subjects. For example, William Stark died as he experimented to determine protein requirements, and, in a different generation, Herbert subjected himself to a folate-deficient diet to determine a mechanism of folate deficiency.

The phrase "on the shoulders of giants" (51) can be no more aptly applied than to the discovery of vitamins. The history of vitamins is not yet ended. Other essential substances are still to be found, other uses for presently known substances recognized, and other false claims documented.

REFERENCES

1. McCollum EV. *A history of nutrition.* Boston: Houghton Mifflin 1957.
2. McCollum EV, Kennedy C. The dietary factors operating in the production of polyneuritis. *J Biol Chem* 1916;24:491–502.

3. Mori M. Uber den Sog. Hik an (xerosis conjunctivae infantum. Keratomalacie) *Jahrb Kinderhlk* 1904;59:175–95.
4. Barker BM, Bender DA. *Vitamins in medicine*, 4th ed. London: William Heinemann, vol I, 1980, vol II, 1982.
5. Wolbach SB, Howe PR. Tissue changes following deprivation of fat soluble A vitamin. *J Exp Med* 1925;42:753–77.
6. McCollum EV, Davis M. Failure of rat growth on cereal grains. *J Biol Chem* 1913;15:167–75.
7. Osborne TB, Mendel LB. Influence of butter fat on growth. *J Biol Chem* 1913;16:423–37.
8. Leung AKC, Carotenemia. *Adv Pediatr* 1987;34:223–48.
9. Wald G. The biochemistry of vision. *Annu Rev Biochem* 1973;23:497–526.
10. Eijkman C. Eine beriberi krankheit der Hakner. *Virchow's Archiv* 1897;148:523–32.
11. Grijns G. Polyneuritis gallinarum. *Tijdschr. Niederland-Indie* 1901;41:3–13.
12. Funk C. The chemical nature of the substance which cures polyneuritis in birds induced by a diet of polished rice. *J Physiol (Lond)* 1911;43:395–400.
13. Jansen BPC, Donath WF. Antineuritisch Vitamine. *Chem Weekblad* 1926;23:201–5.
14. Peters RA, Sinclair HM. Studies on avian carbohydrate metabolism. *Biochem J* 1933;27:1677–86.
15. Brin M. Defects of pyruvate and pentose metabolism in relationship to transketolase activity in rats and man and to the startle response in thiamine deficient rats. In: Wolstenholme GEW, O'Connor M, eds. *Thiamine deficiency*. London: Churchill 1967, 87.
16. Warburg O, Christian W. Ueber ein neues Oxydationferment und sein Adsorptionspektrum. *Biochem Zeitschr* 1932;254:438–7.
17. Gyorgy P, Kuhn R, Wagner-Jauregg T. Ueber dos vitamin B_2. *Klin Wochnschr* 1933;12:1241–5.
18. Goldberger J, Wheeler GA, Lillie RD, Rogers LM. Study of blacktongue—preventive action of 16 foodstuffs with special reference to identity of blacktongue of dogs and pellagra of man. *Pub Health Rep* 1928;43:1385–454.
19. Spies TD, Cooper C, Blankenborn MA. The use of nicotinic acid in the treatment of pellagra. *JAMA* 1938;110:622–7.
20. Elvehjem CA, Madden RJ, Strong FM, Woolley DW. Relation of nicotinic acid and nicotinic acid amide to canine blacktongue. *J Am Chem Soc* 1937;59:1767–8.
21. Goldsmith GA, Miller ON, Unglaub WG. Efficiency of tryptophan as a niacin precursor in man. *J Nutr* 1961;73:172–6.
22. Gyorgy P. The history of vitamin B_6. *Vitam Horm* 1964;22:361–5.
23. Snell EE. Vitamin activities of pyridoxal and pyridoxamine. *J Biol Chem* 1944;154:313–4.
24. Gyorgy P, Eckhart RE. Vitamin B_6 and skin lesions in rats. *Nature* 1939;144:512.
25. Williams RJ, Lyman CM, Goodyear GH, Truesdail JH, Holaday D. Pantothenic aid, a growth determinant of universal biological occurrence. *J Am Chem Soc* 1933;55:2912–27.
26. Lipmann F, Kaplan NO. Report on a coenzyme for acetylation. *Fed Proc* 1946;5:145.
27. Gyorgy P, Rose CS, Hofman K, Melville DB, DuVigneaud V. A further note on the identity of vitamin H with biotin. *Science* 1940;92:609.
28. Kogl F, Tonnis B. Ueber das Bios Problem. *Z Physiol Chem* 1936;242:43–6.
29. DuVigneaud V. The structure of biotin. *Science* 1942;96:455–61.
30. Harris SA, Wolf DE, Mozingo R, Folkers K. Synthetic biotin. *Science* 1943;97:447–8.
31. Wills L. The nature of the hematopoeitic factor in Marmite. *Lancet* 1933;i:1283–6.
32. Mitchell HK, Snell EE, Williams RJ. The concentration of folic acid (Ltr). *J Am Chem Soc* 1941;63:4:2284.
33. Herbert V. Experimental nutritional folate deficiency in man. *Trans Assoc Am Physicians* 1962;75:307–20.
34. Castle WB. Observation on etiological relationship of achylia gastrica to pernicious anemia; effect of administration to patients with pernicious anemia of contents of normal human stomach recovered after ingestion of beef muscle. *Am J Med Sci* 1929;178:748–64.
35. Rickes EL, Brink NG, Konuisy FR, Wood TR, Folkers K. Crystalline vitamin B_{12}. *Science* 1948;107:396–7.
36. Smith EL, Parker LF. Purification of anti-pernicious anemia factor. *Biochem J* 1948;43:VIII.
37. Barness LA, Young D, Mellman WJ, Kahn SB, Williams WJ. Methylmalonate excretion in a patient with pernicious anemia. *N Engl J Med* 1963;268:144–6.
38. Hurley LS. The identification of vitamin C. *J Nutr* 1988;118:1271.
39. Stare FJ, Stare IM. Charles Glen King 1896–1988. *J Nutr* 1988;118:1272–7.
40. Jukes TH. The identification of vitamin C, an historical summary. *J Nutr* 1988;118:1290–3.

41. Holst A, Frolich T. Experimental studies relating to ship beriberi and scurvy. *J Hyg (Camb)* 1907;7:634–71.
42. Szent-Györgyi A. Observations on the function of peroxidase systems and the chemistry of the adrenal cortex: Description of a new carbohydrate derivative. *Biochem J* 1928;22:1387–409.
43. Waugh W A, King CG. Isolation and identification of vitamin C. *J Biol Chem* 1932;97:325–31.
44. Evans HM, Bishop KS. On the existence of a hitherto unrecognized dietary factor essential for reproduction. *Science* 1922;56:650–1.
45. Oski FA, Barness LA. Vitamin E deficiency. A previously unrecognized cause of hemolytic anemia in the premature infant. *J Pediatr* 1967;70:211–20.
46. Sokol RJ, Heubi JE, Iannaccone ST, Bove KE, Balistreri WF. Vitamin E deficiency with normal vitamin E concentrations in children with chronic cholestasis. *N Engl J Med* 1984;310:1209–12.
47. Dam H. Cholesterolinstoffivechsel in Hühnereiern und Hünchen. *Biochem Z* 1929;215:475–92.
48. Dam H, Gerger A, Glavind J, Karrer P, Karrer W, Rothschild E, Salomon H. Isolieurung des vitamins K in hochgereiniger Form. *Helv Chim Acta* 1939;22:310–3.
49. Doisy EA, MacCorquodale D W, Thayer S A, Binkley S B, McKee R W. The isolation and synthesis of vitamin K. *Science* 1939;90:407.
50. Corrigan JJ. The vitamin-K-dependent proteins. *Adv Pediatr* 1981;28:57–98.
51. Bray GA. On the shoulders of giants. *Am J Clin Nutr* 1988;48:929–35.

DISCUSSION

Dr. Stern: I assume that the Cartier you refer to was Jacques Cartier, the discoverer of Canada?

Dr. Barness: He was.

Dr. Stern: On the occasion of the International Physiology Congress in Montreal in 1949, a book was produced entitled *Jacques Cartier et la Grande Maladie* in which he described scurvy. The reason that the Indians told him to use pine needles was that they themselves used birch bark to make tea and they weren't keen on the idea that the French might eat up all their bark. Their descendants, part Indian and part French, found you could prevent scurvy by eating potatoes so long as the skins were left on when they were boiled.

This little book is still around. It makes fascinating reading.

History of Pediatrics 1850–1950, edited by
B.L. Nichols, A. Ballabriga, and N. Kretchmer.
Nestlé Nutrition Workshop Series, Vol. 22. Nestec
Ltd., Vevey/Raven Press, Ltd., New York © 1991.

Anemias

Calvin W. Woodruff

Department of Child Health, University of Missouri-Columbia School of Medicine, Columbia, Missouri 65203, USA

The history of the medicinal uses of iron goes back to the very beginnings of Western medicine, but it was only during this century that the concept of nutritional anemia emerged from the dark ages and became established scientifically. Most of the progress occurred with development of quantitative methods paralleling the progress of chemistry and flowered in the years since 1925. The heyday of chlorosis was the year 1850. To some, this disease was limited to pubertal females, and there was much dispute about the green color. Some authors even interpreted green to mean virginal since they believed that the disease was cured by marriage and pregnancy. The literature on chlorosis is vast and extremely confusing. The spectrum of opinion ranged from equal sex distribution and the constant presence of anemia to an anorexia-nervosa-like illness in adolescent females who may not be anemic or may respond to iron.

The subject will be reviewed in four major categories: methodology, iron deficiency, megaloblastic anemia, and other anemias. Initially, most of the work was done on adults, but the pediatric aspects emerged during the last 50 years of this fascinating century.

METHODOLOGY

By 1850, it was known that blood gives off oxygen when placed in an oxygen-free environment. In 1851, Otto Funk discovered hemoglobin, and Felix Hoppe-Seyler demonstrated its reversible affinity with oxygen in 1866. The first clinical method was that of W.R. Gowers in 1878. Varying dilutions of blood were compared with a single standard of colored glass based on a 1:100 dilution of normal blood.

In 1901, Haldane stated that there had been no satisfactory means of preparing a permanent and, at the same time, definite standard of color for making the comparisons. He pointed out that the colorimetric method is capable of giving extremely exact results, and that both the measurements and the color matching are just as accurate on a small scale as when large quantities of blood are used with the ordinary measuring instruments. He described a technique using carboxyhemoglobin as a more stable standard and defined *normal* as the concentration of hemoglobin that combined with 18.5 volumes % oxygen, 13.8 g/dL according to the latest available data.

Haldane presented replicate normals from both men and animals and showed that properly sealed standards did not change color over time. Each determination was expressed as oxygen-combining capacity, a percentage of normal on the hemoglobin scale, and again as a percentage of normal for the specific group. Unfortunately this excellent work was not generally applied clinically and many levels of oxygen saturation were used as 100% of normal. It would be almost another 40 years before hemoglobin values were universally reported as g/dL rather than % of normal.

According to Gray, the earliest cell count was done on November 16, 1851, by K. Vierordt and published the next year. The average of nine counts on himself was 5.174×10^6. In 1867, Duncan examined red cell size in chlorosis and stated: ''Altogether I have counted 40,000 cells in six cases, three sick and three well. Thereby I found approximately 20,000 for the sick and 20,000 [for] the normals. Since we are dealing with cases whose blood has a color intensity relative to the normal of 1:0.3, 1:0.31, and finally 1:0.37, I came to the conclusion, in the first case, that a reduced number of red cells would surely not be the only cause of the chlorotic color. I would take it to be far more definitely established that in chlorosis every single blood cell contains less pigment than is in the blood corpuscles of healthy individuals.''

At the turn of the century, the 4th edition of Richard C. Cabot's *Clinical Examination of the Blood*, based on 12,000 observations, had accumulated enough data for statistical analysis. It was noted that three-quarters of the blood counts were performed by the interns and that a blood count was routine on every admission to Massachusetts General Hospital.

His instructions for obtaining fresh blood show how much we have learned since 1901 about transmission of disease. ''Gently cleanse the lobe of the patients's ear with a damp cloth and then dry it. All vigorous rubbing or kneading is to be avoided. Attempts to sterilize the skin or to cleanse it with alcohol and ether are a waste of time. A small lancet or bayonet-pointed surgical needle may be used; a sewing needle gives more pain and draws less blood from a given depth of puncture. A steel pen, with one nib broken off, makes a good lancet. The needle need not be sterile. In several thousand blood counts made at Massachusetts General Hospital since 1893 the needles have never been sterilized and no signs of sepsis have been seen in any case.'' Several hemocytometers are described and four hemoglobinometers. The hand-operated Daland hematocrit machine is described, but the use of the hematocrit for determining the volume of the red cells was not advocated. It was said to be too noisy for office use and would be restricted to hospital laboratories! The high red counts in the newborn period and their gradual fall are noted, but no statistical data are presented. Only inanition is mentioned as a cause of secondary anemia in infancy.

L. Emmett Holt's *Diseases of Infancy and Childhood*, published in 1901, is lacking in normal values of a statistical nature. The first effort to establish normal values for infancy and childhood was that of Guest, Brown, and Wing in 1935. They had 1,070 samples on 615 infants from birth to 5 years. None of the infants had received supplemental iron. The hematocrit was included with the red cell count, and the hemoglobin determination and Wintrobe's indices were calculated. It was found that there was a bimodal distribution of mean corpuscular volume (MCV) between 1 and 2 years of age. The microcytosis at 18 months of age, which averaged $70\mu^3$, was noted, but there was no real definition of normal since there was at that time no independent evaluation of iron nutrition. An upper class group of 144 children had higher values than the rest. There was a suggestion that values of hemoglobin less than 10 g/dL might be low after 6 months. Only after independent measures of iron nutrition became available could age- and sex-specific normal values be determined.

IRON DEFICIENCY

Despite all of the confusion concerning the nature of chlorosis in the early nineteenth century, the use of Blaud's pills, often supplemented with a little arsenic, was almost universal. Each pill contained 320 mg of ferrous sulfate ($FeSO_4$) and a like amount of potassium carbonate (K_2CO_3)—64 mg of elemental iron per pill. The dosage was up to 770 mg of iron daily in adults. Despite the assumed formation of ferrous carbonate, the clinical results were excellent, and this pill remained the mainstay of treatment of anemia for nearly 100 years after its introduction in 1832.

In 1855, Bunge, having a great reputation, retarded further experimental approaches for 60 years because he believed, on rather scanty evidence, that animal cells could not synthesize hemoglobin from inorganic iron and that the pathophysiology of chlorosis was an emotionally derived inability to absorb organic iron. In 1893, Stockman showed an adequate hemoglobin response in chlorotic women to parenteral iron. This work was not recognized because the tide of opinion was that the effect of iron was non-specific in chlorosis. Some pediatricians, however, had a much clearer view of iron metabolism in early infancy. In June, 1911, John Howland (see p. 268, Fig. 1) read a paper on nutrition to the American Pediatric Society. "The salts of iron are, however, deficient both in human and especially in cow's milk. The large supply of iron present in the liver and other organs of the newlyborn may gradually be drawn on, and evidently is intended to be drawn on during the first year, but this deficiency of iron is one important reason why an exclusively milk diet should not be persisted in too long."

The modern era in iron deficiency, according to Wintrobe, began in 1925 with a report by Whipple and Robscheit-Robbins, showing that hemoglobin regeneration in phlebotomized dogs followed the oral administration of both iron and liver. They concluded that liver was more potent and, some time later, that the extra potency of liver was solely a result of its iron content. Using balance studies, Heath, Strauss, and Castle showed in 1932 that inorganic iron was incorporated into hemoglobin.

The balance technique continued to be used, and Reiman, Fritsch, and Shick showed in 1936 that replete subjects absorbed little iron and depleted subjects absorbed much iron, half of which appeared in the increased hemoglobin mass. Four years later, Hahn, working with Whipple's group and using the more elegant radioisotopic tracer techniques in dogs, showed that ''as the iron intake is increased the percentage absorption rapidly falls.''

By 1940, then, the pattern of hematologic development was outlined even if the range of normal or optimal values in infancy and childhood was not defined statistically, and the major facts about iron absorption and incorporation into hemoglobin were known. Also about this time there was a beginning of original pediatric work. A great deal of attention was paid to the factors causing variation in the hemoglobin level during the first year of life. In 1933, Helen Mackay used heel-prick blood and the Haldane standard of 13.8 g/dL as 100% but reported her data as hemoglobin values. Her data showed that breast-fed infants had higher hemoglobin values than formula-fed infants. A subsequent paper showed that the largest variable in determining the hemoglobin curve was the birth weight. The fall during the first week was attributed to hemolysis and was greater in the lighter infants. The fall between 1 and 3 months was attributed to decreased production, based on the low reticulocyte counts with evidence for compensation at 2–3 months of age. The rise between 3 and 6 months, greater in the red cell count than in the hemoglobin concentration, was preceded by removal of iron from the liver and spleen. A subsequent fall between 6 and 12 months correlated with the rate of growth and responded to the administration of iron. In retrospect, this careful and conscientious piece of work became a reference point for the refinement of our sense of normal and our criteria for the diagnosis of iron deficiency anemia.

Maternal factors were also the object of study. In 1933, Strauss followed the offspring of women who were quite anemic at the time of delivery and compared them to mothers with normal hemoglobin concentrations. At the end of the first year, the infants of the anemic mothers had significantly lower hemoglobin concentrations than the control group, although they had normal hemoglobin concentrations at birth and there was no obvious difference in feeding between the two groups. This anemia was prevented either by giving iron to the mothers during pregnancy or to the infants. The conclusions were generally accepted until later studies using serum ferritin to measure iron stores showed that there was a preferential transport of iron across the placenta that was not impaired by maternal anemia.

Perhaps one of the first textbooks on pediatric hematology was an article of 144 pages published 50 years ago by Josephs (see p. 270, Fig. 6) in *Medicine*, in which he reviewed exhaustively the literature of the previous 10 years. I shall quote two bits of wisdom from the writing of this thoughtful and critical pediatrician. ''It must be realized that the definitively proven facts concerning iron metabolism are few and that most of our supposed knowledge is inference that has been accepted as fact for so long that it is not appreciated any longer how much of it is not proved.'' There is a modern ring to this conclusion. Also ''The relation of a milk diet to anemia is very striking and has for at least 25 years been used as the starting point for theories of etiology of nutritional anemia.'' Even in 1989, this statement rings true and there is still controversy concerning all of the complex relationships between milk and iron deficiency anemia.

Deprivation of placental blood as a cause of iron deficiency in infants was the subject of a 1941 study by Wilson, Windle, and Alt. Infants whose umbilical cords were clamped immediately after birth had a lower mean corpuscular hemoglobin at 8 to 10 months of age than those whose cords were clamped after the placenta began to descend into the vagina. This study prompted a whole series of approaches over the next decades and it is still confusing to this author what are the ultimate facts and what is the most desirable obstetric practice!

At the end of the century under consideration, Clement Smith performed the first and perhaps the most elegant radioisotope study of iron in infancy, which was first reported at the May, 1950, meeting of the American Pediatric Society although not published for another 5 years. The infants of mothers who received ^{55}Fe during pregnancy were studied for more than 2 years. The quantity of transplacentally acquired iron was greater by some 40%–80% than could be accounted for by the circulating hemoglobin at birth, documenting the presence of stores in the tissues. The specific activity of the circulating hemoglobin was not diluted by exogenous iron until well after the age of 6 months. Even at 2 years of age, about half of the iron in these healthy infants had come across the placenta.

As chemical methods for determining iron in the serum became available, they were applied to pediatric material. Vahlquist published a monumental thesis in 1941 on the serum iron in infancy and childhood in which he described the developmental changes and those in various diseases. At that time, the iron-binding protein was not well characterized. Interpretation of all the serum iron findings was incomplete without this information, which was supplied by Hagberg in 1953.

Widdowson and Spray, using chemical analysis of premature and full-term stillborn infants, determined the concentration of iron in the whole body. They found that the concentration of iron was unchanged during fetal life, averaging about 70 to 80 mg/kg. The amount received by the fetus depended on its size. Some 4%–19% was in the liver and spleen, amounting to 11–51 mg at term. This observation emphasized the fact that the bulk of the iron in the newborn infant was in the circulating hemoglobin, 180–360 mg in six infants weighing over 3000 g.

In 1950, we knew that placental transfer of iron was related to the size of the fetus and that tissue stores were adequate for the first 6 months of life in the full-term infant. Dietary iron would be used when the stores were depleted. Blood loss was rarely considered a factor except for cord clamping practices and in the rapid expansion of the blood volume in preterm infants. Breast feeding was less likely to be associated with iron deficiency anemia than artificial feeding.

Today's perspective is that, in the United States, iron deficiency has become relatively rare, after a huge epidemic in the years 1950 to 1970, the result of both poor iron intakes and occult bleeding due to excessive intakes of fresh cow's milk. A hemoglobin concentration of 9 g/dL today is likely to precipitate a hematology consultation, while 30 years ago house officers were known to treat a microcytic anemia of 3.5 g/dL in the emergency room with intramuscular iron!

MEGALOBLASTIC ANEMIA

Ever since the study of bone marrow in infants began, a syndrome of dystrophy and "pernicious" anemia has been described, often with a sprue-like component. In reviewing the subject in 1926, Glanzmann referred to large numbers of cases in Germany between 1912 and 1915 and again in the post-war period. Many of these infants had been fed goat's milk and the name *goat's milk anemia* was often used. The association with scurvy was noted and he recognized that the anemia at least was not due to scurvy. He fed goat's milk to guinea pigs and found that they developed scurvy and an anemia of a vague character.

In 1935, Paul Gyorgy studied the pathogenesis of a case of goat's milk anemia and found no response to iron, copper, or ascorbic acid. There was a response to liver and to yeast, showing that the missing factor was unlike extrinsic factor. In 1942, Veeneklass updated thinking about the etiology of megaloblastic anemia in infants. He attributed to Matossi (in a dissertation in Zurich in 1928) the observation that goat's milk anemia was unknown in parts of Switzerland where the goats were kept outside and received fresh fodder the better part of the year, compared to areas where the goats were kept in dark stalls and rarely received fresh fodder. Most of his paper relates to the details of the transformation of the megaloblasts to normoblasts during treatment. He also pointed out the presence of leukopenia and thrombocytopenia.

The first major description of megaloblastic anemia in the United States was by Zuelzer and Ogden in the early 1940s. They described 25 infants from Detroit with megaloblastic marrow that responded to folic acid or to crude liver extract. Eleven of them did not receive an antiscorbutic and six had manifest scurvy. The anemia did not respond to ascorbic acid alone. Two infants were breast-fed by anemic mothers, one received goat's milk, and the rest were fed various formulas. Since they responded equally to folic acid and to liver extract, it was assumed that it was the folate in the liver extract that was effective, vitamin B_{12} not being known until 1948.

A comparable series from Italy was reported in 1946 by Amato in infants deprived of good nutrition during and after the end of the war. Shortly after this, Aldrich and Nelson showed that megaloblastic anemia was associated with the feeding of proprietary infant formula that did not contain ascorbic acid. All six of the patients in their series were on such a formula, unsupplemented by ascorbic acid in any form. They all had megaloblastic marrows and responded rapidly to liver extract. This work established beyond doubt the nutritional nature of this anemia and suggested strongly that both ascorbic acid and folic acid were involved in the etiology.

At about this time vitamin B_{12} appeared on the scene and was used by a number of workers in the treatment of megaloblastic anemia, with variable results. The present author was apparently the first to report responses to both folic acid and vitamin B_{12} in the same small series. Scurvy was still a common disease and not all of the cases were in infants fed proprietary formulas.

The relationship between folic acid and ascorbic acid in the pathogenesis of anemia was finally worked out by Charles May in monkeys, which have a dietary requirement for both these vitamins, as does the human. In the fall of 1950 he reported that 7.5 mg of folinic acid, a derivative of folic acid synthesized in the presence of ascorbic acid and probably the actual functioning cofactor, would produce a hematological response in the doubly deficient animal. In restrospect it is clear that milk diets unsupplemented with ascorbic acid did not contain enough folic acid to overcome the lack of conversion to folinic acid. Vitamin B_{12} proved to be occasionally successful as treatment suggesting that, as in pernicious anemia, there is an interrelationship with folic acid.

The formula industry responded to these findings by solving the technical problems of fortifying infant formulas with ascorbic acid, and megaloblastic anemia disappeared in infants fed these formulas, as did scurvy. Scurvy itself became a rare disease at about this time and megaloblastic anemia was seen only in segments of the population having great nutritional deprivation from socioeconomic causes.

OTHER ANEMIAS

Since the anemia of infection has been separated from other causes of microcytic, hypochromic anemia due to iron deficiency at the level of hemoglobin synthesis, there are no clearcut entities to discuss. It should be mentioned that pernicious anemia can occur in infancy and childhood and that the genetic variability in defects in vitamin B_{12} absorption and transport is now better known. Banti's syndrome and other entities, such as achlorhydria, described in earlier texts have virtually disappeared as causes of anemia.

CONCLUSION

The century beginning in 1850 showed the development of the tools of the hematologist in its first half and then a burst of understanding of the etiology of anemias following the discovery of the role of liver in the treatment of pernicious anemia in 1925. By 1950 many of the basic facts concerning iron deficiency were known but it was only later that statistically defined normal values could be based on independent measures of iron nutrition such as serum ferritin determinations. The use of isotopes was just beginning in 1950 and much has been learned about the absorption and metabolism of iron in infants in the last 39 years. The frequent use of iron-fortified formulas has prevented much iron deficiency, so that it is becoming rare in the developed world. Megaloblastic anemia continues to be found in depressed populations. The epidemic of this disease of 1947 has become an object lesson in the development of infant formulas that are truly complete and has taught us how important it is to monitor the use of any change in formulation to detect unsuspected interrelationships between nutrients.

History of Pediatrics 1850–1950, edited by
B.L. Nichols, A. Ballabriga, and N. Kretchmer.
Nestlé Nutrition Workshop Series, Vol. 22. Nestec
Ltd., Vevey/Raven Press, Ltd., New York © 1991.

Salt and Water Disorders

Jack Metcoff

*Department of Pediatrics, University of Oklahoma Health Sciences Center, Oklahoma City,
Oklahoma 73190, USA*

Science, Bronowsky said, is the "act of fusion" derived from the search for unity in hidden likenesses (1). Science is, above all, a process in constant flux, a way of thinking, the formulation of a problem that can be tested, the search for unifying phenomena, for hidden likenesses, for an explanation of the deviation from the expected. The process of science is the creative act. Science is the organization of our knowledge to command more of the hidden potential of nature. It rearranges the disordered events we observe and discovers a new order. The discovery of relationships and the fusion of hitherto unrelated events diminishes ignorance. Science is never static. Theories are proposed that contradict and replace other theories. New evidence supplants or supplements the old. Theories and beliefs once held and strongly defended may not be honored any longer. Science has only one absolute, the continuing search for truth. The boundaries of science are where the soluble meets the insoluble. The battleground is symbolic logic. According to C.P. Snow, science is the use of symbolic systems of thought to understand and control the natural world and to advance knowledge (2). Perhaps nowhere in the evolution of contemporary science does this interpretation find better application than in the story of salt and water disorders.

The story begins early in the morning of August 8th, 1831, when a man named Arnott, about 40 years old, was attacked by a disease closely resembling cholera and died at the end of 12 hours. He was a quarryman in decent circumstances, and resided at Pallion on the River Wear, about two miles from Sunderland. Starting in Bengal in 1826, the disease killed thousands in its relentless migration north through India, Persia, Russia to Moscow, and back through Poland, Scandinavia, Germany, and then to Britain where it reached Sunderland, Newcastle, and Edinburgh in 1831. Four thousand deaths occurred within a year in Great Britain. In Paris, 7,000 died in 18 days. After devastating western Europe, cholera spread to North America and, by the end of the year, had spread widely over the United States and Canada. Between one-third and one-half of those afflicted with the disease died. Ultimately deaths numbered in the millions. Almost every remedy known to medicine at that time was tried, without avail.

The first, unique chapter of the salt and water story was fashioned by three men unknown to each other. After months of collecting and subjecting samples of blood and feces from cholera patients to biochemical analysis, W.B. O'Shaughnessy (see p. 258, Fig. 1), appearing before the Westminister Medical Society in 1831, proposed the intravenous injection of highly oxygenized salts, namely nitrate or chlorate of potash (3). A week later, his brief note, published in the Lancet, described how "the blood had lost a large proportion of its water and of its neutral saline ingredients. The free alkali was often diminished or absent." Although similar observations had been made earlier by several others, O'Shaughnessy concluded that "all the salts deficient in the blood, especially the carbonate of soda, are present in large quantitites in the peculiar white dejected matters" (4). Modifying his opinion, he later recommended that solutions be prepared that contained sodium and chloride, as well as potassium salts and water. This solution was composed to simulate the quantities of salts found in each liter of cholera stool. Knowing that patients in the last stage of cholera could not take fluid by mouth, he recommended that 20–30 pounds of fluid be given by vein to a dying patient, an amount of fluid equivalent to the total amount of stool that had been lost. O'Shaughnessy's report, published on December 31, 1831, compared the results on the composition of blood and stool in cholera with normal values for blood and feces, previously published by Lecanu in France, and with values from patients with bilious diarrhea, and concluded that the ingredients greatly diminished in the blood of malignant cholera patients were present in the dejecta. Based on his observation, he proposed that "the addition of the quantities of salt and water found in the dejecta to the blood, in due proportion, would restore it to its normal constitution." O'Shaughnessy recognized that the loss of salt and water was an effect of the cholera, not its cause, but to that loss attributed the thickening and eventual obstruction of circulation of the blood, leading to gradual wasting, asphyxia and death.

On May 15, 1832, a letter "Injection of saline solutions in extraordinary quantities into the veins in cases of malignant Cholera" was communicated to the editor of Lancet from the Central Board of Health in London. The letter, written by Dr. Robert Lewin of Leith, stated:

> Sir, I perceived it to be my duty to let you know for the information of the Central Board of Health that the great desideratum of restoring the nature current in the veins and arteries, of improving the colour of the blood, and recovering the functions of the lungs of Cholera asphyxia may be accomplished by injecting a weak saline solution into the veins of the patient. To Dr. Thomas Latta of this place is due the merit of first having recourse to this practice. He has tried it in six cases, three of which I have seen and have assisted to treat. The most wonderful and satisfactory effect is the immediate consequence of the injection (5).

On May 23, Dr. Latta wrote to the Secretary of the Central Board of Health:

> Sir, my friend Dr. Lewin has communicated to me your wish for a detailed account of my method of treating Cholera by saline injection into the veins in which I now most willingly comply. . . . Before entering into particulars, I beg leave to premise that the plan which I've put in practice was suggested to me on reading in the Lancet the review of Dr. O'Shaughnessy's report on the chemical pathology of malignant Cholera, by which it appears that in the disease there is a very great deficiency both of the water and saline matter of the blood. Failing to obtain improvement by oral or rectal administra-

tion of water and salts . . . I at length resolved to throw the fluid immediately into the circulation. In this, having no precedent to direct me, I proceeded with caution. . . . The first subject of experiment was an aged female, on whom all the usual remedies had been fully tried. . . . She apparently had reached the last moments of her earthly existence, and now nothing could injure her—indeed, so entirely was she reduced, that I feared I should be unable to get my apparatus ready ere she expired. Having inserted a tube into the basilic vein, cautiously—anxiously, I watched the effects; ounce after ounce was injected but no visible change was produced. Still persevering, I thought she began to breathe less laboriously, soon the sharpened features and sunken eye, and fallen jaw, pale and cold, bearing the manifest impress of death began to glow with returning animation, the pulse, which had long ceased, returned to the wrist; at first small and quick, by degrees it became more and more distinct, fuller, slower, and firmer and in the short space of half an hour when six pints had been injected, she expressed in a firm voice that she was free from all uneasiness . . . her extremities were warm and her every feature bore the aspect of comfort and health. This being my first case, I fancied my patient secure, and . . . left her in charge of the hospital surgeons; but I had not been long gone ere the vomiting and purging recurring, soon reduced her to her former state of disability. I was not apprised of the event, and she sunk in 5-½ hours after I left her. . . . [Latta then described how he] dissolved from 2–3 gms of muriate of soda, 2 of subcarbonate of soda and 6 pints of water and injected it at temperature of 112 degrees Fahrenheit (6) (Fig. 1).

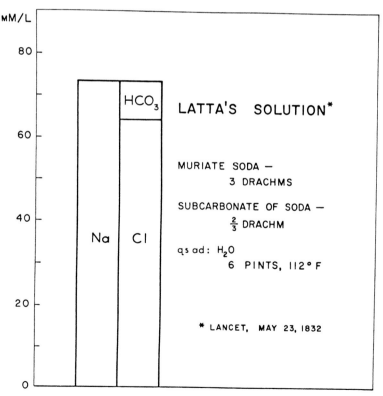

FIG. 1. The figure was constructed from Latta's description in *Lancet*, May 23, 1832.

Latta's remarkable experiment, as is so often the case, was not immediately appreciated (7). It remained for an anonymous editor of the *Lancet* to achieve the act of fusion that concluded this first great episode in the story of salt and water disorders. On June 2, 1832, reviewing the papers that had been published in the *Lancet* relating to O'Shaughnessy's observations and Latta's experiments, an anonymous writer said:

> Now when we contemplate the phenomena of Cholera, when we see the plump and vigorous limbs of youth and adolescence weaken in a few hours to the shrunk dimensions of emaciated old age, it is impossible not to conclude that not only has the blood lost much of its water, as chemistry has so satisfactorily ascertained, but that all of the living solids of the frame, its muscles, nerves, its vascular tunics and membranes, have been robbed of the bulk of fluids essential to the due discharge of their vital functions— to the preservation of their vital condition. The quantity of water to be replaced is therefore immense and bears no relation to the presumed quantity of blood which the human body naturally contains. . . . [Continuing] at length Dr. O'Shaughnessy's experiments have shown the deficiency of water and an occasional diminution of the salts in Cholera blood—having proved that its anatomical structure was preserved, and its capacity for aeration maintained, a more rational principle of treatment was pointed out. It was the necessary inference from these experiments that water *essentially* and salt, *contingently,* should be added to the blood before it could again discharge its functions. It was evident, as stated in Dr. O'Shaughnessy's reported experiments, that water could only be restored in two ways, by absorption or venous injection, and that in the cases in which the power of absorption was irretrievably lost, venous injection left the only hope of a cure. Dr. Latta, of Leith, has now for the first time carried this suggestion into effect. We thank him for the intrepidity, scientific zeal, and assiduity he has displayed. His example has been followed by Drs. Craigie and Macintosh of Edinburgh, and we entertain no doubt that the practice will be repeated all over Great Britain, as a last resource in the desperate cases which have baffled the ordinary methods of treatment and which otherwise would be abandoned to death. (8)

In the following week, numerous reports of the successful application of Latta's solution were published in the Lancet.

With the end of the epidemic, O'Shaughnessy's gift to medical science and Latta's experiments soon were forgotten. To Carl Schmidt, a chemical pathologist at the University of Dorpat, must be attributed the first detailed, complete analyses of the blood in cholera, published in 1850 (9). James L. Gamble (Fig. 2) in his paper on "The Early History of Fluid Replacement Therapy" converted Carl Schmidt's observations on the salt composition of blood serum to our now familiar terminology, expressing the components in milliequivalents per liter (10). The comparison of the values from cholera patients with blood serum values from normal patients, confirmed the results postulated 20 years earlier by O'Shaughnessy.

The story of salt and water disorders is, to paraphase the inimitable prose of James Gamble, like ancient Gaul divided in three parts: It evolves from a conception of the structure of the body fluids, and the regulation of their stability and volume. It is not possible to acknowledge all the observations that comprise our present picture of salt and water disorders. Rather I will attempt to identify a few observations that, in my opinion, provide the foundations on which contemporary therapeutic knowledge is built.

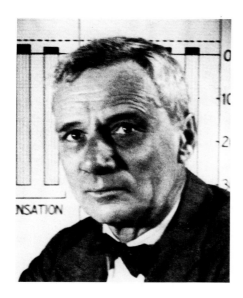

FIG. 2. James L. Gamble, Professor of Pediatrics, Harvard Medical School, Boston, MA. (Photograph by Jack Metcoff, M.D.)

The architecture that preserves the constancy of the environment surrounding the cells and tissues was conceived largely by Lawrence J. Henderson in his physical-chemical description of those components of the blood that are highly adapted to the functions of transporting carbonic acid and oxygen. Coupled with the parameters of the constant k, in the familiar equation describing the relation between carbonic acid (H_2CO_3), and its bicarbonate salt ($BHCO_3$), contributed by Hasselbach in 1909, Henderson proposed the now famous equation describing buffer base balance in his treatise *Fitness of the Environment* (11). The complete description of the carbon dioxide and oxygen dissociation curves in a single specimen of blood then required 135 cc and four investigators working as a team with modified Haldane and Barcroft tonometers. Henderson described an experiment in which "fairly complete information" was obtained by one investigator with only 30 cc of blood (12). Improvements in the blood gas apparatus by Van Slyke (13) permitted Howland and Marriott in 1916 (14) and Schloss and Stetson in 1917 (15) to describe the acidosis of diarrhea in infancy and its correction by the administration of sodium bicarbonate solution. By the first two decades of this century, the rationale for repair of salt and water disorders, then principally cholera and diarrhea, had been demonstrated but still not widely accepted or practiced. In Boston, infants with "summer cholera," i.e., diarrhea, were quarantined on a ship in Boston harbor, "the Boston Floating Hospital," which daily set out to sea with its load of sick babies, returning at nightfall with only one or two survivors for every 10, the others having been duly buried at sea. By the end of the second decade of this century, salt solution was given subcutaneously, or when an urgent need for larger volumes was evident, intraperitoneally, and glucose solution was given simultaneously, intravenously. This "set of fluids" supported structure and volume, and was still common therapy as late as the early 1940s.

Although the practical components for treating the most common abberrations of salt and water were known by 1920, the adaptations by which the kidney, lungs, and cellular fluids defended body composition were not understood. It fell to four epileptic children who were fasted for therapeutic reasons for 15 days and the precisely formulated, simple observations of James L. Gamble, G.S. Ross, and F.F. Tisdall at Johns Hopkins Hospital to introduce the benefits of clinical research, which is the sequel in our story (16). They cited the analyses of cat and fresh human muscle and of blood plasma by Kramer and Tisdall for the relative concentrations of the four fixed bases (sodium, potassium, calcium, and magnesium) and conjectured that the source of the fixed base appearing in the urine of these children during fasting was an adaptation to conserve the structural composition of the extracellular fluids through an economy of base excretion. The interdependence of the values of the structural factors in blood was illustrated by a diagram representing the acid-base composition of the plasma in terms of 0:1 normal acid or base per 100 cc (Fig. 3). They proposed that "The acid substances which are carried bound in the plasma are being conveyed for excretion in the urine." The fixed base was spared by substituting ammonia and titratable acid (base economy) accompanied by structural change in the acid-base balance of the extracellular fluid, characterized by the observed reduction of bicarbonate, and attributed to accumulation of ketoacids from catabolism of protoplasm. A large part of the concentration of bicarbonate found in plasma was considered a consequence of the recession of chloride. The conservation of fixed base, largely sodium, accompanied by a large reduction of chloride, clearly showed

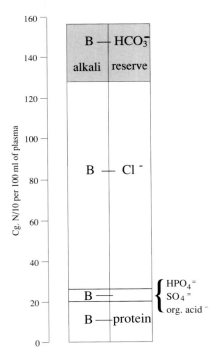

FIG. 3. The first "Gamblegram." From reference 17.

the separate control of the excretion of sodium and chloride. In this early paper, Gamble recognized the important contribution of the intracellular fluid to the preservation of the base economy. By 1932, Gamble with Allen Butler and Charles McKhann had documented the nature of intracellular fluid loss in diarrheal disease (17).

In 1935, Daniel C. Darrow (see p. 115, Fig. 2) with Herbert Yannet, focused on the changes in the distribution of body water that accompanied the change of extracellular electrolytes (18). The restoration of osmotic equality, achieved rapidly, was shown to depend upon the restricted extracellular position of sodium and prompt transfer of water across the cell to produce osmotic equilibrium between the two compartments. Their observations provided a practical basis for repair of hypo- and hypertonicity. Soon afterward, Darrow recognized that potassium, the major structural cation of the intracellular fluid, comprised a significant portion of the salt lost in the diarrheal stools of infants, thus extending studies of stool composition in diarrhea that had been described 30 years earlier by Holt, Courtney, and Fales (1915) (19). By determining the retention of potassium, sodium, and water during recovery from severe diarrhea (which was assumed to correspond with the interval during which it occurred) Darrow estimated the number of days over which infants with diarrhea accumulated the deficits of water, sodium, and potassium at various caloric intakes (20). The balance studies led to investigations of tissue composition that clarified the effect of water and electrolyte disturbances on the composition of the intracellular fluid (21). By 1946, the evidence indicated that potassium chloride, added in limited quantities to solutions containing sodium chloride, sodium lactate, glucose, and water should achieve simultaneous repair of the intracellular and extracellular deficits (22). Dr. Gamble's admiration of the then daring addition of potassium to the intravenous fluid, reminiscent of O'Shaughnessy and Latta, resulted in the famous sobriquet "daring Daniel" (10). Darrow's solution rapidly became a staple of parenteral fluid therapy, and the role of potassium in clinical disturbances of body fluid physiology was established (23).

It is sometimes difficult to maintain perspective, but in the therapy of salt and water disorders it is fitting to recall that Latta's solution, conceived by O'Shaughnessy, reduced mortality in the most severe cases from nearly 100% to 50%–60%. Better understanding of blood and stool losses in such disorders, improvement in technology for analyses, and equipment for delivery of fluids, supplemented by knowledge of the germ theory of the disease, further reduced mortality to about 30%–50%, where it remained until the first decade of this century. As practical methods for dealing with acidosis evolved following the work of Henderson, Howland, and Van Slyke, and the use of ample quantities of sodium chloride, sodium bicarbonate, and water, preceded by infusion of a small amount of blood to support the circulation, became the commonly accepted mode of therapy, only 8–10 infants out of 100 died from severe diarrheal dehydration. Improvements in fluid therapy resulting from Darrow's recognition of the changes induced in the intracellular as well as the extracellular fluids and of the osmotic adjustments that followed, further reduced mortality from severe diarrheal dehydration by another 5%–6% to the present state in which only 1–3 of 100 infants dehydrated from diarrhea is lost. Daniel Darrow had the creative mind, the habit of truth and the sense of human dignity, all qualities that Bronowsky's brilliant essay described as illuminating the deepest meaning of science. That essay profoundly moved Darrow, and I treasure the copy he gave me.

In his Harvey Lectures, Gamble quantified the components of the water exchange and defined the minimal water requirement under conditions of fasting and thirsting for water to remove solute (24). These studies, carried out during the Second World War, were designed to determine the minimal requirements of water and food to support castaways for a limited time on a raft at sea. In parenteral fluid therapy, glucose solution is used to cover water expenditure and to provide some energy. But studies on the life raft ration showed that glucose provided additional physiological services that contributed to the conservation of body fluids; thus, 100 g glucose was found to provide enough energy to achieve maximum sparing of body protein. The losses of extracellular and intracellular water incidental to fasting and breakdown of protoplasm with loss of protein were reduced by half. In the course of these experiments, rather unexpectedly, glucose was found to provide an additional service by sparing sodium excretion and thereby reducing the renal water requirement for removal of solute.

The enormous body of knowledge, gathered with great effort by so many and fused by the creative imagination of a relatively few, succinctly and elegantly summarized in Gamble's syllabus (25) is now effectively employed for repair of salt and water disorders all over the world. But there are several sequels to the story. Among these is the role of the kidney in the regulation of body fluids (see pp. 113–131). I shall not here review the regulation of the *milieu interior* by the kidney, worked out and taught to us by Homer Smith (26) (see p. 117, Fig. 4), but I will comment only briefly on its role in the conservation of volume. The kidney is a most intelligent organ. We have seen how well it manages to conserve fixed base by substituting dispensible cations. Still, the kidney can become confused when acutely confronted by large loads of sodium chloride, which rapidly expand extracellular volume, and responds by removing potassium instead of sodium, at the expense of intracellular volume. The opposite situation occurs when a load of potassium is given. This was first recognized by von Bunge in 1873 (27). It intrigued Dr. Gamble, who recognized the significance of the inverse relation of sodium and potassium in the management of fluid replacement therapy. More refined understanding of how the kidney effects this exchange of cations has emerged in the last quarter century, much of it attributable to the experiments of Smith, Robert Berliner, Robert Pitts, and their associates on Na-K exchange in the nephron. Conservation of volume, however, is limited by the ability of the kidney to conserve water while removing solutes by elaboration of a maximally concentrated urine. The load of solute and the rate of glomerular filtration determine the quantity of water required for removal of excess solute. As the amount of water needed for removal of a given amount of solute increases, the ability of the kidney to conserve and defend volume becomes more limited. At any level of filtration, reducing the solute load reduces the amount of water required to remove it (25). When kidney disease impairs glomerular filtration, body fluid can be conserved by reducing the solute load, but, when the diet contains an amount of salt in excess of water that can be made available from the glomerular filtrate for its removal, edema occurs.

Another limitation of volume control is imposed by the insensible loss of water through skin and lungs. The infant is vulnerable because of a relatively large surface to mass ratio. The fever and increased respiratory rate that often accompany many illnesses contribute to the disadvantage of being small (25). In newborn infants, especially premature, the loops of Henle and proximal tubules are short relative to glomerular size. Henry Barnett and his associates demonstrated that the solute deposited in the interstitium of the kidney, derived from metabolism of the limited amount of protein in the diet of the neonates, has not yet achieved sufficient concentration to permit maximum concentration of urine (28). The inexperienced kidney of the small infant does a remarkable job to reduce the expanded volume with which it is born, described by Friis-Hansen (29), by excretion of a dilute urine. It cannot, however, defend against loss of water from sources it cannot control, e.g., excessive salt intake, insensible water loss, or diarrhea, because of the limited ability to achieve a maximally concentrated urine.

The final sequel concerns body composition. Like science, body composition is not static but is constantly changing. This is exemplified in the growth of the infant. The evolution of our knowledge of the composition of the intracellular fluids began with the whole body chemical analyses that Camerer and Soldner derived from five infants dying at birth from obstetric trauma between 1900 and 1903 (30). To McCance and Widdowson belongs the credit for systematically relating the observations of the excretion of salts and water to the changes in body composition with growth (31). They determined the chemical anatomy of nutrients, including salt and water, in major organ systems of the body from early fetal life to birth and during infancy. They fused their observations of body composition, growth, and renal adaptation to enhance understanding of the interdependence of growth, structure, function, and environment on adaptation of the whole organism.

Finally, it seems appropriate to acknowledge our great debt to the technologies that facilitated measurements of salt and water, thereby allowing prompt, practical identification of structural deviations in the chemical pathology of the body fluids using very small quantities of blood that could be obtained safely from infants. The first practical flame photometer was constructed from a wooden box, a Bunsen burner, and the glass lids of jars used for home canning, by Wallace about 40 years ago, from a design proposed by Befry, Chappell, and Barnes in 1946 (32) (Fig. 4). Wallace then was at Children's Hospital in Boston and responsible for Dr. Gamble's metabolic unit. A few years later, Ernest Cotlove, a research fellow of Gamble and Wallace, developed the simple, rapid electrochemical system for quantification of chloride, displacing the time-consuming, standard titrametric procedure. The freezing-point depression apparatus to quantify solute concentration was superseded by the vapor pressure osmometer, which requires only a drop of blood and few seconds to measure solute concentration. Later, Anderson and Astrup developed instrumentation to measure the partial pressure of CO_2 in a drop of blood, combined with direct determination of hydrogen ion concentration by a glass electrode, which

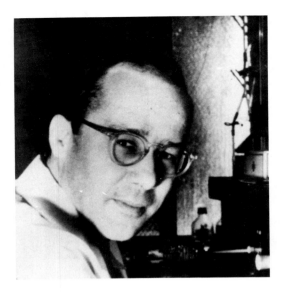

FIG. 4. William Wallace and the first flame photometer, which he built. Circa 1948. (Photograph by Jack Metcoff, M.D.)

permitted computation of the bicarbonate content and the relative quantities of the base excess (33), representing the cationic equivalent of the buffering anions. The buffer-base concept was originally described by Singer and Hastings, who measured bicarbonate content and pH but computed pCO_2 (34). Where technology is limited, and venous infusions are precluded, the knowledge gained in this century now permits rational construction of fluids containing salts, water, and glucose to achieve rehydration by the oral route in infants with diarrheal dehydration (35), completing the therapeutic circle begun more than 150 years ago.

I shall conclude on a note of admiration for James Gamble and Daniel Darrow and the few clinicians and scientists who rearranged the disordered events others had observed and discovered a new order. In a constant search for unity, they found the hidden likenesses; they achieved that act of fusion. Gamble, in particular, through a symbolic system of thought, conveyed these discoveries to us with clarity and elegance. Our contemporary concepts of salt and water disorders are greatly indebted to his genius.

REFERENCES

1. Bronowski J. Science and human values. Harper, New York, 1956.
2. Snow CP. *The two cultures and the scientific revolution.* Cambridge: Cambridge University Press, 1963.
3. O'Shaughnessy WB. Proposal of a new method of treating the blue epidemic cholera by the injection of highly oxygenized salts into the venous system. *Lancet* 1831;1:366–71.

4. O'Shaughnessy WB. Experiments on the blood in cholera. *Lancet* 1831;1:490.
5. Lewin R. Injection of saline solutions in extraordinary quantities into the veins in cases of malignant cholera. *Lancet* 1832;2:243–4.
6. Latta T. Relative to the treatment of cholera by the copius injection of aqueous and saline fluids into the veins. *Lancet* 1832;2:274–7.
7. Central Board of Health, London. Letter of queries addressed to Drs. Lewin and Latta. *Lancet* 1832;1:281–2.
8. Anonymous. Editorial. *Lancet* 1832;1:284–6.
9. Schmidt C. *Charakteristik der epidemischen Cholera gegenuber verwandten transudation sanomalien.* Liepzig, 1850.
10. Gamble JL. Early history of fluid replacement therapy. *Pediatrics* 1953;11:554–67.
11. Henderson LJ. *The fitness of the environment.* Macmillan, New York: 1913.
12. Henderson LJ. *Blood. A study in general physiology.* (Silliman Lecture). New Haven: Yale University Press, 1928.
13. Van Slyke DD, Neill J. Determination of gases in blood and other solutions by vacuum extraction and manometric measurement. *J Biol Chem* 1924;61:523–73.
14. Howland J, Marriott WMcK. Acidosis occurring with diarrhea. *Am J Dis Child* 1916;13:309–25.
15. Schloss OM, Stetson RE. The occurrence of acidosis with severe diarrhea. *Am J Dis Child* 1917;13:218–30.
16. Gamble JL, Ross GS, Tisdall FF. The metabolism of fixed base during fasting. *J Biol Chem* 1923;57:633–95.
17. Butler AM, McKhann CF, Gamble JL. Intracellular fluid loss in diarrhoeal disease. *J Pediatr* 1933;3:84–92.
18. Darrow DC, Yannet H. The changes in the distribution of body water accompanying increase and decrease in extracellular electrolyte. *J Clin Invest* 1935;14:266–75.
19. Holt LE, Courtney AM, Fales HL. The chemical composition of diarrheal as compared with normal stools of infants. *Am J Dis Child* 1915;9:213–24.
20. Darrow DC. Retention of electrolyte during recovery from severe dehydration due to diarrhea. *J Pediatr* 1946;28:515–40.
21. Darrow DC. Body fluid physiology: Relation of tissue composition to problems of water and electrolyte balance. *N Engl J Med* 1945;233:91–7.
22. Govan CD Jr, Darrow DC. The use of potassium chloride in the treatment of the dehydration of diarrhea in infants. *J Pediatr* 1946;28:541–9.
23. Darrow DC. Body fluid physiology: The role of potassium in clinical disturbances of body water and electrolyte. *N Engl J Med* 1950;242:978–83.
24. Gamble JL. Physiological information from studies on the life raft ration. *Harvey Lecture Series* 1946–7;42:247–78.
25. Gamble JL. *Chemical anatomy, physiology and pathology of extracellular fluid. A lecture syllabus.* 6th ed. Cambridge, Mass: Harvard Univ Press, 1954.
26. Smith HW. *The kidney. Structure and function in health and disease.* New York: Oxford University Press, 1951.
27. Von Bunge G. Ueber die Bedeutung des Kochsalzes und das Verhalten der Kalisalze in menschlichen organismus. *Z Biol* 1873;9:104.
28. Edelmann CM, Barnett HL, Troupkou V. Renal concentrating mechanisms in newborn infants. Effects of dietary protein and water content, role of urea, and responsiveness to antidiuretic hormone. *J Clin Invest* 1960;39:1062–9.
29. Friis-Hansen B. Changes in body water compartments during growth. *Acta Paediatr Scand* 1957;Suppl 110:1–68.
30. Camerer W, Soldner JR. *Die chemische zusammer setzung des neugeborenen. Z Biol* 1900;39:173; 1900;40:529; 1902;43:1; 1903;44:61.
31. McCance RN, Widdowson EM. Mineral metabolism of the foetus and newborn. *Br Med Bull* 1961;17:132–6.
32. Befry JW, Chappell DG, Barnes RB. Improved method of flame photometry. *Indust Engin Chem* 1946;18:19–24.
33. Anderson OS, Engle K, Jorgenson E, Astrup P. A micromethod for determination of pH, carbon dioxide tension, base excess and standard bicarbonate in capillary blood. *Scand J Clin Lab Invest* 1960;12:172–6.

34. Singer B, Hastings A B. An improved clinical method for the estimation of disturbances of the acid-base balance of human blood. *Medicine* 1948;27:223–42.
35. Sack R, Santosham M, eds. *Perspectives in oral rehydration therapy.* Proceedings of a Symposium, Washington, New York: Biomed Information Corp, 1986.

DISCUSSION

Dr. Waterlow: The First International Sanitary Conference was held in Paris, in 1851. The question was whether there should be quarantine for cholera. The British delegation was against it because it interfered with trade, and they justified their hostility to the idea by saying that cholera was really a good thing. It purged the bad elements in society—the thieves, ruffians, and the poor (1).

Dr. Guesry: I was fascinated by the description of the rehydration of patients suffering from cholera in 1832. When did it become clear that rehydration could be achieved orally by adding glucose to the solution?

Dr. Metcoff: It was tried in 1831 and 1832 but the patients vomited the fluid and the idea was abandoned for more than a century. It was tried again in a cholera epidemic in the 1960s in what was then East Pakistan, now Bangladesh, as a supplement to intravenous rehydration. Articles began to appear from other developing regions in the late 1960s, and in the 1980s there has been a resurgence of interest in oral rehydration therapy in the developed countries as well as in the Third World.

Dr. Finberg: O'Shaughnessy was about 22 years old when he wrote the letters you referred to. As far as I can tell he never practiced medicine, because he joined the British Raj in India where he served as an administrator and engineer, developing the telegraph system across the subcontinent. He was knighted and eventually retired to England. In the British *Dictionary of National Biography,* you will find no mention about his contribution to the treatment of dehydration. Thomas Latta died a year after his heroic adventure. There is only an occasional reference to him in the medical literature. So what was the most important therapeutic intervention in the history of medicine was unnoticed by the world of learning.

The first scientifically designed oral hydration solutions were produced in Baltimore in 1945 by Dan Darrow and Harold Harrison and were used in Baltimore and New Haven. These gave rise to commercial solutions, although they did not become popular until the work of Phillips on cholera drew attention to the importance of early oral hydration.

Dr. Klish: There has recently been a resurgence of interest in the question of oral refeeding in mild to moderate diarrhea. There have been many recent papers showing that aggressive refeeding in acute diarrhea may be beneficial. However, the first paper supporting this view was written by Chung and Viskarova in 1949. Darrow felt strongly enough about the paper to write a postscript, and, although he did not attack the authors, he appeared to belittle them. I have felt that that postscript was responsible for pediatrics having to wait 20–30 years before refeeding of diarrhea became an acceptable practice.

Dr. Stern: One problem in rehydrating infants in the early 1930s was the difficulty in finding adequate veins. Allen Ross, my chairman at McGill, told me the story of how Sam Karelitz first suggested using a vein in the scalp for this purpose, and how he (Ross), Clement Smith (who died recently) and Sam Karelitz, who were interns together at the time, put it into practice. For the first 6 months after they started doing this, they used to sit beside the infant with their fingers on the needle, until one of them, I do not know who, decided that you could put a piece of tape over the needle and go away and leave it.

Dr. Visakorpi: We have already heard about the European origins of American pediatrics, but we should not forget that after the Second World War the development of modern European pediatrics owed much to American influence. James Gamble was one of the most influential teachers and taught many European scientists. My own teacher, Nilo Hallman, was one of these. He brought modern pediatrics (including the new advances in the treatment of fluid and electrolyte disturbances) to Finland in the difficult years after the war. This was very important considering the high infant mortality at that time.

REFERENCE

1. Howard-Jones N. The scientific background of the International Sanitary Conferences, 1851–1938. *WHO Chron* 1974;28:159–71.

History of Pediatrics 1850–1950, edited by
B.L. Nichols, A. Ballabriga, and N. Kretchmer.
Nestlé Nutrition Workshop Series, Vol. 22. Nestec
Ltd., Vevey/Raven Press, Ltd., New York © 199

Energy Metabolism

Paul R. Swyer

Department of Pediatrics, University of Toronto, and The Research Institute, Division of Neonatology, The Hospital for Sick Children, Toronto, Ontario M5G 1X8, Canada

To put the history of energy metabolism in its proper perspective, it is necessary to deal briefly with the period before 1850, because the discoveries of the late seventeenth and early eighteenth centuries were the essential bases for the phenomenal progress made between 1850 and 1950. There are four fairly distinct eras. The first, or *Pre-scientific Era*, lasted to about 1773 AD when oxygen was discovered, ushering in the *Scientific Era*. This lasted until 1840–1850, when the *Physiological Era* began and with which I shall mainly be concerned. Finally, around 1950–1960 we entered the *Modern Molecular Biological Era*.

In the late Pre-Scientific Era there were some surprisingly accurate forecasts concerning the connection between respiration and metabolism. Galenos (131–201 AD), Greek physician to the Roman Emperor, Marcus Aurelius, described his theory of Three Pneumas (Spirits)—*Psychikon* (brain), *Physikon* (liver), and *Xotikon* (heart). He postulated transfer of some vital substance from the air in the lungs to the *Xotikon* in the heart that was then necessary for the renewal of the *Physikon* and *Psychikon* and predicted that one day this vital substance in the air would be discovered. It took almost 1500 years before Robert Boyle (1627–1691) showed that air was necessary for animal life and his contemporary, John Mayow (1643–1679) demonstrated the simultaneous extinction of both an animal and a candle in a closed vessel, speculating that they both removed similar particles from the enclosed air (1).

These discoveries laid the foundation for the Scientific Era of energy metabolism, which began in 1774 with the identification of "dephlogisticated air," or oxygen, by Joseph Priestley (1733–1804) and independently and simultaneously by C.W. Scheele, a Swedish chemist (2). Priestley also recognized the connection between combustion and the evolution of animal heat. At Priestley's suggestion, Adam Crawford (1788) (3) constructed a combustion calorimeter to measure the heat evolved when "pure" and "inflammable air" (oxygen and hydrogen) were burned together or when living animals were placed within. The heat evolved was deduced by measuring the increase in temperature of a known volume of water in a surrounding jacket insulated with eiderdown. This apparatus embodied the principle of direct calorimetry. Antoine Lavoisier (1743–1794) subsequently characterized this "pure" gas of Priestley as the element, oxygen, dismantling the complicated and erroneous *Phlogiston* theory.

Lavoisier's experiments proved the equivalence of chemical energy and animal heat energy in compliance with the First Law of Thermodynamics. They initiated the application of physico-chemical principles to the investigation of the quantitative relationships between the macronutrients ingested, gas exchange, and the evolution of energy as heat.

Lavoisier and the mathematician, Laplace (1780), examined the comparative heat production of fed animals and of direct combustion of food, using an ice calorimeter in which the heat produced in each process is measured by the amount of ice melted (4). They formulated the unitary theory of oxidation in which they postulated that the chemical reactions of burning and production of animal heat were similar. These reactions involved the combination of oxygen with organic substance and the formation of carbon dioxide in precise proportions. In 1784, Lavoisier made the first measurements of respiratory gas exchange. The experiment was elegant in its simplicity. A guinea pig was introduced into a bell jar through a mercury seal and the mercury level noted. After a period of about 10 hours, the new level was noted and the animal was rescued. A small piece of sodium hydroxide was then introduced to absorb the carbon dioxide, and the level again recorded after aligning the mercury inside and outside the jar. In this way, both the oxygen consumed and the carbon dioxide (CO_2) produced by the animal were measured. Essentially this is the principle of closed circuit indirect calorimetry.

Lavoisier and Laplace also conducted experiments in small animals and man. The results were outlined briefly in a letter from Lavoisier to Black in Edinburgh in 1790 (5) in which it was stated that energy production varied inversely with external temperature and was increased by exercise and during the digestion of food. These are all still valid observations. Lavoisier's work was of the greatest importance to nutritional science as it rendered possible the quantitative study of biological energetics. Lavoisier was guillotined on May 8, 1794 during the French Revolution.

At the beginning of the nineteenth century, John Dalton (1766–1844) conceived the Atomic Theory of Matter that offered a simple explanation for the laws of chemical combination. Between 1845 and 1850, fundamental laws of physics were discovered by Mayer, Helmholtz and Hess, defining the interrelationships of chemical energy, heat, and mechanical energy, and the fundamental Laws of Thermodynamics were formulated. These discoveries were the essential bases for further progress in the understanding of energy metabolism.

During the 1840s, two chemists, J. B. A. Dumas and Justus von Liebig (see p. 50, Fig. 1), had advanced a theory of the physiology of nutrition (later called metabolism) asserting that valid conclusions could be drawn from the comparison of the substances taken up by the living organism with the substances isolated from the tissues, fluids, and excreta. These hypotheses were contested by Claude Bernard (1813–1878), who by 1860 (6) had accepted that all animal heat originated from the combustion of organic substances. He objected on the ground that such analyses told nothing about the intermediate steps by which nutrients were converted to tissue and excretory components. Nevertheless this lead was pursued in both France and Germany, and the stage was then set for the Physiological Era beginning around the mid-nineteenth century.

There ensued a most productive period in which the evolution of animal heat was related to macronutrient oxidation and thermoregulation by means of increasingly sophisticated direct and indirect calorimetry. Max Rubner (1854–1932) was the most important contributor to this era.

In 1849, Regnault and Reiset (7) described an improved apparatus for measuring gaseous exchange according to the closed circuit principle with a circulating air pump and a CO_2 absorber but dependent on changes in pressure in the system for measurement. Other modifications of the closed circuit principle are shown in Fig. 1. This was closely followed by the open circuit apparatus of Pettenkofer and Voit in 1862 (8) in which CO_2 and water vapor production were measured, and later O_2 uptake. Other modifications followed, for example, the Douglas bag, which was a valved, semi-open system depending on analysis of expired gases, and which permitted mobility in the subject.

Bernard had argued against Lavoisier's assumption that animals are "chemical furnaces," because such explanations disregarded the neural control of body temperature. It is therefore to the credit of the German school of physiologists, initiated by Carl Voit and led by Max Rubner, that they followed up this lead from Lavoisier's discoveries and, without becoming bogged down in the complexities of intermediary metabolism, they concentrated on the nutrient input and the end-product excretion. In this approach, the heat produced by the animal was related to the oxygen uptake and the amount and chemical nature of the food and excreta, and/or ex-

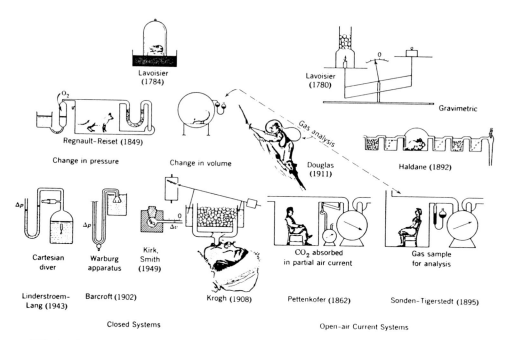

FIG. 1. Closed and open circuit indirect calorimeters. (Reproduced with permission from Kleiber, ref. 1, p. 63. Copyright © 1961, John Wiley & Sons, Inc.)

pired CO_2. Thus the study of energy metabolism by indirect calorimetry was pursued using the new knowledge of the fundamental nature and relationships of energy and matter.

The scientific "genealogy" of the eighteenth- and nineteenth-century schools of nutritional research is given by Graham Lusk (9). Max Rubner (see p. 274, Fig. 2) was the outstanding contributor in the second half of the nineteenth and early twentieth century. He was born in Munich in 1854. At first the pupil of Carl von Voit, he was later associated with Pettenkofer, Lusk, Atwater, and others during the laboratory's most productive period. From 1885 to 1891, he was Professor of Hygiene at Marburg, where he built his own calorimeter and demonstrated that the first Law of Thermodynamics applied to living organisms. In 1891, he moved to the Chair of Hygiene in Berlin, succeeding Koch. In 1909, he assumed the Chair of Physiology in Berlin until he retired in 1924 at the age of 70. He died in 1932. His book *The Laws of Energy Consumption in Nutrition* was translated into English (10) in 1968.

Rubner's major contributions have been summarized as follows:

1. Confirmation of the Isodynamic Law that protein, carbohydrates, and fat may replace each other in accordance with their heat producing value (Table 1).

2. Delineation of the energy value of the major macronutrients.

3. Formulation of the law of constancy of metabolic rate in relation to surface area (Table 2).

TABLE 1. *Rubner's isodynamic law*

	Equivalent energy value	Rubner's standard value (kCal/g)
Fat	100 g	9.3 Fat
Starch	232 g	4.1 Carbohydrate
Cane sugar	234 g	
Dry meat	243 g	4.1 Protein

From ref. 10.

TABLE 2. *Rubner's surface area law*

	Weight (kg)	kCal/m$_2$
Pig	128.0	1078
Human	64.0	1042
Dog	15.0	1039
Rabbit	2.3	917
Goose	3.5	967
Chicken	2.0	943
Mouse	0.018	1188

From ref. 10, after E. Voit.

4. Demonstration of the validity of the law of conservation of energy using a combined direct/indirect calorimeter.

5. The concept of the Specific Dynamic Effect of food.

6. The discovery of non-shivering thermogenesis.

7. The first precise work on evaporative and convective-conductive heat loss of the animal body.

8. The discovery of the critical (thermoneutral) temperature of animals.

9. The first quantitative work on the effect of insulation (fur, hair, clothing) on animals and men exposed to a cold environment.

A major purpose of this workshop that is the subject of this book is to honor the memory of Max Rubner by the dedication of a Library in his name. I would like to quote the concluding paragraph in a tribute by his distinguished colleague, Graham Lusk, (11). Lusk too died following surgery before this tribute appeared.

> I have tried to draw in its varied aspects a picture of a great scientific man. It is happy to think that we may all learn many lessons from the life of such a man as Max Rubner. For the whole of the individual life in health and in disease depends upon the energy metabolism. And the whole of the life of the state, for weal or for woe, depends upon the ability to furnish sufficient Calories in food to maintain the individuals composing the state.

The first half of the twentieth century saw the application of improved apparatus, especially in the study of the metabolism of newborn and premature infants. Rubner was again prominent, with Heubner and Langstein (12–15) in a series of studies of newborn metabolism from 1898 to 1915. John Howland (see p. 268, Fig. 1), whom we are also honoring, performed studies on infants between 1910 and 1913 (16–19) using a combined direct/indirect calorimeter to obtain information on newborn energy metabolism, its relation to surface area, and the comparability of indirect and direct calorimetry. He confirmed the applicability of Rubner's Surface Law to growing infants.

Also at this time, Benedict, following construction of his indirect calorimeter in 1912, collaborated with Talbot and others in metabolic investigations of 94 infants (20).

In 1924, Graham Lusk (21) (see p. 52, Fig. 2) produced a table from data obtained by Zuntz and Schumberg (1901) (22) on the energy value of a liter of oxygen when various mixtures of carbohydrate and fat were oxidized. This table is still in use for calculation of the relative proportion of carbohydrate and fat oxidized when the protein-free respiratory quotient (RQ) and the amount of oxygen consumed per gram of substrate oxidized are measured.

During the latter part of the first half of the twentieth century, many able investigators (among whom were Gordon, Levine, and their collaborators who published a series of studies from 1929 to 1940 [23]) added to our knowledge of energy metabolism in infancy. Day and co-workers (24), also in a series of studies, made fundamental observations on thermoregulation and energy metabolism in relation to environmental temperature for prematures, using both indirect and direct calorimetry. Karlberg in 1952 (25), using a closed circuit incorporating Krogh's spirometer (26,27), examined 60 infants according to their "standard metabolism", i.e., resting metabolic rate. The results confirmed those of Benedict-Talbot (20) and Gordon-Levine (23). Karlberg also measured surface area by an electrical capacitance method and was able to construct a regression equation of metabolic rate on surface area rather than relating metabolic rate to body weight, body weight and length, or formulas designed to predict metabolic rate from some function of weight and/or length.

Reference standards for metabolism are still controversial, and there seems no entirely satisfactory reference standard that will take account of differences in body composition, proportion, age, and sex.

Work in the first half of the twentieth century (Brody (28), Kleiber (1)) indicates that metabolic rate in homeotherms, in size from mice to cattle, is more nearly proportional to the ¾ power of body weight than to its ⅔ power (analogous to surface area) as stated by Rubner's Surface Area Law. Under standard conditions, the metabolic rate of adult homeotherms is $292.9 \text{ kJ} \cdot \text{body weight}^{3/4}$ per day. The difference between the two standards is shown in Fig. 2. Nevertheless as a close approximation of the physiological rules relating energy metabolism to body size, Rubner's insight has proved most valuable in comparative studies of energy metabolism over the years.

The mid twentieth century marks the beginning of the modern period of study of energy metabolism. Rapid and accurate gas analysis by physical methods and min-

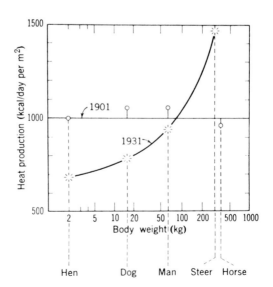

FIG. 2. Heat production in relation to body weight for different sized species illustrating the differences in energy production as described in 1931 compared with earlier findings in 1901 when Rubner's surface area law was the conventional wisdom. (Reproduced with permission from Kleiber, ref. 1. Copyright © 1961, John Wiley & Sons, Inc.)

iaturization allied to computerized measurement techniques enable study of pathological states in prematures, newborns, infants, and adults, that had hitherto been technically impossible. Thus the derangements in energy metabolism in conditions such as sepsis, trauma, obesity, and extreme prematurity are being explored.

The advent of radio- and stable-isotope technology has offered new tools for the understanding of intermediary energy metabolism (29,30) and the interconversion of the basic nutrients. Non-invasive methods of chemical imaging by nuclear magnetic resonance are throwing new light on the energy metabolism of inaccessible sites such as the brain (31).

Thus are we building on the solid foundation laid for us by such as Lavoisier, Rubner, Howland, and our other illustrious forebears since the discovery of oxygen in 1780.

REFERENCES

1. Kleiber M. *The fire of life*. New York: John Wiley & Sons, 1961.
2. Weeks ME. Discovery of the elements, 6th ed. Easton, Pennsylvania: *J Chemical Education,* 1956.
3. Crawford A. *Experiments and observations on animal heat and the inflammation of combustible bodies,* 2nd ed. London, 1788.
4. Lavoisier AL, Laplace P de, Mémoire sur la chaleur. *Mémoires de l'Academic Royale,* 1780a:355. *Oeuvres de Lavoisier,* vol 2. Paris: Imprimérie Impériale, 1862:283. *Ostwald's Klassiker 40,* Leipzig: Wilhelm Engelmann, 1892.
5. Report of the British Association for the Advancement of Science. Edinburgh, 1871:189.
6. Bernard CC. *Leçons sur la chaleur animale*. Paris: JB Baillière and Son, 1856.
7. Regnault V, Reiset J. Récherches chimiques sur la respiration des animaux. *Ann Chim Phys* 1849, Ser 3;26:299–519.
8. Pettenkofer M. Uber die Respiration. *Ann Chemie Pharm* 1862;Suppl 2:1–52.
9. Lusk G. *The science of nutrition.* 4th ed. 1928, Philadelphia: WB Saunders Co, 1928:12.
10. Rubner M. *Die Gesetze des Energieverbrauchs bei der Ernährung.* Leipzig: Franz Deuticke, 1902. Translated and reprinted by the United States Army Research Institute of Environmental Medicine, Natick, Massachusetts, 1968.
11. Lusk G. Contributions to the science of nutrition. A tribute to the life and work of Max Rubner. *Science* 1932;76:129–35.
12. Rubner M, Heubner O. Die Ernahrung Naturliche eines Sauglings. *Z Biol* 1898;36:1.
13. Rubner M, Heubner O. Die Kunstliche Ernahrung eines Normalen und eines Atrophischen Sauglings. *Z Biol* 1899;38:315.
14. Rubner M, Heubner O. Zur Kenntniss der naturlichen ernahrung des Sauglings. *Z Exp Pathol Therap* 1904/05;1:1.
15. Rubner M, Langstein L. Energie- und Stoffwechsel zweier Frühgeborener Säuglinge. *Arch Anat Physiol* 1915;39:39.
16. Howland J. The metabolism, directly determined, of healthy children during sleep. *Proc Soc Exp Biol Med* 1910/11;8:63.
17. Howland J. Der Chemismus und Energieumsatz bei Schlafenden Kindern. *Z Physiol Chem* 1911;74:1.
18. Howland J. Direct calorimetry of infants, with a comparison of the results obtained by this and other methods. Transactions of the 15th International Congress on Hygiene and Demography, Washington 1912, vol 2;438.
19. Howland J, Dana AT. A formula for the determination of surface area in infants. *Am J Dis Child* 1913;6:33.
20. Benedict FG, Talbot FB. *The physiology of the newborn infant. Character and amount of the katabolism.* Publication 233, Carnegie Institute of Washington, 1915.
21. Lusk G. Analysis of the oxidation of mixtures of carbohydrate and fat. *J Biol Chem* 1924;54:41–2.

22. Zuntz N, Schumberg L. *Studie zu einer Physiologie des Marsches.* Berlin: A. Hirschwald, 1901:361; quoted in (20).
23. Gordon HH, Levine SZ, Deamer WC, McNamara H. The respiratory metabolism in infancy and in childhood. 23. Daily energy requirements of premature infants. *Am J Dis Child* 1940;59:1185.
24. Day R, Curtis J, Kelly M. Respiratory metabolism in infancy and childhood. 27. Regulation of body temperature in premature infants. *Am J Dis Child* 1943;65:376–98.
25. Karlberg P. Determinations of standard energy metabolism (basal metabolism) in normal infants. *Acta Paediatr Scand (Suppl 89)* 100;41:151.
26. Krogh A. The respiratory exchange of animals and man. London: Longmans, Green, 1916:40.
27. Krogh A. Ein Respirationsapparat zur klinischen Bestimmung des Energieumsatz des Menschen. *Wien klin Wochenschr* 1922;35:290.
28. Brody S. *Bioenergetics and growth, with special reference to the efficiency complex in domestic animals.* New York: Reinhold Publishing Corp, 1945.
29. Sauer PJJ, Van Aerde JEE, Pencharz PB, *et al.* Glucose oxidation rates in newborn infants measured with indirect calorimetry and (U^{13}C)-glucose. *Clin Sci* 1986;70:587–93.
30. Winthrop AL, Jones PJH, Schoeller DA, *et al.* Doubly labelled water method for measurement of energy expenditure in post surgical infants. *Surg Forum* 1986;37:88–90.
31. Leonard JC, Younkin DP, Chance B, *et al.* Nuclear magnetic resonance: an overview of its spectroscopic and imaging applications in pediatric patients. *J Pediatr* 1985;106:756–61.

DISCUSSION

Dr. Holliday: I came across a passage in Homer Smith's book in which he alludes to the change in glomerular filtration rate during the first two years of life and showed that, when expressed in terms of weight to the 0.75 power, the values diverged considerably from those expressed in terms of surface area. We have tended to be preoccupied by surface area laws when in fact surface area should be regarded as a convenient biological resolution with a fair amount of variation around it. You can't expect the law to hold up rigorously and specifically, especially in the first 2 years of life.

Dr. Swyer: It is simple-minded to think that we can describe such a varied proportionality of the body in terms of a single function.

Dr. Waterlow: I find it extraordinary that the metabolic processes of oxygen turnover and protein turnover that are vital to life proceed at different rates per gram in animals of different sizes, nevertheless all sum up to just what is needed to keep the body at the right temperature.

Dr. Swyer: I believe this is due to the physics of heat transfer—the requirement to move the quantity of the heat necessary for internal metabolism to the exterior in the most effective way, given the circulatory system, the insulation, the demands of the environmental temperature and the activity of the animal.

Dr. Friis-Hansen: If one tries to compare energy metabolism to any body measurement, one should take body composition into account. For example, the liver, heart, and brain together amount to only about 10% of the body weight, but between them they account for two-thirds of the energy expenditure. So if you compare different animals of a different size you should be aware that if you use weight as a factor the result obtained will depend on the internal distribution of the organ weight.

Dr. Swyer: The relatively large size of the brain in relation to the rest of the body in small-for-gestation infants is thought to be the reason for their hypermetabolic states. People have tried to refer their metabolic standards to lean body mass or to total body potassium content, but it may not be helpful to try to find a single standard of comparison.

History of Pediatrics 1850–1950, edited by
B.L. Nichols, A. Ballabriga, and N. Kretchmer.
Nestlé Nutrition Workshop Series, Vol. 22. Nestec
Ltd., Vevey/Raven Press, Ltd., New York © 1991.

Amino Acid Requirements

Selma E. Snyderman

Department of Pediatrics, New York University Medical Center, New York City, New York 10016 USA

The role of nitrogen in the diet was first recognized by Magendie in 1816 after a series of studies in dogs; those fed either fat or carbohydrate died after a few weeks, but those fed only cheese or eggs survived indefinitely. As early as 1840, differences in the quality of protein were appreciated by Liebig (1) who found that animals fed a gelatin diet died of starvation. Some 20 years later, Voit (2) performed the first precise nitrogen balance studies and together with Bishop demonstrated that a gelatin diet did not permit nitrogen equilibrium in dogs (3). Individual amino acids were first prepared by hydrolysis of proteins in 1820, but knowledge of their existence seems to have preceded this, since in 1810 Wollaston (4) found cystine in urinary stones of patients suffering from cystinuria. The existence of quantitative differences in the amino acid content of different proteins was demonstrated in the beginning of this century. The importance of this finding was first appreciated by Willcock and Hopkins who were able to prolong the survival of mice fed zein by adding tryptophan to the diet (5). Several years later, Osborne and Mendel (6) supplemented zein with lysine as well as tryptophan and obtained good growth in mice, thereby demonstrating that these two amino acids were essential. This led Mendel (7) to formulate the concept that the law of the minimum applied to amino acids. He stated, ''growth is limited by the supply of each essential amino acid. It matters not whether this is exhibited as such or in the guise of protein; in either case the law of the minimum is exemplified.''

The discovery of threonine in 1935 made it possible for Rose to use mixtures of amino acids to determine which were required by the growing rat. This was soon followed by similar studies in young men (8). At approximately the same period of time, L. Emmett Holt, Jr. used casein hydrolysates prepared to be deficient in a single amino acid in order to study amino acid requirements (9). He demonstrated that tryptophan, lysine, and methionine were essential for young adult men, and obtained a quantitative requirement for tryptophan. His study of arginine deficiency was of special interest. He performed sperm counts, since this tissue is high in arginine, and found that the count fell when arginine was omitted and returned to control values when it was reintroduced. However, the usual sign of amino acid deficiency, negative nitrogen balance, did not develop. This finding was not confirmed by Rose who regarded arginine as unessential. The relationship of arginine to spermatogenesis is still controversial. The studies of Rose in young men were soon followed by a series of similar studies in young women (10). These resulted in requirement values that were somewhat higher than those of men, and this difference has been attributed to different criteria for setting the minimum requirements.

The first study of an amino acid requirement in an infant was performed by Levine and his group in 1943 (11). They concluded that tyrosine could not replace phenylalanine in the diet of the premature infant. Just after 1950, L. Emmett Holt, Jr. (Fig. 1) initiated a series of studies at New York University Medical Center that explored a number of facets of amino acid requirements of infants. These studies lasted for the next decade. The first were designed to determine quantitative requirements. These studies utilized a mixture of L-amino acids in the same proportion as they occur in human milk. Carbohydrate was provided by dextrimaltose and fat by corn oil. This was supplemented by a vitamin and mineral mixture. The intake of the amino acid under study was either removed or greatly reduced and then increased in a stepwise fashion until the rate of weight gain and the amount of nitrogen retained were equivalent to that of the control period when the full quota of the amino acid was included. Rate gain and nitrogen retention on the control diet were equal to that on the evaporated milk formula that was the standard infant feeding at that time. The subjects were all male infants whose age ranged from 2 weeks to 4 months at the onset of the studies. Several had been premature infants but were several months of age and growing well. Quantitative requirements for each of the essential amino acids were obtained (12).

Our attention was next directed to two amino acids whose essentiality had been disputed: histidine and arginine. The original studies of histidine in adults had shown that it was not essential; however it had been found to be essential for a num-

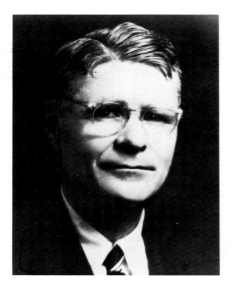

FIG. 1. L. Emmett Holt, Jr. (b. 1895). Photograph courtesy of United States National Library of Medicine.

ber of growing animals. Our studies definitely established it as a dietary essential for the human infant: weight gain was either reduced or absent, and the amount of nitrogen retained fell whenever it was removed from the diet. In addition, a rash developed that had the appearance of infantile eczema although it was pathologically different (13). The protocol of one of these studies is illustrated in Fig. 2. We have data suggesting that histidine continues to be essential for at least the first year, but we do not know how much longer it is required. Recently there has been some information suggesting that histidine is at least partially essential for the adult. When deprived of histidine for more prolonged periods than in the original studies, subjects became anemic and this is probably the result of the high histidine content of hemoglobin. The adult uremic patient also seems to require histidine.

Our studies of arginine did not show any evidence of an obligatory requirement (14). Growth continued at the same rate and the retention of nitrogen continued to be good when arginine was omitted for as long as a month. However, there are more recent data showing a need for this amino acid under specific circumstances. It cor-

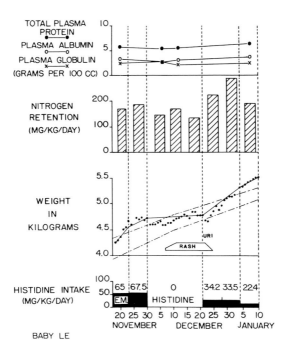

HISTIDINE REQUIREMENT OF THE NORMAL INFANT

FIG. 2. Protocol of a study of the histidine requirement. Weight gain and nitrogen retention were reduced when histidine was omitted, however, the rash responded promptly to the reintroduction of histidine. This infant's histidine requirement was between 34 and 22 mg/kg/day.

rected the hyperammonemia that was a frequent occurrence during the early days of complete intravenous alimentation. This hyperammonemia resulted from the use of excessive amounts of amino acid solutions and it was compounded by the amino acid imbalance of these solutions. However, there is still the possibility that arginine may be at least partially essential if other criteria (such as an increase in orotic acid excretion) are used. In addition, arginine is a dietary essential for those with inherited defects in the urea cycle.

Several interesting findings arose from our studies of the amino acid requirements of premature infants. They showed that all the requirements were significantly higher than those of the full-term infant: approximately one-third more was required. Quantitative techniques for amino acid analyses of small samples of blood became available at this time, and they were included as a criterion of adequacy. The smallest amount that was adequate for the full-term infant was the lowest amount that was studied in the premature. The results obtained on the effect of amino acid intake on blood concentrations were of special interest. There was a significant drop in blood concentration whenever the intake was insufficient according to the other two parameters. However, in a number of instances, the intake that permitted normal weight gain and nitrogen retention did not bring the blood concentration back to normal. More of the amino acid was required.

Two amino acids not required by the full-term infant are, at least partially, essential for the premature infant. The requirements for tyrosine and cystine are the result of delayed development of the enzymes necessary for their synthesis from their precursors, phenylalanine and methionine. This may explain the variability of the results obtained. One-half of the infants studied on cystine-free diets had some evidence of deficiency. The studies on the tyrosine requirement did not include determination of nitrogen retention. Eight were studied on tyrosine-free diets. There was impairment of weight gain in five and a fall in the blood tyrosine level in six.

Some of the studies on the requirements of the full-term infants were repeated with blood amino acid concentrations. They again show that more of the amino acid is needed to bring the blood level back to normal than is required to permit normal weight gain and nitrogen retention.

Amino acid requirements, when expressed in terms of body weight, drop precipitously during the first months of life and then more gradually during childhood. They are directly related to the growth rate. The relationship of amino acid requirement to age and growth rate is illustrated in the Fig. 3. It compares our requirements for premature and full term infants with those obtained in the Japanese investigations (15) in 12- to 14-year old boys and a composite obtained from several investigations in adults. All of these studies were similar in that the nitrogen moiety of the diet was a mixture of amino acids.

The marked fall in amino acid requirements during the early months of life is also seen in the treatment of children who have inborn errors of amino acid metabolism. If the amino acid requirement is defined as the minimum sufficient for tissue repair, specific functions, and normal growth, then the requirement is similar for the normal and the affected individual of the same age. The only difference is in the handling of the excess above the requirement. The normal individual can take care of

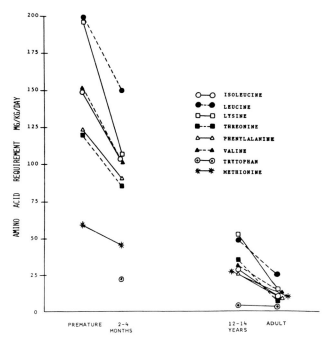

FIG. 3. The relationship of age to amino acid requirements expressed in terms of body weight.

an excess at least several times the requirement without any elevation of plasma level. In the patient with an anomaly of amino acid metabolism, any intake above requirement will be manifested as an elevation of the plasma concentration as a result of a disturbance in the pathway that maintains homeostasis in the normal individual. Thus, information about amino acid requirements can be obtained if the effort is made to maintain the plasma concentration in the normal range by alterations in intake. Figure 4 shows the phenylalanine requirement of 150 phenylketonuric children. The phenylalanine requirement of this group between 2 and 4 months of age is similar to the requirement in the normal infant. There was a similar finding from a study of twenty infants with histidinemia.

One of the concerns of the requirement studies based on mixtures of amino acids is that the requirement may be different if natural protein is used. The results with the phenylketonuric and histidinemic children are somewhat reassuring since a casein hydrolysate provided the nitrogen moiety for most of these children, and natural protein, usually milk, was used to provide the phenylalanine or the histidine requirement. In addition, there are studies by Fomon *et al.* (16), who employed soybean or milk as the protein source and derived figures for essential amino acid intake. They ''assumed that the requirements of protein and essential amino acids of these infants was not greater than the amount consumed.'' These figures, with the exception of methionine, fall within the same range as those obtained with the mixture of amino acids as the nitrogen source. Filer et al. (17), in a more recent study

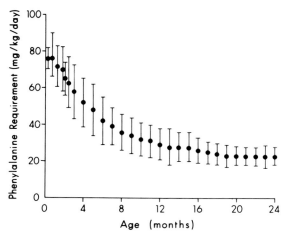

FIG. 4. The phenylalanine requirement of 150 phenylketonuric infants. This illustrates the rapid fall in requirement during the first months of life (mean and 1 standard above and below the mean).

using casein hydrolysate and casein and whey mixtures, found the tyrosine requirement of premature infants to be similar to that found by our group.

Another study (18), which we undertook for a different purpose, also supplied information about the validity of these requirement figures. The intake of cow's milk protein was gradually reduced while maintaining a constant caloric intake until there was decline of weight gain and a reduction of nitrogen retention. At this point there were two possibilities: a deficiency of unessential nitrogen, or a deficiency of one or more essential amino acids. Addition of unessential nitrogen as either glycine or urea resulted in the resumption of normal weight gain and nitrogen retention. This occurred at intakes of milk protein of 1.1 and 1.3 g/kg. Calculation of the intake of essential amino acids contained in these quantities of protein gives values very close to those obtained with the amino acid diets.

In 1950, there were a number of problems concerning the understanding of amino acid requirements, and there are probably even more today. The degree of individual variability in these requirements is still largely unknown, the majority of studies having been performed in a small number of individuals from a homogeneous population. Agencies such as Food and Agriculture Organization/World Health Organization (FAO/WHO) (19) have attacked the problem by suggesting the use of various factors, but exact data are not yet available. Another criticism of studies using amino acid mixtures has been the suggestion that more energy is required than with whole protein; however, this has not been consistent and has never really been evaluated in a systematic way. There are still no studies in children between 2 and 12 years of age and none during adolescence; these are very important gaps in knowledge. There is a need for more information about the requirements of very small premature infants, those weighing less than 1000 g at birth—a group with a very low survival rate until recently.

The majority of requirement figures have been determined after only a short period of study. There is little information about whether they are still valid for prolonged periods of time. Practically all studies have employed nitrogen balance as the criterion of adequacy, but sources of error inherent in the techniques, especially after infancy, have been pointed out by a number of observers. There is a need for better criteria for establishing requirements; plasma amino acid concentrations may be more reliable. The use of kinetic studies that measure the rate of whole-body protein turnover has been proposed (20), but thus far, in adults, they have shown that greater amounts of amino acids are required to maintain a high rate of whole-body protein turnover than are required to meet other criteria of adequacy. However, at present we have no information about whether there is a nutritional advantage to a higher turnover rate.

There have been very important advances in our knowledge of amino acid requirements during the past 100 years. The coming years should bring more precise figures for all age groups and a better understanding of their relationship to amino acid and protein metabolism and to all phases of nutrition.

REFERENCES

1. Liebig J Von. *Animal chemistry or organic chemistry in its application to physiology and pathology* (trans. W. Gregory). London: Taylor and Walton, 1842.
2. Voit G. Ueber die verschiedenheiten der eiweissaersetzung beim hungern. *Z Biol* 1866;2:308–65.
3. Bischoff TLW, Voit C. *Die Gesetze der Ernahrung des Fleischfressers*. Leipzig: Winter, 1860.
4. Wollaston, WH. On cystic oxide, a new species of urinary calculus. *Phil Trans B* 1810;100:223–30.
5. Willcock EG, Hopkins FG. The importance of individual amino acids in metabolism. Observations on the effect of adding tryptophan to a dietary in which zein is the sole nitrogenous constituent. *J Physiol (Lond)* 1906;35:88–102.
6. Osborne TB, Mendel LB. Amino acids in nutrition and growth. *J Biol Chem* 1914;17:325–49.
7. Mendel LB. Nutrition and growth. *Harvey Lectures* 1914–1915;10:101–31.
8. Rose WC. The amino acid requirements of adult man. *Nutr Abst Rev* 1957;27:631–47.
9. Holt LE, Albanese AA. Observations on amino acid deficiencies in man. *Trans Assoc Am Physicians* 1944;58:143–57.
10. Swendseid ME, Dunn MS. Amino acid requirements of young women based on nitrogen balance data. II. Studies on isoleucine and on minimum amounts of eight essential amino acids fed simultaneously. *J Nutr* 1956;58:507–17.
11. Levine SZ, Dann M, Marpes E. A defect in the metabolism of tyrosine and phenylalanine in premature infants. 3. Demonstration of the irreversible conversion of phenylalanine to tyrosine in the human organism. *J Clin Invest* 1943;22:551–62.
12. Snyderman SE. The amino acid requirements of the infant. In: Nyhan WL, ed. *Heritable disorders of amino acid metabolism*. New York: John Wiley and Sons, 1974.
13. Snyderman SE, Boyer A, Roitman E, Holt LE, Prose PH. The histidine requirement of the infant. *Pediatrics* 1963;31:786–801.
14. Snyderman SE, Boyer A, Holt LE. The arginine requirement of the infant. *J Dis Child* 1959;97:192–5.
15. Nakagawa I, Takahashi T, Suzuki T, Kobayashi K. Amino acid requirements of children: nitrogen balance at the minimal level of essential amino acids. *J Nutr* 1964;83:115–8.
16. Fomon SJ, Thomas LN, Filer LJ, Anderson TA, Bergmann KE. Requirements for protein and essential amino acids in early infancy. *Acta Paediatr Scand* 1973;62:33–45.
17. Filer LJ, Stegink L, Chandramouli B. Effect of diet on plasma aminograms of low birth weight infants. *Am J Clin Nutr* 1977;30:1036–43.
18. Snyderman SE, Holt LE, Dancis J, Roitman E. Boyer A, Balis ME. Unessential nitrogen: a limiting factor for human growth. *J Nutr* 1962;78:57–72.

19. FAO/WHO/UNV. *Expert Consultation on Energy and Protein Requirements.* Tech Rept Ser No 724. Geneva: World Health Organization, 1985, pp. 1–206.
20. Young VR, Bier DM. A kinetic approach to the determination of human amino acid requirements. *Nutr Rev* 1987;45:289–98.

DISCUSSION

Dr. Visakorpi: What is your opinion about taurine? Should we add it to infant formulas?

Dr. Snyderman: I did not mention taurine since it is not a component of protein and the need for it is still in doubt. It has been difficult to demonstrate a deficiency state in children although minor manifestations of taurine deficiency have been observed in children maintained on intravenous therapy for prolonged periods. Young infants who are fed milk formulas tend to have lower blood taurine levels than breast-fed infants, and this has been construed to be an indication for taurine supplementation.

Dr. Waterlow: Kwashiorkor varies in its characteristics in different parts of the world. When it became possible to measure plasma amino acid concentrations, Dr. Emmett Holt got the idea that perhaps these differences were due to different amino acids being limiting in different countries. He made a collaborative study of plasma aminograms in several countries including Jamaica, in which we took part (1). The patterns were all the same, the only differences being related to their severity. This showed that the limiting factor was total nitrogen and not any single amino acid.

Dr. Hansen: I take issue with Professor Waterlow. We used the same type of balance study described by Dr. Snyderman and, when using maize or corn as the sole source of protein, we got different effects on nitrogen balance, blood chemistry, and growth from those in infants on milk protein diets. I believe it is not the total nitrogen intake but the amino acid quality of the protein.

Dr. Snyderman: There were changes in the plasma amino acids of the kwashiorkor children we studied. However, the changes were similar in children from various areas of the world who received different diets and were similar to those of children fed low protein diets of good quality. In the milder cases, alterations included elevation of certain of the nonessential amino acids, especially glycine and alanine, and some reduction in the essential amino acids. All the amino acids were decreased in the more severe cases. The most striking decrease was in the branched-chain amino acids, while phenylalanine and lysine tended to fall the least.

The fact that the changes in plasma amino acids were similar, despite the different types of protein ingested, led us to believe that total nitrogen was the first limiting factor. They were observed in infants fed on limited amounts of good quality protein who were, at the same time, receiving an adequate caloric intake.

REFERENCES

1. Holt LE, Snyderman SE, Norton PM, Roitman E, Finch J. The plasma aminogram in kwashiorkor. *Lancet* 1963;11:1343–8.

History of Pediatrics 1850–1950, edited by
B.L. Nichols, A. Ballabriga, and N. Kretchmer.
Nestlé Nutrition Workshop Series, Vol. 22. Nestec
Ltd., Vevey/Raven Press, Ltd., New York © 1991.

Marasmus

John D. L. Hansen

*Department of Pediatrics and Child Health, University of the Witwatersrand,
Johannesburg, South Africa*

DEFINITION AND NOMENCLATURE

In the 1850–1950 era, wasted, emaciated, or marasmic infants had various clinical names attached to them such as the *hypothrepsie,* or *dystrophy,* of the French and German texts. Some authors, for example, Marriot (1923) (1), Marfan (1930) (2), and Finkelstein (1938) (3), classified their cases according to the severity of the wasting of body tissues, and others such as Czerny and Keller (4) proposed an etiological classification. It is confusing for those accustomed to the classifications of the modern day. Kerpel-Fronius, the well-known Hungarian pediatric investigator who bridged the pre- and post-1950 eras, has joined, in his book *The Pathophysiology of Infantile Malnutrition,* the old and the new nomenclature, *protein energy malnutrition* (5). He has pointed out that the terminology used in pediatrics to describe malnourished states is so rich as to provoke confusion. He found that the great wealth of early clinical information pubished by the German and French pediatricians at a time when infantile malnutrition was still frequent in Europe has been ignored. The contradictions in the terminology of the 1850–1950 era was rooted in regional differences, age of weaning, local foods, and the prevalence of infections. Problems of nomenclature arose because of the variable degrees of wasting, the unsatisfactory definition of the severity of malnutrition, and the misunderstandings that occurred when marasmus was defined only by the loss of subcutaneous fat and the absence of edema. Kerpel-Fronius classified the various types of malnutrition in the following way:

1. Hypoalbuminemic forms:
    i. Edematous
        a. Kwashiorkor
        b. Mehlnährschaden
    ii. Hypoalbuminemic forms without edema
2. Dry forms without hypoalbuminemia:
    i. Underweight (dystrophic) infants
        a. Stationary stage
        b. Repairing stage, with retardation in height—stunted infants

   ii. Marasmus (atrophy)
      a. Moderately severe
      b. Severe forms
  iii. Severest form in young infants aggravated by diarrhea and dehydration. This is the athrepsia, or *dekomposition,* of the classic texts of pediatrics.

This classification assists the identification of the malnourished children described in various case reports, articles, and books of the 1850–1950 time period. This chapter is confined to the non-edematous forms of malnutrition.

A description of the clinical signs of what is now called *marasmus* is given in a speech by Charles Dickens at a fund-raising dinner for the Hospital for Sick Children on February 9, 1858 (6). After enumerating the tens of thousands of children who died because of poverty and sickness, he described a tour of the worst-lodged inhabitants of the old town of Edinburgh. In one of the most wretched dwellings "there lay, in an old egg box, which the mother had begged from a shop, a little feeble, wasted, wan sick child. With his little wasted face and his little hot worn hands folded over on his breast and his little bright attentive eyes looking steadily at us." By 1950, marasmus resulting from poverty and sickness had become very rare in Europe and North America and was largely a problem of the developing countries. But it had been a major problem in all developed countries and countries affected by war and famine throughout the latter part of the nineteenth century and the first half of the twentieth. The causes of marasmus were similar wherever it occurred—lack of hygiene, infection, overcrowding, ignorance, illiteracy, and poverty, or low living standards (5).

CLINICAL DESCRIPTIONS OF MARASMUS

The American textbook, *Abt's Pediatrics* (1924) (7), describes marasmus under the heading "atrophy or decomposition," stating that it is a severe nutritional disturbance characterized by emaciation and weakening of the body. The temperature is subnormal, the pulse is slow, and breathing irregular. Various acute and chronic infections, malignant diseases, and blood diseases may be followed by marasmus. In most cases, it occurred gradually following a succession of nutritional disorders. Abt considered that underfeeding played a causal part in its etiology, aggravated by diarrhea and the therapeutic error of reducing food intake in the treatment of diarrhea. The English textbook, *Sick Children,* by Paterson (1947) (8) states that out of 100 cases of marasmus, 84 were underfed. These textbook descriptions of marasmus approximate our current understanding. However, different views of the pathogenesis were held at the time. Finkelstein considered the condition to be dependent upon abnormal chemical processes in the intestines, and that death was caused by loss of water and salt from the body (7). Czerny believed that atrophy was due to a low assimilative capacity for fat. Malabsorbed fatty acids were thought to combine with the alkalis of the body tissues, and the potassium and sodium salts were lost as soap in stools (7). There was agreement that the most severe and quickly progressing forms appeared in connection with enteral infections (5). The clinical signs were so striking that Parrot (1877) (9), Marriot (1923) (1), Marfan (1930) (2) and Finkelstein (1938) (3) described this clinical entity under the name *athrepsia*, or *decomposition*. It was one of the scourges of the hospitals. Kerpel-Fronius (5) quotes Marfan, writing in 1930, as saying that he had seen in his long career only three recoveries from "geniune" athrepsia. Kerpel-Fronius, in linking this unfamiliar terminology with modern thought, describes the clinical picture in one sentence: "diarrheal dehydration superimposed on marasmus of a young infant suffering a great acceleration of wasting of somatic tissues" (5). Certainly all writers considered diarrhea as a major complication of marasmus and that hospitals were a typical source of diarrheal disease in a time before pathogenic bacteria could be identified. Marfan warned pediatricians not to admit marasmic infants to the hospital because they die there in athrepsia (2). Henoch, as quoted by Peiper (1958) (10), gave similar advice to his successor Heubner (1894) in the famous Charité Clinic in Berlin.

Currently, marasmus is diagnosed when the weight is ≤60% of the 50th percentile, National Center for Health Statistics (NCHS) standards. This definition as suggested by Jelliff (11) has general acceptance, especially since the publication of the Wellcome classification in 1970 (12). Kerpel-Fronius writes in 1947 that, on the basis of prewar literature, if the degree of wasting reaches 35% to 40% of the average body weight, recovery is impossible (13). Marfan (2) emphasized the importance of the thinning of the skinfolds and a sequence of loss of fat first from the abdomen, then from the trunk, then from the extremities, and finally from the face. When pinching up a skinfold on the abdomen, it is found that the subcutaneous fat is entirely gone, according to Marfan's expression "one has between the fingers something like a piece of taffeta."

In 1948, Waterlow published the monograph, *Fatty Liver Disease* (14). In this he distinguished between his cases of "fatty liver disease" and those who were undernourished but had no evidence of liver damage. The clinical manifestations of the second group were failure of growth and loss of body fat and resemblance to the condition known in Europe as infantile atrophy, athrepsia, or marasmus. This was an important description of marasmus in a tropical country and drew the clinical distinction between marasmus and kwashiorkor. His cases of marasmus were mostly below 60% expected weight for age.

PREVALENCE OF MARASMUS

Marasmus must have been a leading cause of the high morbidity and mortality among infants and pre-school children in the latter half of the last century and the early part of this one, both in Europe and North America. Exact figures are difficult to obtain because of the confusion of nomenclature and diagnosis. Peiper's book, *Chronik der Kinderheilkunde* (10) states that a large percentage were illegitimate foundlings, who numbered 15% to 45% of all newborn infants in most European capitals. Their destiny was the foundlings' home, where mortality due to poor hygienic conditions reached 30% to 90% during the first year of life. There was a similar mortality in North American institutions: Chapin (15) quotes a death rate in 11 foundling institutions in New York State of 422 per 1,000 in children under 2 years compared with a community figure of 87 per 1,000. Another alternative was nursing in private homes, but most foster mothers were poor, ignorant, and unscrupulous "makers of angels," and foster children died more often than not from malnutrition. With the two World Wars, the scourge of the past reappeared in Europe, especially in besieged cities such as Warsaw, Leningrad, and Budapest.

As a further example of the situation in North America in 1921, in the annual report of the Infants Hospital, Boston, Schloss, the new medical director, called attention to "the frequent relationships of both malnutrition and acute infections to infant deaths" and stressed their importance as fields for research (16). In lists of diagnosis of admissions in the year 1883–1913, marasmus or atrophy does not appear, but figures for debility, dysentery, and diarrhea are high. In 1882, more than a one-third of admissions were for "debility".

RESEARCH ON MARASMUS

Hypothermia, BMR, and Hypoglycemia

Hypothermia is a common feature of severe infantile malnutrition, and Parrot in 1877 published a number of cases presenting with rectal temperatures as low as 27°C (9). In 1921, Talbot (17) measured heat production, that is, the basic metabolic rate (BMR) in marasmic infants under basal conditions and found that there was no change in metabolism until there was a 20% loss of body weight. Beyond this point there was an increase in heat production (loss) per kg of body weight. He believed that this was due to loss of the insulating layer of subcutaneous fat and larger body surface in relation to weight of marasmic infants. When heat loss became greater than heat production, there was a loss of body temperature. The infants developed a state known to the clinicians of the time as *vita parva* (5), showing no interest in their surroundings, and tolerating injections without crying. In the extreme cases, oxygen consumption and temperature would fall, and the infants would become unconscious.

In 1928, Levine et al. (18), in an excellent review of previous work and theories preceding their own investigations, established the BMR of marasmic infants as 72–82 kcal/kg compared to 51–63 in normal infants. They reasoned that the loss of metabolically inactive fat could account for the higher BMR in marasmus and that there was no abnormal metabolic process in the active metabolic tissue. The fact that the BMR depended on the stage of malnutrition in infants was further studied by Kerpel-Fronius and Frank in 1949 (5), who emphasized that malnutrition in growing individuals had markedly differing effects on various organs. Thus the metabolically active brain, kidney, and heart were much less reduced in size in malnutrition than was muscle or fat, and this in itself would raise the BMR expressed in relation to body weight or surface area.

Hypoglycemia was known frequently to supervene in marasmus. Kerpel-Fronius in 1953 claimed that hypoglycemia caused respiratory paralysis that was relieved by glucose (5). Coblimer in Germany in 1911, and Jaso in 1932, called attention to the poor prognostic significance of falling blood sugar levels (5). In 1950, Aballi (19) stated that 4 of 20 marasmic infants younger than 9 months of age had one or several hypoglycemic attacks.

Marasmus and Infection

Early in this century, German and French pediatricians stressed that the fate of undernourished infants depended on whether they escaped infection. Wertheimer and Wolf in 1920 (20) described how, in severely undernourished infants, in contrast to healthy breast-fed infants, influenzal infections dragged on, often ending in death. There were many other recorded instances, and the problem of infectious diarrhea in marasmus has already been mentioned. The French and German texts pointed out that a rapid decline in the weight curve ending in an extreme state of marasmus could seldom be caused by simple semi-starvation (5). In 1922, McCann (21) showed that urinary nitrogen excretion was markedly increased in tuberculosis. Scrimshaw et al. (22) cite similar findings in typhoid (Vogel (1854), Traub (1855)). Although diarrhea was a regular feature, nitrogen absorption was little affected. In 1915, Holt and associates (23) noted that, even in severe diarrhea, nitrogen absorption rarely fell below 75%.

Body Composition

In 1905, Steinitz and Weigert performed direct analysis of the bodies of three young marasmic infants. Kerpel-Fronius has compared these data with those of Sommerfeld's (1900) analysis of a near-normal infant of the same age (5). The striking difference was the fat content of the marasmic infants, which was 1.7% of body weight in comparison to 13.1% in normals (Table 1). Similar figures found by Steinitz in 1904 are quoted by Levine (18). Klose in 1920 (quoted by Talbot) (17) found 1.4% fat in skin of marasmics compared to 47% in normals. Body water was increased from 70% in normals to 80% in marasmus. These findings are comparable with the in vivo body composition studies done after 1950.

With regard to extracellular water in malnutrition, the first study of the "thiocyanate space" was done by Kerpel-Fronius and Kovach in 1948 (24), and showed an increase in this space from 25% in normals to 50% in the undernourished. Kerpel-Fronius and Frank went on to demonstrate that brain, kidneys, and skeleton were relatively preserved in marasmus (5).

TABLE 1. *Composition of body in malnutrition*

	Control (3 months)	Malnourished (3 months)
Weight g	4340	2583 (60% expected wt.)
Fat %	13.11	1.74
Water %	70.15	80.20
Protein %	14.18	14.60
Ash %	2.73	3.09

Electrolyte Metabolism

Papers relating to water and salt metabolism in marasmus are few in the 1850 to 1950 era. Abt in 1924, in his text book of pediatrics (7) advocated intraperitoneal injections of saline, and quoted Donelly's (1921) recommendation that 10% glucose be given intravenously at the same time.

In 1947, Kerpel-Fronius (Fig. 1) reported on infantile mortality in Budapest during the siege of 1945. With the availability of drugs, milk, and blood and plasma transfusions, he was able to save many children's lives even though their weight was only 40% of the ideal—a level at which recovery had been thought impossible before the war (13).

Potassium had been found to be low relative to nitrogen in postmortem analyses of undernourished children before World War I (5). Holt in 1915 showed losses of

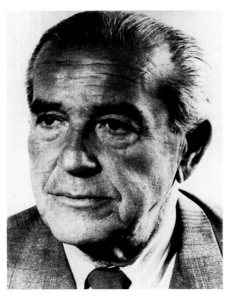

FIG. 1. Eugen Kerpel-Fronius. (Courtesy of CNRC Archives; gift of Gyula Soltesz.)

potassium in diarrheal stools in atrophic infants, and subsequent work by Darrow in the 1930s and 1940s established the value of potassium in the treatment of diarrhea (25,26), so often a complication of marasmus.

Edema

Kerpel-Fronius stated that edema was exceptional in wasted infants because edema-promoting factors, e.g., dietary starch and salt, were mostly absent from the diets of these infants (5). This was because, in most cases, wasting was due to insufficient energy intake. Edema occurred in the 1- to 3-year age group—mainly gypsy children who had hypoalbuminemia. Lack of animal proteins, especially milk, in diet was more serious in these edematous children. Kerpel-Fronius concluded that wasting without hypoalbuminemia was never accompanied by edema.

Vitamins

Currently, there is an increased interest in vitamin A deficiency in malnutrition. Of relevance is an early observation of Bloch (1920–1921) (27) who pointed to the prime importance of food intake in the etiology of keratomalacia. In Denmark in 1918–1919, due to butter exportation, children were fed with vegetable margarine and xerophthalmia made its appearance. Rickets and scurvy in children occurred frequently among the poor in 1850–1950 era (28,29), and many such children must also have been marasmic.

Endocrine Glands

Early in the century it was stated (Lucien 1908, Jackson 1925) (5) that in athrepsia all glands diminish in weight—the thymus practically disappears, the pituitary, the thyroid, and adrenals are greatly reduced, although in some cases the adrenals were hypertrophic (Nicolaeff, 1923) (5). In 1940, investigators working on rats coined the concept of pseudohypophysectomy in starvation (30) because weight loss of adrenals and ovaries could be prevented by pituitary implants. This hypothesis was tested in the post-1950 era and found to be wanting.

TREATMENT OF MARASMUS

Infant feeding was a main preoccupation of pediatricians at the turn of the century and up to 1950, and the treatment of marasmus centered around the feeding practices of the time.

Rotch, in his 1906 edition of *Pediatrics,* stated that atrophy was susceptible to treatment with breast milk or modified cow's milk (1% protein, 32 calories/100 ml) and that if the child did not die there was complete recovery. Among other measures, he recommended that the patients be kept warm by external warmth and stimulants, and that small doses of brandy could be given for weeks with benefit! (31).

The Rubner and Heubner paper on the metabolism and average daily energy needs of the normal and atrophic infant appeared in 1898 (32), the atrophic infant being said to need 120 kcal/kg body weight compared with 100 kcal for the normal infant. It was possible for the first time to feed infants according to energy needs, and this early work has relevance to this day. It was believed by some that the deficiency of energy in cases of marasmus resulted mainly from withholding sugar from markedly diluted milk formulas (5). Edema occurred when the diet was rich in carbohydrates. Heubner in 1907 thought that overfeeding played a great part in the causation of diarrhea and vomiting (33).

The most widely accepted advance in treatment of marasmus came from the school of Finkelstein (34,35). He postulated that wrong feeding (Fehlernärung) lowered tolerance to food. This in turn would lead to chronic diseases of alimentation including dystrophy and dekomposition.

The principal cause of wrong feeding he believed to be an excess of carbohydrate and fat in the diet. All manifestations could be reversed by "protein milk" and the prognosis of "atrophy" changed for the better after his papers were published beginning in 1907. This milk contained 3% protein (mostly casein), 2.5% fat, and 1.5% lactose (40 kcal/100 ml). It was rendered acid by conversion of lactose to lactic acid by the lactobacillus. In 1910, by administering this milk to 41 cases of dekomposition he had only five deaths (12%), which was outstanding at the time since mortality from previous low protein formulas had been very high (36). From that time onward there was a steady decline in the death rates from marasmus in developed countries. Between 1907 and 1950, there was much discussion (often heated) in the pediatric literature on why protein milk was successful. By 1950, it had been replaced by more modern formulas that contained more carbohydrate, but in retrospect its value lay in its protein content. Its energy value was only half that of whole milk and Finkelstein and Meyer (36) recommended that it should always be supplemented with 1%–3% sugar if there were no weight gain.

The value of human milk in the treatment of chronic diarrhea, a scourge of marasmus, is mentioned in the research carried out in the Boston Floating Hospital (37) and also by Cameron in the United Kingdom (38). The contribution of Howland and Marriott in 1915 in showing that dehydrated infants had acidosis (39), and Marriott's demonstration, in 1919 (40) of anhydremia set the scene for acute replacement of fluid and electrolyte loss. In 1910, dextrose saline infusions were used for collapsed and depleted cases, including infantile atrophy, as recorded in the article by Beavan on the activities of the Boston Floating Hospital (37). Darrow, (25) pointed out that the presence of potassium loss as well as losses of sodium and chloride in diarrhea had been demonstrated by Schmidt in 1850, Meyer in 1910, Tobler in 1911, and Jundell in 1913. He commented that the great schools of pediatrics in Germany, under the leadership of Czerny and Finkelstein, appreciated that the loss of potassium occurred in relative excess over nitrogen in "malignant diarrhea." They believed that the rapid terminal loss of nitrogen was a consequence of the loss of alkali. Their assumption that the process could not be reversed by replacement therapy, however, was incorrect. In the United States Holt, Courtney, and Fales (23) published in 1915 on electrolyte losses in normal and loose stools of infants. They showed increased water, fat, chloride, sodium, and potassium losses in loose stools. Of 21 cases studied by Holt et al., eight (38%) were cases of marasmus as judged by the modern criterion of weight that is less than 60% of expected. At the conclusion of their paper, the authors say: "In attempting to supply their loss [of electrolytes] by hypodermochysis it should be remembered that not only are water and sodium needed but potassium and magnesium as well." It took until 1946 for this advice with regard to potassium to be followed, when Darrow showed that the loss of intracellular potassium in diarrhea could be corrected safely by the administration of potassium chloride (25). The decrease in mortality from diarrhea was dramatic—6% compared to 32% of controls—when potassium was added to conventional sodium chloride, sodium lactate, and glucose solutions (26). Many cases of marasmus with dehydration benefited from this new form of therapy. However, as Kerpel-Fronius observed in 1947 (13), the lowering of infantile mortality is not so much a medical as a social and financial problem.

SOCIAL AND POLITICAL IMPLICATIONS OF MARASMUS

During the nineteenth century in the industrial towns of Europe and North America, marasmus resulting from poor diets and numerous infections probably took as large a toll of infant lives as it does today in many Asian, African, and South American towns (5,41). The Industrial Revolution of the last century produced multitudes of a new urban proletariat who were uprooted from their rural origins and packed around factories in bad housing. In 1900, infant mortality rates were over 100 per 1,000 births in many towns in Europe and North America as a result of poor hygiene and malnutrition (5,28,29). Women were employed extensively in factories, and they farmed their children out to wet nurses, foster homes, or creches. In France, about 20,000 infants were sent out in this way, with a mortality of 75%. A point made by Levy (1912) is that, in the Franco-Prussian War (1870–1871) the factories closed down and the mothers went home, resulting in a reduction of infant mortality in Paris of 40% (42). He stressed that maternal nursing is the most important factor in reducing infant mortality—more important than ignorance, illiteracy, overcrowding, and poor ventilation. In 1874, Roussel introduced the famous *loi Roussel* for the protection of infants sent to the provinces from Paris for wet nursing (43). This law required government inspection of all places where infants under 2 years were farmed out. The ruling principle of Roussel's life had been to translate charitable sentiment into enacted law, and he was a pioneer in promoting child health. With regard to the relationship of poverty to malnutrition, Orr showed clearly in 1936 the relationship between food, growth, health, and income (44). Only in the twentieth century did governments begin to assume responsibility for seeing that the poorer and more underprivileged sections of society received enough of the right types of food (29).

After considerable improvement during the earlier part of the twentieth century, marasmus again became a problem during World Wars I and II in areas of Europe and Asia (5). The effects of war in causing marasmus can also have long-term political consequences or implications. This is well illustrated in my own country by the British camps for women and children in the Boer War, 1899–1902. There was marasmus and a high mortality of young Boer (Afrikaner) children in these camps from measles and from repeated diarrhea, due to the poor sanitary conditions and diet (Fig. 2). Hobhouse (1902) (45) wrote, when describing conditions in the camps, "No child can thrive on a diet consisting of ½ pound of flour and one bottle of watery milk daily, and that is what all children under five get." She goes on to quote a Mrs. Dickenson from the South Australian Advertiser: "I saw some terrible instances of emaciation amongst children which could only be matched by the famine stricken people of India." The Nazi concentration camps and ghettos produced marasmus and are a recent example of deliberate genocide during wartime (46,47).

These are but two tragic examples of marasmus occurring during political upheaval and war. That the world had become shocked into consciousness of these effects was partly responsible for the Declaration of the Rights of the Child of the United Nations in 1959 (48). However, we should all be aware that 30 years later there are still political upheavals causing famine and marasmus.

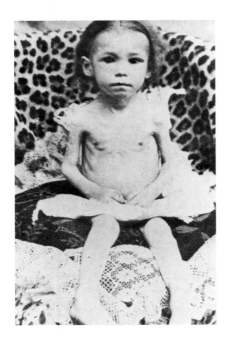

FIG. 2. Marasmic Boer child in British concentration camp during the Boer War, 1899–1902. (Reproduced with permission from *South African Medical Journal* vol. 74:9, Nov. 5, 1988. Copyright © War Museum of Boer Republics, Bloemfontein.)

REFERENCES

1. Marriot MW. Anhydraemia. *Physiol Rev* 1923;3:275. (Quoted by Kerpel-Fronius, 5.)
2. Marfan AB. *Les affections des voies digestives.* II. Paris: Masson, 1930. (Quoted by Kerpel-Fronius, 5.)
3. Finkelstein H. *Säuglingskrankheiten.* Amsterdam: Elsevier, 1938. (Quoted by Kerpel-Fronius, 5.)
4. Czerny A, Keller A. *Des Kindes Ernährung, Ernährungstörungen und Ernährungstherapie.* Vol 2, Leipzig: Deuticke, 1928. (Quoted by Kerpel-Fronius, 5.)
5. Kerpel-Fronius E. *The pathophysiology of infantile malnutrition, protein energy malnutrition and failure to thrive.* Budapest: Akademiai Kiado, 1983.
6. Dickens C. Speech on behalf of The Hospital for Sick Children, 1858. Printed by Fulkard and Son, London, 1867. Reprinted *J Pediatr* 1956;49,607.
7. Abt IA. In: *Abt's Pediatrics,* Vol III. Philadelphia: WB Saunders and Company, 1924:263.
8. Paterson D. In: Paterson D, ed. *Sick children,* 6th ed. London: Russell and Co, 1947:81.
9. Parrot J. *L'athrepsie.* Paris: Masson, 1877. (Quoted by Kerpel-Fronius, 5.)
10. Peiper A. *Chronik der Kinderheilkunde.* 3rd ed., Thieme, Liepzig: 1958. (Quoted by Kerpel-Fronius, 5.)
11. Jelliffe DB. Protein-calorie malnutrition in tropical pre-school children; a review of recent knowledge. *J Pediatr* 1959;54:227–56.
12. Wellcome Trust Working Party. *Lancet* ii;1970:302.
13. Kerpel-Fronius E. Infantile mortality in Budapest in the year 1945. *J Pediatr* 1947;30:244–9.
14. Waterlow JC. *Fatty liver disease in the British West Indies.* London: MRC Special Report Ser No 263, HM Stationery Office, 1948.
15. Chapin HD. A plea for accurate statistics in infants' institutions. *Arch Pediatr* 1915;32:724–6.
16. Smith CA. *The Children's Hospital of Boston.* Boston: Little Brown and Co, 1983.
17. Talbot FB. Severe infantile malnutrition. *Am J Dis Child* 1921;22:358–70.
18. Levine SZ, Wilson JR, Gottschall AB. The respiratory metabolism in infancy and childhood. *Am J Dis Child* 1928;35:615–30.
19. Aballi A. Disturbances of carbohydrate metabolism in infantile malnutrition. *Rev Cubana Pediatr* 1950;22:509. (Quoted by Kerpel-Fronius, 5.)
20. Wertheimer E, Wolf E. Ermährungszustand und Infection. *Z Kinderheilkd* 1920;28:295. (Quoted by Kerpel-Fronius, 5.)
21. McCann WS. The protein requirement in tuberculosis. *Arch Intern Med* 1922;29:33. (Quoted by Schrimshaw, 22.)
22. Scrimshaw MS, Taylor CE, Gordon JE. *Interactions of nutrition and infection.* Geneva: WHO, 1968.
23. Holt LE, Courtney AM, Fales HE. The chemical composition of diarrheal as compared with normal stools in infants. *Am J Dis Child* 1915;9:213–24.
24. Kerpel-Fronius E, Kovach S. Volume of extracellular fluids in infantile malnutrition. *Pediatrics* 1948;2:21–3.
25. Darrow DC. The retention of electrolytes during recovery from severe dehydration due to diarrhea. *J Pediatr* 1946;28:515–40.
26. Govan CD, Darrow DC. The use of potassium chloride in the treatment of the dehydration of diarrhea in infants. *J Pediatr* 1946;28:541–9.
27. Bloch CE. Observations on xerophthalmia in Denmark during 1918 and 1919. *J Hyg* 1920–21;19:301. (Quoted by Kerpel-Fronius, 5.)
28. Cone TE. *History of American pediatrics.* Boston: Little Brown and Co, 1979.
29. Passmore R. In: McLaren DS, ed. *Nutrition in the community,* ch. 2. London: John Wiley, 1983.
30. Mulinos MG, Pomerantz L. Pseudohypophysectomy—a condition resembling hypophysectomy produced by malnutrition. *J Nutr* 1940;19:493–504.
31. Rotch TM. *Pediatrics,* 5th ed. Philadelphia: Lippincott, 1906, 341.
32. Rubner M, Heubner O. Die Natürliche Ernährung Eines Säuglings. *J Biol* 1898;36:1. (Quoted by Cone, 28.)
33. Heubner O, Thomas JJ. The importance of the estimation of the caloric values of infant food. *Arch Pediatr* 1907;24:81–5.
34. Finkelstein H. Alimentary intoxication in infants (Abstr). Arch Pediatr 1907;24:871–2. *Jahrbuch fur Kinderhk,* March 1, 1907, p. 263.

35. Leopold JS. The Finkelstein-Meyer method of infant feeding by casein milk. *Archiv Pediatr* 1910;27:603.
36. Finkelstein H, Meyer LF. "Eiweissmilch". *Jahrbuch fur Kinderhk, May/June, 1910. Abs Archiv Pediat* 1910;27:363–8.
37. Beaven P. A history of the Boston Floating Hospital. *Pediatrics* 1957;19:629–38.
38. Cameron HC. *Diet and disease in infancy.* London: Churchill, 1915.
39. Howland J, Marriott W McK. Indications for treatment of severe diarrhea in infancy. *Trans Am Pediatr Soc* 1915;27:201. (Quoted by Cone, 28.)
40. Marriott W McK. The pathogenesis of certain nutritional disorders. *Trans Am Pediatr Soc* 1919;31:34. (Quoted by Cone, 28.)
41. Passmore R. In: Passmore R, Eastwood MA, eds. *Human nutrition and dietetics.* Edinburgh: Churchill Livingstone, 1986:280.
42. Levy J. The relation of social and economic conditions to infant morbidity and mortality. *Arch Pediatr* 1912;29:46–54.
43. Abt AF, ed. *Abt-Garrison. History of pediatrics* Philadelphia: WB Saunders, 1965:154.
44. Orr JB. *Food, health and income.* London: MacMillan, 1936.
45. Hobhouse E. *The brunt of the war.* London: Methuen, 1902.
46. Berger N. *Chapters from South African history* (Jewish and general, book 2). Johannesburg: Kayor Publishers, 1986.
47. Gilbert M. *The Holocaust.* London: Collins, 1986.
48. United Nations General Assembly. The Declaration of the Rights of the Child, 1959.

DISCUSSION

Dr. Ballabriga: German authors at the beginning of the century described the condition *Mehlnährschaden* in which, although there was edema, skin lesions of the kwashiorkor type were not seen. I am not sure whether this corresponds to what we now call *kwashiorkor*. In the forms of kwashiorkor that were seen at the end of the Second World War in Greece, Italy, and Spain, cutaneous lesions were usual. The disorder described as *Milchnährschaden* corresponds to the dystrophies associated with excess ingestion of milk and deficiency of carbohydrate. "Hunger dystrophy" was also described by Rominger.

"Decomposition" differed from atrophy in that the loss of weight was intense, progressive, and accompanied by metabolic breakdown. This was a classical concept in the German literature. Decomposition was the last stage, when all mechanisms of metabolic regulation had failed. To the concept of dystrophy, that of *dysergia* was also added, which encompassed the immunological defect conditioned by the nutritional disorder.

Dr. Nichols: Finkelstein differentiated between the atrophic child with diarrhea and without diarrhea.

Dr. Ballabriga: Yes, but decomposition almost always occurred as a continuation of or as a termination of enteritis, as described by Kerpel-Fronius.

Dr. Rossi: Mehlnährschaden was not the same as kwashiorkor. It was a clinical picture, of a marasmus with edema, but skin lesions as in kwashiorkor were never described.

Dr. Hansen: The critical factor in relation to the question of the presence or absence of skin lesions in kwashiorkor is the protein composition of the flour on which the children were fed. Wheat flour protein contains the amino acid tryptophan, which is absent from corn and maize protein. Our work in Cape Town showed that when children had been on a corn or maize diet there were no nicotinamide in the urine and these were the children with skin lesions. Children who had been fed on bread or wheat starch had nicotinamide in the urine and no skin lesions. I believe the reason why some European children had edema but no skin lesions is that they were getting enough tryptophan.

Dr. Nichols: What did Kerpel-Fronius teach about the intestinal component of malnutrition?

Dr. Ballabriga: Mucosal lesions observed at post-mortem could be due to autolytic changes and in vivo intestinal biopsy was not available at the time, so it was difficult to be sure about the intestinal lesions. It was for this reason that Kerpel-Fronius did not consider this subject in his last book, "The Pathophysiology of Infantile Malnutrition."

Dr. Suskind: In the United States and Europe the term, *failure to thrive* has superseded *malnourished child*. Nevertheless the child with failure to thrive has malnutrition, whether it be primary or secondary.

Dr. Kretchmer: Discussion and commentary on acute and chronic forms of malnutrition and on questions of definition relating to skin lesions miss the most important consideration. This is that malnutrition is a disease of ignorance and politics. Our efforts should be directed toward those quarters, for prevention.

History of Pediatrics 1850–1950, edited by
B.L. Nichols, A. Ballabriga, and N. Kretchmer.
Nestlé Nutrition Workshop Series, Vol. 22. Nestec
Ltd., Vevey/Raven Press, Ltd., New York © 1991.

Kwashiorkor

John C. Waterlow

London School of Hygiene and Tropical Medicine, London WC1E 7HT, United Kingdom

NAMES

Names are important and can influence the growth of knowledge. A wise physician, Asher (1), has written that a disease does not exist until it has a name. In the case of kwashiorkor, the history of the disease and the history of the name form two threads that cannot easily be disentangled, and it is difficult to describe the unfolding story in a logical way, without repetition.

The names that are given to diseases are of two kinds. The first kind is descriptive; it implies recognition of a syndrome and, as it were, brings the disease into existence. I call such a description a *code* name. It either recalls the discoverer, e.g., Still's disease, or it is an attempt to describe a syndrome by its essential features, for example, pellagra (rough skin).

The second kind of name is causal and tends to take over from the descriptive name once the cause has been established, so that now we talk about ascorbic acid deficiency rather than scurvy. A descriptive name conjures up a clinical picture. Therefore it makes no sense to talk of *subclinical* scurvy, but it does make sense to talk of *subclinical vitamin C deficiency.*

One feels that causal names are more "scientific", but it is important to get the cause right. In the early 1950s, it seemed that the causal name *protein malnutrition* would supersede and make redundant the code name, kwashiorkor. Then it was realized that the diets that produce the syndrome are deficient in energy as well as in protein, so that protein malnutrition was superseded by *protein-calorie, or protein-energy malnutrition* (PEM) (2,3).

From the point of view of cause, therefore, the nomenclature is still confused. However, this group of names has made possible, perhaps even stimulated, an important transition: a shift of interest from children with severe cases of malnutrition as seen in hospital—the "tip of the iceberg"—to the more numerous children with mild or moderate malnutrition in the community. Why, then, is the name *kwashiorkor* still used more than 50 years after it was first proposed (4)? The answer is that clinicians still see these cases and need a name to describe what is seen.

One may ask: If a descriptive or code-name is needed, why *kwashiorkor*? The name was introduced by Williams (Fig. 1) in the *Lancet* in 1935 (4), where she says:

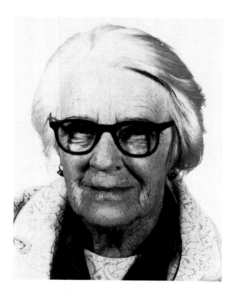

FIG. 1. Dr. Cicely D. Williams, who introduced the name *kwashiorkor* in 1935, when she was Lady Medical Officer, Colonial Medical Service, Gold Coast.

"The name *kwashiorkor* indicates the disease the deposed baby gets when the next one is born, and is the local name in the Gold Coast for a nutritional disease of children, associated with a maize diet." Later (5) she elaborated: "The word comes from the Ga language of Accra, Ghana. . . . It indicates 'the disease of the deposed baby when the next one is born.' It has a connotation of jealousy between siblings, as well as of a physical sickness. The etymology of the word is not quite certain. One of my Ga friends told me that *kwashiorkor* used to be a ritual name given to a second child." An idea arose that *kwashiorkor* means "red boy". This misconception probably derived from a paper by Lieurade in 1932 (6), who described a condition in the French Cameroons that he called *enfants rouges* because of the children's gross depigmentation. These cases, which were characterized by massive ascites, seem more likely to have been examples of Senecio poisoning (veno-occlusive disease of Jamaica (7,8)), since ascites is seldom, if ever, seen in kwashiorkor.

Trowell (Fig. 2), in his history of kwashiorkor published in 1954 (9) lists 31 vernacular names used in tropical Africa, and more from other countries. Why has *kwashiorkor* survived and all the others disappeared? For example, Dricot, writing from the Congo (10) abandoned the local name *M'Buaki* and adopted kwashiorkor. There are three reasons: first, Williams gave a full and clear description, not only of the clinical picture but of the circumstances in which it appeared. The second reason is the language: earlier accounts in Spanish, Portuguese, or French were simply ignored in the English-speaking world. As recently as 1979, Fondu, working in Kivu, has written: "We sometimes feel that papers of non-English speaking people are systematically ignored by some authors (11)." The third reason is the journal. The early accounts appeared in local journals, pediatric journals, or journals of tropical medicine. Williams' second paper (4), in which she introduced the name, was pub-

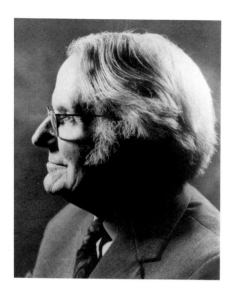

FIG. 2. The Rev. Dr. H.C. Trowell, formerly Chief Physician, Mulago Hospital, Kampala, Uganda and co-author of the book, *Kwashiorkor* (1954).

lished in the *Lancet*. In 1935, the *Lancet* was 100 years old, and was an international journal. One might add to Asher's dictum that a disease does not exist until it has been described, a further dictum: a description does not really exist until it has been published in a widely read journal!

EARLY ACCOUNTS OF KWASHIORKOR

Since this is a pediatric workshop the discussion shall be confined to children. It is not clear whether famine edema in adults (the history of which has been described by McCance (12)) is the same disease as kwashiorkor in children. The childhood picture in Europe during and after the two World Wars seems to be different from that in India, where hypoalbuminemia was more common (13). I shall also at this stage mention only descriptions from the Third World. Trowell's review (9), covers the history up to about 1950.

The first known account was by Hinojosa in Mexico in 1865 (14). He described a condition that came on at weaning, at 1–2 years of age, starting with diarrhea and followed by edema of the feet, which soon became generalized. There were also lesions of the skin. The description resembles that by Williams in 1933 (15) (Table 1). Our story moves on to the present century and the period between the wars. In the 1930s, an increasing number of accounts appeared of what was obviously kwashiorkor, although many different names were used. A selection of these reports is listed in Table 2. Various views were advanced about essential characteristics and causes. The Latin American authors regarded it as a multiple deficiency state, with special emphasis on vitamin deficiencies. This was in keeping with the philosophy of the

TABLE 1. *Characteristics of kwashiorkor as described by Williams, 1933*

Age   1–4 years
History of an "abnormal" diet: breast-feeding by an old or pregnant woman with supplementary feeds of maize paps
Edema
Wasting
Diarrhea
Sores of mucous membranes
Desquamation of skin on legs and forearms
"Diffluent" fatty liver
Uniformly fatal unless treated

From ref. 15.

time. E. V. McCollum, carried away by advances in our understanding of the biochemistry of the vitamins, in a well-known textbook published in 1939 (34), expressed the view that the nutritional problems of the world were all but solved. Williams' work pointed to protein deficiency, but it was only later that she stated this view explicitly. One of the early pioneers of the theory of protein deficiency was the French physician Normet, working in Indochina. In 1926, he published a

TABLE 2. *Some early accounts of kwashiorkor in Third World countries before 1946*

			Reference
Latin America and Caribbean			
1865	Hinojosa	Mexico	14
1927	Payne and Payne	Haiti	16
1934	Gil	Mexico	17
1935	Castellanos	Cuba	18
	Goenz	San Salvador	19
1938	Ubico and Klee	Guatemala	20
1938	Chavarria	Costa Rica	21
1943	Umaña	Colombia	22
1945	Carvalho	Brazil	23
Africa			
1933	Williams	Ghana	15
	Gillan	Kenya	24
1937	Trowell	Uganda	25
1938	Van Daele	Congo	26
1938	Trolli (see FLD)	Congo	27
1938	Shukry *et al.*	Egypt	28
1943	Kark	Basutoland	29
1946	Pieraerts	Congo	30
Asia			
1926	Normet	Annam	31
1930	Weech	China	32
1942	Chen	China	33

paper (31) proposing that the condition called *la bouffissure d'Annam* resulted from a deficiency of dietary protein, because he found that the 24-hour urea output was very low. This was probably the first application of biochemistry to the study of kwashiorkor.

Except for the work of Normet and some accounts of nutritional edema in children in China (32,33), the early reports came from Latin America and Africa. A series of papers from the Belgian Congo, listed by Trowell (9) appeared, which were independent of the work of Williams. By 1939, kwashiorkor was recognized in some parts of the world as a widespread and serious nutritional disease of children.

Why did this recognition come so late? Britain had for a long time been responsible for the medical services of large parts of Africa and Asia. How could the doctors have missed a condition that was very common and striking? As far as the indigenous populations were concerned, a major objective of the medical services was to understand and control communicable diseases. The reasons for the neglect of malnutrition were partly economic, partly that malaria, cholera, etc., have no respect for position or race. With the exception of the work of McCarrison in India, nutrition received little attention. It was not until 1934 that the Secretary of State commissioned a report on "Nutrition in the Colonial Empire" (35). The secretary of the committee that compiled that report was B.S. Platt (Fig. 3), my first chief and one of the pioneers in Britain of interest in Third World nutrition. Trained as a chemist, Platt qualified in medicine and went to work at the Henry Lester Institute in Shanghai. When the Japanese invaded China, Platt returned to England where he was befriended by Mellanby, at that time Secretary of the Medical Research Council (MRC). He was made director of a new MRC unit for research on human nutrition, and after the war extended it to an out-station in the Gambia. This was the origin of the MRC Unit in that country, which is still active. Platt was appointed as the first

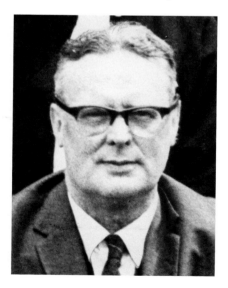

FIG. 3. Professor B.S. Platt, formerly Director of the Medical Research Council's Human Nutrition Research Unit in London, and first Professor of Human Nutrition at the London School of Hygiene and Tropical Medicine.

Professor of Human Nutrition in the London School of Hygiene and Tropical Medicine, and in that capacity influenced and encouraged many young workers from the Third World. I worked under him in the year immediately after the war and succeeded him when he died in 1970. Cicely Williams was, for a time, a senior lecturer in his department. Until recently, of all the schools of Tropical Medicine in Europe, that in London was the only one to have a department of nutrition.

THE DEVELOPMENT OF WORK ON KWASHIORKOR AFTER WORLD WAR II

The Second World War slowed down the research stimulated by the early papers, but after it ended there was a flowering of interest all over the world. In Uganda, Trowell, a general physician, had continued to publish on kwashiorkor throughout the war, and his book with Davies, a pathologist, and Dean, a pediatrician, is one of the classics of our subject (9,36). In many departments of pediatrics all over the world, malnutrition became a main topic of research. Examples are the groups of Gomez (see p. 270, Fig. 4) in Mexico, of Meneghello, and later Monckeberg in Chile, of Hansen in Cape Town, Gabr in Cairo, and Gürson in Istanbul. Elsewhere, nutrition research institutes, such as the National Institute of Nutrition in India and the Instituto de Nutricion de Centro America y Panama (INCAP) in Central America, which had previously been concerned with population surveys, turned their attention to investigation of childhood malnutrition. Developed countries supported units or groups set up for work on malnutrition. These included the British Medical Research Council Units in Uganda and Jamaica, both established in 1954 through

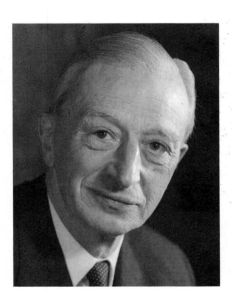

FIG. 4. Sir Harold Himsworth, who, as Secretary of the British Medical Research Council, was responsible for establishing units for research on childhood malnutrition in Uganda and Jamaica in 1954.

the stimulus of Sir Harold Himsworth (Fig. 4), Secretary of the Medical Research Council; the Rockefeller-funded institute in Chiang Mai, Thailand; the research groups led by Graham in Peru and by McLaren in Beirut. Work on kwashiorkor was going on in the Congo in the 1930s (Table 2), and has continued since independence, in association with Vis and his colleagues in Brussels. Another long association continues today between workers in Sweden and Ethiopia.

The United Nations' agencies were quick to recognize the importance of the problem. In the early 1950s, the Food and Agriculture Organization (FAO) organized the mission under Brock and Autret that culminated in the report "Kwashiorkor in Africa" (37). The World Health Organization (WHO) followed suit with reports on kwashiorkor in Central America (38), Brazil (39) and South India (40).

As a result of this interest and support, the 25 years from 1950 to 1975 represent the golden era of clinical research on PEM and kwashiorkor. During this period, the foundations were laid of our knowledge and understanding of the physiological, biochemical, pathological, and psychological changes. This knowledge has been brought together in books and reviews (41–44). In the last decade there have been important contributions, in immunology (45), membrane function (46,47), trace element deficiency (48) and free radical damage (49). The fact remains, however, that the volume of basic research is less, although it cannot be said that all the problems have been solved (50). The emphasis has shifted from the ward to the field, from clinical to community research. Cicely Williams questioned the need for "scientific" research on kwashiorkor, since the condition was well recognized and the cause known (51). This view was reflected in Kretchmer's discussion in the last chapter. Prevention, is better than cure, but preventive programs are unlikely to succeed unless firmly founded on basic knowledge.

WORLDWIDE INCIDENCE OF KWASHIORKOR

After the Second World War it was recognized that kwashiorkor was found throughout the developing world, although with varying frequency from one region to another. It is puzzling that kwashiorkor was not described earlier in India, perhaps for the reasons suggested above. The first Indian publication was in 1950 (52), followed by one from Gopalan and coworkers at the National Institute of Nutrition in 1951 (53). Gopalan had returned to India about 1948 after completing his PhD with Platt in London. Thus he and I share a common lineage through Platt.

When communications in Europe were restored after the war, we began to realize that kwashiorkor could not be considered a purely tropical disease. When conditions were bad enough it appeared in Europe. At the first meeting on the subject that I attended, a paper was given by Professor Frontali, describing cases of kwashiorkor in Italy during the German occupation (54). Cases were also reported from Hungary by Kerpel-Fronius (55) and by Veghelyi (56). It was then natural to ask: Has this condition always been present in Europe under another name? Looking into this question (57) I found that in 1906 the German pediatricians Czerny and Keller had described the condition called *mehlnährschaden* (flour-feeding injury) characterized by edema and fatty liver that occurred in babies with prolonged diarrhea who had been fed on starchy paps. Surely this was kwashiorkor, even though there was no mention of skin or hair lesions. Gürson's review (58) notes Czerny's work but makes no mention of earlier descriptions of edematous malnutrition. In fact, there were sporadic reports of edema in malnourished children in the German, French, and English literature at the turn of the century. Some of these reports emphasize that edema appeared after a long period of intractable diarrhea (e.g., 59). This would correspond to "marasmic kwashiorkor" in our current terminology. It is possible that there are two etiologically distinct kinds of edema in malnourished children. In any case, it must be concluded that kwashiorkor may appear in any part of the world, and this recognition is important for our ideas about etiology.

KWASHIORKOR AND MARASMUS

Kwashiorkor in its fully developed form is a dramatic condition, and for a time it occupied the centre of the stage, diverting attention from the equally severe form of childhood malnutrition that we now refer to as marasmus. As Hansen's chapter in this workshop shows, marasmus under a variety of names had been familiar to European pediatricians for a very long time. Gürson (58) traces written knowledge of it to the sixteenth century. There was a need, therefore, for a synthesis of European and tropical experience. Table 3 reproduces my first effort in this direction (60). We began to think that, from the clinical point of view, kwashiorkor and marasmus represented the two ends of a spectrum. This made necessary the invention of a new ge-

TABLE 3. *An early attempt to distinguish systematically between kwashiorkor and marasmus*

	Fatty liver disease	Undernourished, without liver damage
Number	15	21
With BSP retention[a]	14	0
Weight, percent of standard	68	50
Number with: palpable liver	14	5
edema	11	1
glossitis	11	5
angular stomatitis	7	1
cheilosis	8	2
"mosaic" skin	6	3
raised serum bilirubin	8	1
Hemoglobin (% of Haldane standard)	56	60
Serum total protein, g/100 ml	4.5	5.7
Serum phosphatase, KA units	19.7	19.4
Liver fat, percent of wet weight	40.2 (4 cases)	4.6 (6 cases)

From Waterlow, 1948, ref. 60.
[a]Bromsulphalein test of liver function.

neric name, protein-calorie malnutrition (PCM) or protein-energy malnutrition (PEM). It also stimulated attempts to draw diagnostic boundaries. In the 1950s and 1960s, arguments arose about which of the signs described by Williams and others were essential for the diagnosis of kwashiorkor: were the skin changes (61), the hair changes (37), the fatty liver (60), etc., essential? To achieve some agreement, an international working party was organized by the Wellcome Trust, which produced the Wellcome classification (Table 4) (62). According to this, the essential diagnostic criterion, apart from weight deficit, is edema. This brings us back to the early European accounts. The main purpose of this classification was to make possible comparable studies of the relative frequencies of kwashiorkor and marasmus in different regions. Even if it could be obtained only at the hospital level, such information would be of interest. McLaren, for example, even before the Wellcome classification was published, had pointed out that in the Middle East marasmus was far more common than kwashiorkor (63). Unfortunately few studies have been published that comply with the diagnostic criteria, in spite of their importance for our understanding of the epidemiology of PEM.

Finally, it must not be forgotten that a kwashiorkor-like syndrome occurs also in adults. It was described by Trowell in 1954 (36), and there have been a number of reports from India under the name *nutritional edema* (e.g., 64). If *kwashiorkor* means *the deposed child,* it is an inappropriate classification for adults; this was another reason for introducing the term *PEM.*

DEVELOPMENT OF IDEAS ABOUT THE CAUSE OF KWASHIORKOR

In some the original accounts, ascariasis was suggested as the cause of kwashiorkor. The early Latin American workers regarded it as a multiple nutritional deficiency state, although the idea that the edema was a form of wet beri-beri has not stood the test of time. It has long been recognized that children with kwashiorkor may be deficient in many nutrients, since no natural deficiency is pure, and that the picture varies according to region, with deficiencies of vitamin A, riboflavin, and folic acid being important in some parts of the world. To these a number of minerals have been added in recent years, in particular zinc.

TABLE 4. *The Wellcome classification of severe protein-energy malnutrition*

Weight for age, percent of expected[a]	Edema	
	Present	**Absent**
80–60	Kwashiorkor	Undernutrition
<60	Marasmic kwashiorkor	Marasmus

From ref. 62.
[a]Expected weight for age by Harvard standards.

If the essential characteristic of kwashiorkor is edema, the key question is what is the cause of edema? I will end by summarizing briefly the theories put forward.

Protein Deficiency

As already mentioned, Normet (31) was the first proponent, against much opposition, of the idea that edema in malnourished children was caused by protein deficiency. The work of Williams gave the protein deficiency theory strong support, because of the conditions under which kwashiorkor occurred—displacement of the child from the breast and cure by milk. Brock and Hansen (65) provided evidence when they showed that loss of edema could be initiated by treatment with a mixture of purified amino acids, without vitamins and containing potassium.

The protein deficiency theory was widely accepted until the mid-1960s. Thus Dean and Whitehead (66), writing in 1954, stated: "Our experience has convinced us that the chief cause of kwashiorkor in Uganda is lack of protein in the diet." This belief led to attempts of the United Nations agencies to develop low-cost, high-protein weaning foods (67). Too much emphasis was given to *high* protein content. The difference between adequate and inadequate protein intakes may be quite small, say between 7% and 5% protein to energy. By 1975, when McLaren published his paper "The protein fiasco" (68), the pendulum had begun to swing the other way.

The "protein fiasco" did much to discredit protein deficiency as a cause of kwashiorkor. The theory has been described as "effete" (69) but is still alive. I have discussed elsewhere the biochemical evidence for such a mechanism (70). Some of the discrepancies observed at the clinical level, such as the lack of correspondence between hypoalbuminemia and the presence or degree of edema may be explained by the potassium deficiency demonstrated by Hansen (71). He had returned to work with Brock in Cape Town, after pediatric training in the United States, where he absorbed the teachings of Gamble and Darrow. Hansen's important work on electrolytes thus represents a direct link with the pioneers whose contributions are described in this volume by Holliday and others (72). Potassium and protein are found together in foods and potassium deficiency is an acknowledged cause of edema.

Dysadaptation

The first major blow to the protein deficiency theory was struck by Gopalan (73) in a paper at a meeting organized by McCance. On the basis of animal experiments, McCance was a firm believer in the existence of distinct syndromes of protein deficiency and calorie deficiency.

Dietary intake studies showed that the previous energy intakes of children with kwashiorkor were clearly inadequate by current standards, more inadequate than those of protein. Gopalan described a prospective study in which, in a population of children with marginal intakes, some developed kwashiorkor and some marasmus. No quantitative or qualitative differences could be detected in the preceding diets. Gopalan therefore proposed that kwashiorkor developed as a consequence of the failure of some children to adapt to low intakes. It was later suggested that this failure resulted from differences in endocrine responses (74). Whitehead and coworkers have shown that there are differences in the patterns of insulin and cortisol in children developing kwashiorkor and marasmus (75,76). The question is, which is the cart and which the horse? Do the endocrine changes cause the so-called dysadaptation, or are they responses to different dietary conditions?

Free Radical Damage

Golden and coworkers have formulated a theory that breaks with tradition and asserts that kwashiorkor and marasmus do not form a continuum but are etiologically different (77). In both there is a background of dietary deficiency and nutrient depletion. The distinguishing feature in the production of kwashiorkor is the impact of harmful factors or "noxae", such as infections, toxins, (e.g., aflatoxins (78)), and perhaps solar radiation. The noxae stimulate the production of free radicals, which through oxidation have effects on biological membranes, lipids, and other body components. In a malnourished child the defenses against free radical damage are impaired. Many of the defensive mechanisms depend on metallo-enzymes, the activity of which may be compromised by deficiencies of trace elements such as zinc, copper, and selenium. It is not possible in a short space to give a proper account of the theory or of the extensive evidence that has been obtained in support of it. As to the mechanism by which free radical attack leads to edema, the proposal suggests that free radicals damage cell membranes and alter the activity of the sodium pump.

CONCLUSION

It is important formally that these differences about the etiology of kwashiorkor should be resolved, because there are practical implications. If the protein deficiency theory is correct, we must look again at our estimates of children's protein requirements, and we must examine in more detail the intakes of children in regions where kwashiorkor is common or uncommon. I know of no study of this question since that of Annegers (79) in West Africa, who claimed that the relative frequency of kwashiorkor increased as one moved south from the Sahel to the sea, in parallel with a decrease in the protein-energy ratio of the prevailing diet.

It is impossible to prove or disprove theories of this kind. The best that can be done is to weigh the evidence and to try to get more of it. Some evidence may come from experimental work in animals but some must also be derived from studies on children with severe PEM. It is therefore a cause for concern that facilities for such studies are available now in only a small number of places. No one should think that the problem is solved, if only because mortality rates, even in hospitals, remain unacceptably high (80,81). Perhaps this challenge will be recognized, and the 1990s will provide a new chapter in the history of research on kwashiorkor.

REFERENCES

1. Asher R. *Talking sense,* Sir Francis Avery Jones, ed. London: Churchill Livingstone, 1986.
2. Jelliffe DB. Protein-calorie malnutrition in tropical pre-school children. *J Pediatr* 1959;54:227–56.
3. WHO. Joint FAO/WHO Expert Committee on Nutrition, 6th Report. Tech Rep Ser no 245. Geneva: WHO, 1962.
4. Williams CD. Kwashiorkor: a nutritional disease of children associated with a maize diet. *Lancet* 1935;ii:1151–2.
5. Williams CD. The story of kwashiorkor. *Courier* 1963;13:361. Reprinted in: *Nutr Rev* 1973; 31:334–40.
6. Lieurade M. Les enfants rouges du Camerouns. *Bull Soc Pathol Exot Filiales* 1932;25:46–8.
7. Bras GA, Hill KR. Veno-occlusive diseases of the liver: essential pathology. *Lancet* 1956;ii:161–3.
8. Rhodes K. Two types of liver disease in Jamaican children. *W Ind Med J* 1957;6:1–161.
9. Trowell HC, Davies JNP, Dean RFA. Kwashiorkor: Part I. *Reports of kwashiorkor in children and a discussion of terminology.* Part II. *The history of kwashiorkor.* London: Edward Arnold, 1954. Reprinted by the Nutrition Foundations. New York and London: Academic Press, 1982.
10. Dricot C, Beheyt P, Charles P. Contribution à l'étude du kwashiorkor (Mbuaki du Kwango). *Ann Soc Belg Méd Trop* 1951;31:581–630.
11. Fondu P, Mandelbaum IM, Vis HL. The erythrocyte membrane in protein-energy malnutrition. *Am J Clin Nutr* 1979;31:717–9.
12. McCance RA. The history, significance and aetiology of hunger edema. In: *Studies of Undernutrition, Wuppertal, 1946–9.* MRC Special Report Series no. 275. London: HMSO, 1951.
13. Bose JP, Dev N, Mukerjee P. A preliminary study of the biochemical changes in starvation cases. *Ind J Med Res* 1946;34:143–50.
14. Hinojosa F. Apuntes sobre una enfermedad del pueblo de la Magdalena. *Gacéta Médica de Mexico* 1865;1:137–9.
15. Williams CD. A nutritional disease of childhood associated with a maize diet. *Arch Dis Child* 1933;8:423–33.
16. Payne GC, Payne FK. The incidence of an edema disease among children in the Republic of Haiti. *Am J Hygiene* 1927;7:73–83.
17. Gil AC. Manifestaciones raras de avitaminosis en los niños de Yucatan. *Rev Méd Yucatàn* 1934;17:467–73.
18. Castellanos A. Contribución al estudio clínico de las avitaminosis 'B' en Cuba. El sindrome pelagroide-beri-bérico. *Bol Soc Cubana de Pediatria* 1935;7:5–68.
19. Goenz, AR. 1935. (Quoted in reference 21.)
20. Ubico CE, Klée GI. Memoria del V. Congreso Medico Centroamericano, 1938. San Salvador, 1942:543.
21. Peña Chavarria A, Rotter W. Edema avitaminósico de la infancia. *Rev Med Latinoam* 1937–38;23:1027–41.
22. Umaña CT. Los corpúsculos sanguineos en el edema distrófico. *Bul Soc Cub Pediatr* 1943;15:775–85.
23. Carvalho M, Pinto AG, Schmidt MM, Potsch N, Costa N. Distrofia pluricarencial hidropigénica. *J Pediatr (Rio de Janeiro)* 1945;11:395–439.
24. Gillan RU. An investigation into certain cases of oedema occurring among Kikuyu children and adults. *E Afr Med J* 1934;11:88–98.
25. Trowell HC. Pellagra in African children. *Arch Dis Child* 1937;12:193–212.
26. Van Daele G. Sur une affection de carence et de déséquilibre diététique observée au Congo (Buaki des indigènes). *Ann Soc Belge Méd Trop* 1938;18:653–70.
27. Trolli G. *Résumé des observations réunies au Kwango au sujet de deux affections d'origine indéterminée.* Brussels: Impr des Travs Publics, 1938.
28. Shukry H, Mahdi MA, El Gholmy AA. Nutritional oedema in children in Egypt. *Arch Dis Child* 1938;13:254–7.

29. Kark SL. Adult and infant pellagra in South African Bantu. *S Afr J Med Sci* 1943;8:106–14.
30. Pieraerts G. Etude sur la syndrome depigmentation-oedeme au Kassai. *Bull Soc Pathol Exot Filiales* 1946;39:226–35.
31. Normet L. La "boufissure d'Annam." *Bull Soc Pathol Exot Filiales* 1926;19:207–13.
32. Chen J. Nutritional oedema in children. *Am J Dis Child* 1942;63:552–80.
33. Weech AA. Association of keratomalacia with other deficiency diseases. *Am J Dis Child* 1930;39:1153–66.
34. McCollum EV, Orent-Keiles E, Day HG. *The newer knowledge of nutrition.* 5th ed. New York: Macmillan, 1939.
35. Economic Advisory Council: Committee on Nutrition in The Colonial Empire. First Report. London: HMSO, 1939.
36. Trowell HC, Davies JNP, Dean RFA. *Kwashiorkor.* Part III: *Kwashiorkor in children.* Part IV: *Protein malnutrition in adults.* London: Edward Arnold, 1954.
37. Brock JF, Autret M. Kwashiorkor in Africa. World Health Organization Monograph Series no. 8, Geneva: WHO, 1952.
38. Autret M. Behar M. *Le syndrome de polycarence en Amérique Centrale (kwashiorkor).* FAO Nutrition Studies no 13. Rome: FAO, 1955.
39. Waterlow J, Vergara A. *Protein malnutrition in Brazil.* FAO Nutrition Studies no 14. Rome: FAO, 1956.
40. Someswara Rao K, Swaminathan MC, Swarup S, Patwardhan VN. Protein malnutrition in South India. *Bull WHO* 1959;20:603–39.
41. Olson RE, ed. *Protein-calorie malnutrition.* New York: Academic Press, 1975.
42. Alleyne GAO, Hay RW, Picou DI, Stanfield JP, Whitehead RG. *Protein-energy malnutrition.* London: Edward Arnold, 1977.
43. Waterlow JC, Cravioto J, Stephen JML. Protein malnutrition in man. *Adv Prot Chem* 1960;15:131–238.
44. Waterlow JC, Alleyne GAO. Protein malnutrition in children: advances in knowledge in the last ten years. In: *Adv Prot Chem* 1971;25:117–235.
45. Suskind RM, ed. *Malnutrition and the immune response.* New York: Raven Press, 1977.
46. Patrick J, Golden MHN. Leucocyte electrolytes and sodium transport in protein energy malnutrition. *Am J Clin Nutr* 1977;30:1478–81.
47. Kaplan SS. Na$^+$ 'pump' and cell energetics in protein-energy malnutrition. *Nutr Res* 1984;4:935–48.
48. Golden MHN, Golden BE, Bennett FI. Relationship of trace element deficiency to malnutrition. In: RK Chandra, ed. *Trace elements in nutrition of children.* New York: Raven Press, 1985:185–207.
49. Golden MHN, Ramdath D. Free radicals in the pathogenesis of kwashiorkor. *Proc Nutr Soc* 1987;46:53–68.
50. Waterlow JC. Emerging priorities for the nutritional sciences. In: *Nutrition issues in developing countries for the 1980s and 1990s.* Washington, DC: National Academy of Sciences, 1986:43–56.
51. Williams CD. On that fiasco. *Lancet* 1975;i:793–4.
52. Achar ST. Nutritional dystrophy among children in Madras. *Br Med J* 1950;i:701–3.
53. Gopalan C, Patwardhan VN. Some observations on the "nutritional oedema syndrome." *Ind J Med Sci* 1951;5:312–7.
54. Frontali G. Malnutrition from protein deficiency. *Sci Med Italica* 1955;4:275–305.
55. Kerpel-Fronius E, Varga F. The problem of oedema in infantile malnutrition. *Acta Paediatr Scand* 1953;42:256–64.
56. Veghelyi P. Nutritional edema. *Ann Paediatr* 1950;175:349–377.
57. Czerny A, Keller A. *Des Kinde Ernährung. Ernährungstörungen und Ernährungstherapie* 2nd ed. Leipzig: Franz Deuticke, 1925–28.
58. Gürson CT, Saner GT. Historical introduction. In: McLaren DS, Burman, D, eds. *Textbook of paediatric nutrition,* 1st ed. Edinburgh: Churchill-Livingstone, 1976:3–17.
59. Still GF. *Common disorders and diseases of childhood,* 1st ed. London: Oxford University Press, 1909.
60. Waterlow JC. *Fatty liver disease in infants in the British West Indies.* MRC Special Report Series No 263. London: HMSO, 1948.
61. Trowell HC. Infantile pellagra. *Trans R Soc Trop Med Hyg* 1941;33:389–404.
62. Wellcome Trust Working Party. Classification of infantile malnutrition. *Lancet* 1970;ii:302–3.
63. McLaren DS. A fresh look at protein-calorie malnutrition. *Lancet* 1966;ii:485–8.
64. Gopalan C, Venkatachalam PS, Srikantia SG. Body composition in nutritional edema. *Metabolism* 1953;11:335–43.

65. Brock JF, Hansen JDL, Howe EE, Pretorius PJ, Davel JGA, Hendrickse RG. Kwashiorkor and protein malnutrition: a dietary therapeutic trial. *Lancet* 1955;ii:355–60.
66. Dean RFA, Whitehead RG. Plasma aminogram in kwashiorkor. *Lancet* 1964;ii:98–9.
67. United Nations. *International action to avert the impending protein crisis.* Report to the Economic and Social Council of the Advisory Committee on the Application of Science and Technology to Development. New York: United Nations, 1968.
68. McLaren DS. The protein fiasco. *Lancet* 1975;ii:93–6.
69. Landman J, Jackson AA. The role of protein deficiency in the aetiology of kwashiorkor. *W Ind Med J* 1980;29:229–38.
70. Waterlow JC. Kwashiorkor revisited: the pathogenesis of oedema in kwashiorkor and its significance. *Trans R Soc Trop Med Hyg* 1984;78:436–41.
71. Hansen JDL. Electrolyte and nitrogen metabolism in kwashiorkor. *S Afr J Lab Clin Med* 1956;2:206–31.
72. Holliday MA. Pediatric nephrology, 1915–1985. In: Nicols BL Jr, Ballabriga A, Kretchmer N, eds. *History of pediatrics,* New York: Raven Press, 1991:113–121.
73. Gopalan C. Kwashiorkor and marasmus. Evolution and distinguishing features. In: McCance RA, Widdowson EM, eds. *Caloric deficiencies and protein deficiencies.* London: Churchill, 1968:49–58.
74. Rao KSJ. Hypothesis: marasmus and kwashiorkor. *Lancet* 1974;i:709–11.
75. Whitehead RG, Coward WA, Lunn PG, Rutishauser I. A comparison of the pathogenesis of protein-energy malnutrition in Uganda and The Gambia. *Trans R Soc Trop Med Hyg* 1977;71:189–95.
76. Lunn PG, Whitehead RG, Coward WA. Two pathways to kwashiorkor? *Trans R Soc Trop Med Hyg* 1979;73:438–44.
77. Golden M. The consequences of protein deficiency in man and its relationship to the features of kwashiorkor. In: Blaxter KL, Waterlow JC, eds. *Nutritional adaptation in man.* London: John Libbey, 1985:169–88.
78. Hendrickse RG. The influence of aflatoxins on child health in the tropics with particular reference to kwashiorkor. *Trans R Soc Trop Med Hyg* 1984;78:427–35.
79. Annegers JF. Ecology of dietary patterns and nutritional status in West Africa. *Ecol Food Nutr* 1973;2:107–19.
80. Tolboom JJM, Ralitapole-Maraping AP, Kabir H, Molatseli P, Anderson J. Severe protein-energy malnutrition in Lesotho, death and survival in hospital, clinical findings. *Trop Geograph Med* 1986;38:351–8.
81. Waterlow JC. Elimination of severe PEM by the year 2000? Paper presented at the ACC Subcommittee of Nutrition, 13th Session. Washington, DC, 1987.

DISCUSSION

Dr. Hansen: It is important to emphasize the similarities as well as the differences between kwashiorkor and marasmus. All affected children come from a poor background, all show growth failure, and in all a good diet is necessary for recovery. Differences can be explained on the basis of factors such as age, quality and quantity of diet, infection, and environmental and family stress, as has been determined in research units around the world.

When I returned to Cape Town after Professor Brock had published his FAO/WHO report in 1952 he summoned me into his office to discuss possible research projects on kwashiorkor. Holding a can of dried milk powder he said that the thing in his tour around Africa that had impressed him the most was the fact that children with kwashiorkor responded to a milk diet. He suggested that I should find out what it was in skimmed milk that initiated a cure. This is how our research in kwashiorkor began.

Dr. Waterlow: Even in the 1980s the mortality from severe malnutrition in good hospitals in countries such as Nigeria (1) or Bangladesh (2) is as high as 20% or more. I believe that it can be reduced to practically zero, in the light of the knowledge that we have, without elaborate facilities.

I agree with Professor Hansen about the similarities between marasmus and kwashiorkor except that if you believe, as I do, that the particular features of kwashiorkor are due to a predominant protein deficiency (3), then this has public health implications.

Dr. Barness: I came across a quotation from an article in the early 1920s suggesting that the disease we now call kwashiorkor was due to a poison. Last year I read a paper suggesting that kwashiorkor was caused by aflatoxins.

Dr. Waterlow: You are referring to the work of Hendrickse (4). However, the epidemiological evidence does not fit.

Dr. Benakoppa: Dr. Gopalan is a leading nutritionist in India and South East Asia. For many years he worked as director of the National Institute of Nutrition in Hyderabad and at present he heads the Nutrition Foundation of India. He was influential in the view that malnutrition was not due to protein deficiency alone and that lack of calories was a most important aspect. He coined the terms *food gap* and *calorie gap* and in 1968 he introduced the concept of *dysadaptation*, whereby kwashiorkor represented a disorder of failure of adaptation, while at the opposite pole marasmus represented an extreme degree of adaptation.

Dr. Frenk: In 1946, Federico Gómez proposed the Spanish word *desnutrición* as the generic term for the whole array of names that have been given to the various clinical pictures that are called (not entirely correctly) *malnutrition* in English. One of the best of these names, which has not been mentioned in this workshop, is *cacochymia,* which denotes the profound distortion of tissue chemical composition that characterizes advanced cases of the syndrome. Gómez's viewpoint, soon shared by Gopalan and many others, was that the different clinical appearances represent a spectorum, with young normoalbuminemic marasmic infants at one extreme and hypoalbuminemic one- to four-year-old toddlers at the other, regardless of whether their kwashiorkor was "marasmic" (i.e., cachectic) or not.

Dr. Darby: There are three further names that deserve a mention because of their foresight in sponsoring some of the earliest studies in this area. They are Fred Clements of Australia, who was the first director of nutrition for the World Health Organization; his successor, Jim Burgess; and Wallace Aykroyd, who was head of nutrition in the FAO.

Dr. Metcoff: We should mention fetal malnutrition. Prior to 1950, Stuart and Clifford, in Boston, described the "dystrophic" newborn because such infants appeared malnourished. Some were postmature and underweight, others just underweight. Later, when the relation of birthweight to gestational age became part of the clinical assessment of the newborn, and intrauterine growth curves such as those of Lubchencko became standard in most nurseries, babies who were too small for their gestational age were labeled *SGA* (small-for-gestational age). However their clinical appearance, i.e., whether they seemed malnourished or not, was largely ignored. Malnourished infants are born almost every day in every large nursery; yet malnutrition in newborn infants is not often recognized. It is important that pediatricians realize that fetal malnutrition is not uncommon and is not confined to the Third World.

REFERENCES

1. Laditan AAO, Tineimebwa G. The protein-energy malnourished child in a Nigerian teaching hospital. *J Trop Pediatr* 1983;29:61–4.
2. Brown KH, Gilman RH, Gaffar A, et al. Infections associated with severe PEM in hospitalized infants. *Nutr Res* 1981;1:33–46.
3. Waterlow JC. Kwashiorkor and its significance. *Trans R Soc Trop Med Hyg* 1984;78:436–41.
4. Hendrickse RG. The influence of aflatoxins on child health in the tropics with particular reference to kwashiorkor. *Trans R Soc Trop Med Hyg* 1984;78:427–35.

History of Pediatrics 1850–1950, edited by
B.L. Nichols, A. Ballabriga, and N. Kretchmer.
Nestlé Nutrition Workshop Series, Vol. 22. Nestec
Ltd., Vevey/Raven Press, Ltd., New York © 1991.

Body Composition

Gilbert B. Forbes[1]

Departments of Pediatrics and Biophysics, University of Rochester School of Medicine and Dentistry, Rochester, New York 14642, USA

Among the biological sciences, anatomy held the stage until the early years of the nineteenth century, when it was overtaken by the rapidly developing science of chemistry. Much later emerged the modern technologies we now use in body composition studies, to make possible the evaluation of living human beings. We can today effectively measure the chemical anatomy of the living human body to study the nature of growth.

TISSUE AND WHOLE BODY COMPOSITION

As a student, Liebig (see p. 50, Fig. 1) obtained a travel grant from the Duke of Hesse-Darmstadt to study chemistry in Paris under Gay-Lussac, a former student of Lavoisier, and in 1824 he returned as Professor of Chemistry at Giessen. Then he obtained another grant that he used to set up what was to be the first well-equipped student laboratory in Germany and proceeded to establish himself as the founder of organic chemistry. He proved that body heat was the product of the combustion of carbohydrate and fat, not carbon and hydrogen, and, based on his analyses of plants and soils, he established the importance of chemical fertilizers. He analyzed animal tissues and found that blood plasma composition differed from that of body tissues, the former being rich in sodium, the latter rich in potassium. Of interest to infant nutritionists was Liebig's development in 1867 of the first infant formula, which was widely advertised in the United States. It was composed of wheat flour, milk, and malt flour cooked with potassium bicarbonate (1).

Schmidt's book, published in 1850, provided information on the chemical composition of digestive secretions, and his values for electrolytes and protein in blood plasma are strikingly similar to modern values. He found that the blood of cholera patients had reduced levels of sodium and chloride, and increased amounts of protein (2). However, large quantities of blood—as much as 200 ml—were required for his analyses, and it was not until many years later that methods suitable for infants were to become available.

---

[1]Because of illness in the Forbes family, the manuscript was read by Kenneth J. Ellis.

Bezold, a young German student, discovered that growth in animals was accompanied by a decrease in water content and an increase in ash content (3), which marked a beginning of the science of developmental biochemistry. Lawes and Gilbert (4) demonstrated an increase in body fat content as well as some increase in lean tissue, as meat animals were fed for market; incidentally, they noted that body water varied inversely with fat content.[2] Later on, Pfeiffer (5) reported that the variability in the water content of animal bodies could be greatly reduced if the data were expressed on a fat-free basis.

Fehling (6) and Camerer and Söldner (7) established the changes in human body composition during fetal life, and their work was extended by Iob and Swanson (8) and by Widdowson and her co-workers (9). Fetal growth in man was found to be associated with an increase in Ca, P, and N contents per unit body weight, and a decline in water, Na, and Cl contents. By the mid-1950s, several adult human specimens had been analyzed for major elements (9–11), and others had assayed various individual tissues for a number of trace elements (12).

Drawing on data from the literature, Moulton announced in 1923 the concept of *chemical maturity,* that stage of life when body composition approaches the adult value and hence is considered *mature* (13). He concluded that mammals reach chemical maturity at about 4% of their life span. If this holds for humans, the age would be about 3 years.

FAT-FREE BASIS FOR EXPRESSING TISSUE COMPOSITION

Earlier mention was made of Pfeiffer's finding that the variability of tissue water content was greatly reduced when calculated on a fat-free basis. These and other data led Magnus-Levy to announce in 1906 that the fat-poor muscle of a starved animal cannot be compared directly to one normally nourished and rich in fat. Organs can be compared only on a fat-free basis (14). This concept underlies most methods for estimating the body fat content of living subjects. The total body water, densitometric, and total body potassium techniques for estimating lean body mass (LBM) and body fat all depend on the assumption of the constancy of LBM composition.

In 1905, Magnus-Levy (Fig. 1) was appointed Professor of Medicine at Berlin, a position that he held until 1922, when he entered private practice in order to have more time for research. His accomplishments were many: he found that the basal metabolic rate (BMR) was elevated in patients with thyrotoxicosis and depressed in cretins and in malnutrition, and that BMR was higher per unit weight in children than in adults. He isolated β-hydroxybutyric acid from the blood of diabetics, and his skill at analyzing human tissues for electrolytes was such that at least one physiologist from the United States sent tissue samples to him for analysis.

---

[2]Of more than passing interest is an experiment performed by these investigators. They fed sheep a low fat diet and, in finding that these animals put on the usual amounts of body fat, concluded, quite rightly, that carbohydrate could be converted to fat—a remarkable insight for those days when enzymes and intermediary metabolism were unknown.

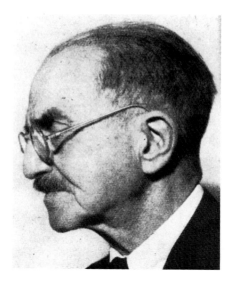

FIG. 1. Adolph Magnus-Levy, 1865–1955.

THE METABOLIC BALANCE TECHNIQUE

Once methods for analysis of food and excreta for nitrogen and minerals had been developed, physiologists began to apply them to the study of human metabolism. By analyzing the food and drink consumed, and feces and urine for the element in question, intake and output are determined: When intake exceeds output, the subject's body is being enriched with the particular element under study; and when output exceeds intake, body content is impoverished. The former state is spoken of as positive, the latter as negative, metabolic balance.

This technique appears to have been in common use by the early 1900s. Examples are Cathcart's (15) demonstration of loss of body nitrogen during fasting, and Benjamin's (16) finding that infants retained nitrogen as they grew. Later nutritionists used this technique as a means of estimating dietary protein and mineral requirements. It should be remembered that the metabolic balance technique can detect only *changes* in body content of a number of elements, not body content per se. Moreover, in quantitative terms, it has limitations: skin losses are difficult to measure, a fore-period of adjustment is needed whenever intake is altered, positive balances tend to be overestimated, and negative balances underestimated. Benjamin (16), for example, found that the calculated increase in body protein in growing infants was much greater than expected, especially when cow's milk was fed. The uncritical use of the balance method has led to spuriously high estimates of protein requirements for infants, pregnant women, and adults by nutritionists (17).

Since sodium is the predominant cation and chloride the predominant anion of extracellular fluid (ECF) and, since most of the body potassium is located in intracellular fluid (ICF), Gamble and Peters and van Slyke were able to deduce the relative changes in ECF volume and ICF volume from the magnitudes of Na, Cl, and potassium (K) balances (18,19). Gamble (see p. 193, Fig. 2) developed the concept of the companionship of water and electrolyte in body fluid economy (20). He was to improve greatly our understanding of body fluid electrolytes by depicting cations and anions in terms of milliequivalents rather than milligrams per liter, thus emphasizing the electroneutrality of the body fluids.

Using the metabolic balance technique, Darrow (see p. 115, Fig. 2) was able to show that infantile diarrhea was accompanied by potassium losses sufficient to require treatment with potassium salts (21). Mention should be made of Darrow's demonstration of the occurrence of shifts in ECF and ICF volumes in response to changes in ECF osmolality; osmotic equilibrium is achieved by the transfer of water between these two fluid compartments (22). The balance technique has broadened our knowledge of human body composition.

THE CONCEPT OF BODY FLUID VOLUME

The demonstration in 1832 by the Scottish physician Latta (2) that cholera patients could be revived by infusing saline and bicarbonate solutions intravenously apparently did not find favor with physicians until many years later (or perhaps they tried it only to be dissuaded by the occurrence of serious complications). Later there were attempts to treat acidosis in cholera patients with intravenous sodium bicarbonate. These were largely unsuccessful due to the failure to realize that dehydration and acidosis were both involved. We now know that correction of the latter without correcting the former could not be expected to restore the patient to normal. Pediatric textbooks published around the turn of the century mention the use of subcutaneous saline solutions in the treatment of cholera infantum, but only very briefly, the major emphasis being placed on other medications such as cathartics, opium, bismuth, etc.

The work of Keith, Rowntree, and Geraghty (23) on the determination of blood volume by the dilution of dyes (Vital Red, Congo Red) stimulated a resurgence of interest in body fluid volume as an important physiological variable. Their method was widely used in studies of patients with various disorders, including shock in wounded World War I soldiers.

Although trained as a biochemist, Marriott (see p. 141, Fig. 4) managed to take enough courses at Cornell to earn an M.D. degree. In 1910, he went to St. Louis with Philip Shaffer to develop the Department of Biochemistry at Washington University School of Medicine. There he met Howland who, after his removal to Johns Hopkins, invited Marriott to join him; then in 1917, despite having had rather limited clinical experience, he was called to the Chair of Pediatrics at Washington University, where he was able to put his biochemical training to good use.

At Marriott's suggestion, Utheim studied blood flow in infants with severe diarrhea and found it to be greatly reduced. For this purpose, Utheim used a calorimetric technique: a limb is immersed in a measured volume of water at a known temperature somewhat below that of the body. The rise in temperature after a 10 minute period is proportional to the amount of blood passing through the extremity per unit time.

Earlier, Howland and Marriott (24) had found that infants with diarrhea were acidotic. Marriott (25) now correctly deduced that the prime disturbance in severe infantile diarrhea was dehydration and diminished blood volume, which led to compromise of the circulation, concentration of the blood, failure of organ function, and acidosis. His analysis of the situation put to rest the concept of *alimentary intoxication,* so long a favorite of Continental physicians. The problem was not production of unidentified toxins, but of loss of body fluids. Together with contributions by Schloss, Blackfan, and Karelitz, the stage was set for the science of parenteral fluid therapy.

Marriott showed the different features of weight loss due to diarrhea and athrepsia: the former being due to loss of water from the body, the latter to lack of proper nourishment. He and Jeans published a book on infant nutrition (26) that served as a standard work for several years. This work was based on their own clinical experience.

It was the Hungarian physicist, von Hevesy (Fig. 2), who was first to use deuterium to estimate total body water by the principle of isotopic dilution (27). He was also among the first to use radioactive isotopes as tracers for the study of mineral absorption by plants and the metabolism of phosphorus. Later, methods were developed for the estimation of ECF volume. McCance and Widdowson (28) estimated body fluid volumes in malnourished individuals, and were able to show that relative ECF volume was increased, and that it diminished, in relative terms, as the patients recovered. Similar findings were reported by Cokington et al. (29) for malnourished

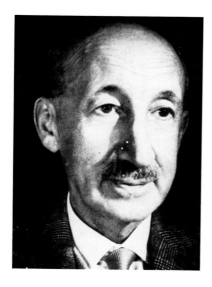

FIG. 2. Georg von Hevesy, 1886–1966.

infants. Cheek documented the changes in body fluid volumes during growth in infancy and childhood (30).

REGIONAL BODY COMPOSITION

Studies of regional composition include the measurement of subcutaneous tissue plus skin thickness (''skinfold thickness'') by calipers, roentgenographic measurements of bone widths and muscle widths, various body circumferences, and more recently the use of single or dual photon absorptiometry to assess bone mineral content. Urinary creatinine excretion is an index of muscle mass. There are now a vast amount of data for individuals of all ages, and for patients with various disorders (see (17)).

MODERN TECHNIQUES

Although there had been a few earlier attempts, it was left to Behnke (31) to make full use of the densitometric technique for estimating total body fat and lean mass. He used the Archimedean principle that the amounts of two components of differing but known density could be determined by measuring the density of the entire system. Assuming a constant density for the fat-free mass, and with the knowledge that body fat has a different density, one can calculate the relative proportions of fat and lean in the entire body from the observed body density. The most commonly used technique is to weigh the subject in air and again under water. Keys and Brozek (32) then proceeded to put this technique on a sound footing.

Moore (33) used the isotopic dilution method to estimate total body water (D_2O), total exchangeable sodium (^{24}Na) and total exchangeable potassium (^{42}K). He then developed the concept of body cell mass as ''the working, energy-metabolizing portion of the human body in relation to its supporting structures,'' defined as *total exchangeable K multiplied by the reciprocal of the average intracellular K concentration* (34).

A number of long-lived radioisotopes were formed at the time of the great nuclear fire that led to the formation of terrestrial matter several billions of years ago. Among these is potassium-40 (^{40}K), present wherever potassium is found. Sixty years ago, Schlundt (35) found that the human body gave off radioactive emissions. At first this was ascribed to radium, a known contaminant of bone. With the development of high resolution gamma-ray spectrometers, it was later determined that these emissions were largely due to ^{40}K, present in sufficient quantities to permit quantitation by specially constructed external scintillation counters. From the recorded radioactive emissions from ^{40}K one can calculate total body potassium, and, as is the case for total body water, an estimate of LBM can be made and, by subtraction, total body fat (36,17).

These three methods (density, total body water, and total body K) all rely on the principle of compositional constancy of the lean body mass. Such an assumption is a reasonable one for the years from late adolescence up to old age; however, there are differences in the elderly and in infancy and early childhood.

These techniques have been widely used in studies of growth and aging, nutritional excess and deficiency, response to trauma, and in various disease states. It has been established that obese individuals usually have an increased lean weight as well as a larger amount of body fat, that LBM and fat both decrease when energy intake is subnormal, and that both increase in response to energy surfeit. There seems to be a companionship for these two body components: a change in one is accompanied by a change in the other, albeit in variable proportions. In other situations, such as androgen administration, the feeding of low-protein high-energy diets, and in experimental hypothalamic obesity, an increase in one component is accompanied by a decrease in the other. The finding of a decreased LBM in experimental obesity serves to set it firmly apart from the human condition.

The protective value of body fat has been demonstrated. During dietary-induced weight loss, thin individuals lose relatively large amounts of lean tissue compared to fat, whereas the obese lose proportionally more fat and thus tend to conserve lean. This is why obese individuals tolerate starvation better than those who are thin (37).

It has been known for many years that neutron bombardment serves to transmute a number of elements, which then become radioactive and can be assayed by radiation detectors. This technique was first used by Anderson and co-workers in London about 25 years ago (38), and then elaborated by Cohn at the Brookhaven National Laboratories, and by investigators in Great Britain, Canada, Australia, and the United States. By this means, total body Ca, P, N, Na, and Cl can be estimated. Although the radiation dose to the subject is very small ($\sim$30 mrad), there has been a reluctance to employ this technique with infants.

Other techniques are currently under study: lean weight by total body electrical conductivity and bioelectrical impedance, skeletal size by dual-photon absorptiometry, body fat distribution and organ size by computed tomography and nuclear magnetic resonance. We now have a wide array of techniques at our disposal for the assessment of human body composition during growth.

REFERENCES

1. Cone TE. *History of American pediatrics.* Boston: Little, Brown and Co, 1979.
2. Gamble JL. Early history of fluid replacement therapy. *Pediatrics* 1953;11:554–67.
3. von Bezold A. Untersuchungen über die Vertheilung von Wasser, organischer Materie und anorganischen Verbindungen im Thierreiche. *Z Wissensch Zool* 1857;8:487–524.
4. Lawes JB, Gilbert JH. Experimental inquiry into the composition of some of the animals fed and slaughtered as human food. *Philos Trans R Soc Lond (Biol)* 1859;149:493–680.
5. Pfeiffer L. Über den Fettgehalt des Körpers und verschiedener Theile desselben bei mageren und fetten Thieren. *Z Biol* 1887;23:340–80.
6. Fehling H. Beitrage zur Physiologie de placentaren Stoffverkehrs. *Arch Gynaekol* 1876;11:523.
7. Camerer W, Söldner. Die chemische Zusammensetzung des Neugeborenen. *Z Biol* 1900;39:173–92.
8. Iob V, Swanson WW. Mineral growth. *Growth* 1938;2:252–6.

9. Widdowson EM, Dickerson JWT. Chemical composition of the body. In: Comar CL, Bronner F, eds. *Mineral metabolism,* vol 2, part A. London: Academic Press, 1964:2–247.
10. Forbes RM, Cooper AR, Mitchell HH. The composition of the human body as determined by chemical analysis. *J Biol Chem* 1953;203:359–66.
11. Forbes GB, Lewis A. Total sodium, potassium, and chloride in adult man. *J Clin Invest* 1956; 35:596–600.
12. International Commission on Radiological Protection, No. 23. *Report of the task group on reference man.* Oxford: Pergamon Press, 1975.
13. Moulton CR. Age and chemical development in mammals. *J Biol Chem* 1923;57:79–97.
14. Magnus-Levy A. Physiologie des Stoffwechsels. In: von Noorden C, ed. *Handbuch der Pathologie des Stoffwechsels.* Berlin: Hirschwald, 1906:446.
15. Cathcart EP. Über die Zusammensetzung des Hungerharms. *Biochem Z* 1907;6:109–48.
16. Benjamin E. Der Eiweissnährschaden des Säuglings. *Z Kinderheilkunde* 1914;10:185–302.
17. Forbes GB. *Human body composition: growth, aging, nutrition, and activity.* New York: Springer-Verlag, 1987.
18. Gamble JL, Ross SG, Tisdall FF. The metabolism of fixed base during fasting. *J Biol Chem* 1923;57:633–95.
19. Peters JP, Van Slyke DD. *Quantitative clinical chemistry,* vol 1. Baltimore: Williams and Wilkins Co, 1946.
20. Gamble JL. *Companionship of water and electrolytes in organization of body fluids* (Lane Medical Lecture). Stanford University Press, 1951.
21. Govan DC, Jr, Darrow DC. The use of potassium chloride in the treatment of the dehydration of diarrhea in infants. *J Pediatr* 1946;28:541–9.
22. Darrow DC, Yannet H. The changes in the distribution of body water accompanying increase and decrease in extracellular electrolyte. *J Clin Invest* 1935;14:266–75.
23. Keith NM, Rowntree LG, Geraghty JT. A method for the determination of plasma and blood volume. *Arch Intern Med* 1915;16:547–76.
24. Howland J, Marriott WK. Acidosis occurring with diarrhea. *Am J Dis Child* 1916;11:309–25.
25. Marriott WMcK. Some phases of the pathology of nutrition in infancy. *Harvey Lectures* 1919–1920;15:121–51.
26. Marriott WM, Jeans PC. *Infant nutrition.* 3rd ed. St. Louis: CV Mosby Co, 1941.
27. von Hevesy G, Hofer E. Die Verweilzeit des Wassers im menschlichen Körper, untersucht mit Hilfe von "Schwerem" Wasser als Indicator. *Klin Wochenschr* 1934;13:1524–6.
28. McCance RA, Widdowson EM. A method of breaking down the body weights of living persons into terms of extracellular fluid, cell mass and fat, and some applications of it to physiology and medicine. *Proc R Soc Land, Series B* 1951;138:115–30.
29. Cokington L, Hanna FM, Jackson RL. Changes in body composition of malnourished infants during repletion. *Ann NY Acad Sci* 1963;110:849–60.
30. Cheek DB. *Human growth: body composition, cell growth, energy and intelligence.* Philadelphia: Lea & Febiger, 1968.
31. Behnke AR, Feen BG, Welham WC. The specific gravity of healthy men. *JAMA* 1942;118:495–8.
32. Keys A, Brozek J. Body fat in adult man. *Physiol Rev* 1953;33:245–345.
33. Moore FD. Determination of total body water and solids with isotopes. *Science* 1946;104:157–60.
34. Moore FD, Olesen KH, McMurray JD, Parker HV, Ball MR, Boyden CM. *The body cell mass and its supporting environment.* Philadelphia: WB Saunders Co, 1963.
35. Schlundt H, Barker HH, Flinn FB. The detection and estimation of radium and mesothorium in living persons. *Am J Roentgenol* 1929;21:345–54.
36. Forbes GB, Hursh J, Gallup J. Estimation of total body fat from potassium-40 content. *Science* 1961;133:101–2.
37. Forbes GB. Lean body mass-body fat interrelationships in man: dietary changes induce changes in both body compartments. *Nutr Rev* 1987;45:225–31.
38. Anderson J, Osborn SB, Tomlinson RWS, et al. Neutron-activation analysis in man in vivo: a new technique in medical investigation. *Lancet* 1964;ii:1201–5.

History of Pediatrics 1850–1950, edited by
B.L. Nichols, A. Ballabriga, and N. Kretchmer.
Nestlé Nutrition Workshop Series, Vol. 22. Nestec
Ltd., Vevey/Raven Press, Ltd., New York © 1991.

Salt and Water Therapy

Bent Friis-Hansen

*Department of Neonatology, University of Copenhagen, Rigshospitalet, Copenhagen,
Denmark*

We have just seen the outside of a foundling home. It looked nice and tidy but the
outcome was disastrous for the infants. In Paris the mortality rate was above 90%,
mainly due to gastroenteritis which was endemic—and no treatment was available.

In the years 1830–1836, a terrifying cholera epidemic spread over Europe. The
physicians tried many remedies, but with little success. One of the most effective
was simple administration of salt solutions. Actually this was so simple that many
doctors fought against it, and, as the epidemic subsided, the method was soon forgotten only to be rediscovered at a later epidemic in Naples in 1884.

By the early 1950s, intravenous (IV) fluid therapy was well established in the developed world as the treatment for dehydrated children, and it may well have
reached a state where it became an art in itself. This may have delayed the treatment
of infants suffering from diarrhea throughout the developing world. The recent
worldwide use of simple oral rehydration solutions has been a giant step forward—
in spite of the fact that the composition of these fluids is quite similar to that recommended 150 years ago. It is this cycle of therapy that I shall describe.

Preceding chapters have described some of the central figures in the development
of water and electrolyte therapy: O'Shaughnessy (Fig. 1) and Latta, and later Marriott, Gamble, and Darrow. I shall here give the background of their work and introduce a few of the other early pioneers in this field.

O'Shaughnessy was not the first to study the chemical composition of the blood.
Around 1806–1810, Berzelius (2) in Stockholm and, in 1830, LeCanu (3) in Paris
had studied the composition of animal blood. In 1829, Clanny (4) published a description of an apparatus for sampling the composition of the blood in health and
disease. Figure 2 shows the multiple applications of a similar syringe used by Latta
(5). It could also be used to draw blood from a patient. The capacity was 200 ml, so
repeated examinations in children were out of the question.

In 1817, the severe cholera epidemic began in the Ganges delta in India, slowly
spreading north to Russia and from there to the rest of Europe. The mortality was
high at 60%–90%, and it must have been dramatic for physicians to follow the
spread of the disease.

Early attempts had been made to investigate the composition of blood from cholera patients in Warsaw and Moscow but without remarkable results. Then on No-

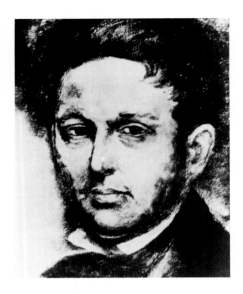

FIG. 1. Sir William B. O'Shaughnessy. (From ref. 5.)

vember 19, 1831, indicating the grave concern with which cholera was regarded, the *Lancet* published a special issue of 30 pages under the title: *History of the Rise, Progress, Ravages etc. of the Blue Cholera of India.* On December 29, O'Shaughnessy (6) published a letter in the *Lancet,* and two days later W.R. Clanny (7) published similar results.

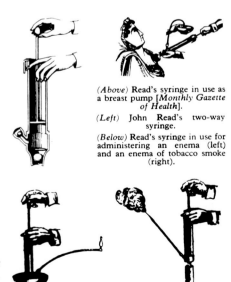

(*Above*) Read's syringe in use as a breast pump [*Monthly Gazette of Health*].

(*Left*) John Read's two-way syringe.

(*Below*) Read's syringe in use for administering an enema (left) and an enema of tobacco smoke (right).

FIG. 2. The infusion apparatus used by Thomas A. Latta, designed by John Read. (From ref. 5.)

O'Shaughnessy became interested in chemistry early in his career. His first paper was on confectionary poisoned with lead, copper, and other heavy metals (8). His main achievement was to demonstrate the biochemical changes found in the blood of cholera patients and to conclude that ''all the salts deficient in the blood . . . are present in large quantities in the peculiar white dejected matter.'' Later he became a surgeon in Bengal and wrote a manual of chemistry. Ultimately, he was made professor at the Medical School in Calcutta and wrote the Bengal *Pharmacopoeia*. His main interest was in electricity and in the newly invented telegraph. He became director of the Indian Telegraphic Society and was later knighted for his achievement of establishing telegraph lines over great areas of India.

William Reid Clanny was born in Ireland. He became a surgeon, served under Nelson, and was later private doctor to the Duke of Sussex. In 1813 he constructed an early safety lamp to be used in the English coal mines.

A few months after the papers by O'Shaughnessy and Clanny, Latta (9), in the *Lancet*, described the effect of intravenous infusions of sodium chloride and sodium bicarbonate to severely sick patients suffering from cholera. The first patient died, but to the second he gave a total of 10 liters of 0.5% sodium chloride and 0.2% sodium bicarbonate over a period of 10 hours. The patient, a woman, woke up from coma, started to smoke her pipe and was cured. This represents a turning point in the history of medicine, since the treatment of diarrhea had for centuries been carried out according to Paracelsus, with bloodletting and the administration of a mixture of emetics and vitriolic acids. If that did not help, a red-hot iron was applied to the neck as close as possible to the brain. But now, for the first time in the history of medicine, treatment based upon scientific observations was carried out successfully.

Latta and O'Shaughnessy were presumably inspired by the work of William Stevens. He is an important but often overlooked figure in the early history of water and electrolyte therapy. He was born in Scotland in 1786 and, by 1810, was settled as a general practitioner in the West Indies, on the Danish Island of St. Croix, which was temporarily occupied by the English during the Napoleonic wars. He was an able surgeon and was the first to perform a ligation of the internal iliac artery, in 1813, in a woman with a large aneurysm. He traveled often and became a member of the Royal College of Physicians in 1814. He is described as a gentle man with a wry sense of humor, but he must also have been a man with a hot temperament since in 1820 he took part in a duel. He was shot in the thigh and removed the bullet himself.

Very early on, he became interested in the treatment of tropical fevers (yellow fever and cholera) with salt, and in 1829 he returned to Europe where he gave a paper, ''Observations on the blood,'' to the Royal Colleges of Physicians in 1830, over a year before the paper by O'Shaughnessy in the *Lancet*. It was published as a book in London in 1832 with the title *Observations on the Healthy and Diseased Properties of the Blood* (10). In it he states, ''It can be clearly proved that in the West Indian Fevers the patients that are left entirely to themselves have a much better chance of recovery than those who are treated with emetics, calomel or antimony, opium or acids, and that these remedies instead of being useful aggravate the suffering of the patients . . . and add greatly to the mortality from fevers in hot climates.''

Stevens understood that not only the blood but the whole body had lost salt and water and that these losses should be restored. His book received poor notices in the *Lancet,* the *Medicochirugical Review* and the *London Medical Gazette.* Nevertheless his method was used in an epidemic of cholera in the Cold Bath Fields prison in London, and the mortality dropped from 50% to 3%. It was claimed, however, that most of the patients did not suffer from cholera, and the chairman of the Board of Health in London, Barry, wrote a report published in the *Lancet* and *London Medical Gazette* in which he claimed that Stevens was a quack, since he would only treat cholera patients with ordinary ''culinary salt'' and that he even failed to give the standard treatment. In spite of this, the Central Board of Health sent questionnaires to a number of doctors and some doctors supported the new treatment. The results were ambiguous, presumably because too little salt and water was given, often together with the old remedies.

In 1833, Stevens visited Copenhagen, where he published a book *Anvisning til den Asiatiske Koleras Behandling* (11) that was translated into English as *Observations on the Treatment of Cholera, Copenhagen 1833* (12). Translations of his book appeared in Sweden and France in 1833 and 1836. He was also interested in respiration and wrote a paper on the theory of respiration (13).

His treatment was introduced with good results in Moscow, and he became internationally famous. The Tzar even gave him a diamond ring.

The next cholera epidemic spread over Europe from the Baltic countries around 1848. In 1850, Schmidt from Dorpat wrote a book, *Charakteristik der epidemischen Cholera.* His figures on the composition of normal blood and blood from cholera patients confirmed low sodium and very low bicarbonate values (14).

In 1853, Stevens published a new book, *The Nature and the Treatment of the Asiatic Cholera* (15), and again the reviews, particularly in the *Lancet,* were very poor, perhaps in response to his attacks against the English health system and ''. . . their self ignorance that even to this day they do not know what true knowledge is.'' Stevens died in 1868 and an obituary in the *British Medical Journal* praised his scientific and clinical activities and mentioned his many honors. The *Lancet* passed the event in silence.

In his many publications, Stevens pointed out that salt and water should be given early—at the beginning of the cholera. Once the patients had collapsed, the chances of saving them were poor. He therefore also advocated intravenous treatment.

A complete list of his publications is found in the Danish *Yearbook of Medical History,* 1976 (16).

In 1884, a new epidemic of cholera spread over Europe and again electrolyte therapy was introduced, this time by Arnoldi Cantani from Naples (17). He gave subcutaneous infusions of 0.4% sodium chloride and 0.3% sodium bicarbonate, but only in small amounts (1–1½ liters per day), and furthermore he did not consider acidosis important in these patients. By this time, the concept of water and electrolyte metabolism was better understood, since Claude Bernard had already introduced the concept of the *milieu intérieur* in 1859 (18), stating that "the maintenance of the stability of the *milieu intérieur* was necessary for the maintenance of all the conditions necessary to the life of the element."

DEHYDRATION AND TOXICOSIS

During the latter part of the nineteenth century, an expansion of biochemistry took place in Germany, and German pediatricians led the field in the growth of pediatrics. However, from the early part of this century, leadership slowly passed to the United States. Henderson (19) wrote his book, *The Fitness of the Environment* in 1913, and in 1917 the Henderson-Hasselbalch equation was formulated (20), stating that the pH of the blood is dependent on the equilibrium between bicarbonate and pCO_2.

Gastroenteritis in an infant or young child can develop into a life-threatening condition with vomiting, diarrhea and consequent dehydration. The infant may become progressively comatose. This condition was named *toxikosis,* or *coma dyspepticum* in Germany. This gave the impression that some toxin was present—an idea further supported by the liver necrosis often observed at autopsy. Chemical changes were found in the blood that were called *dekomposition*. This was a misleading name that seemed to give an explanation of the condition of the infants. Much time was lost in search of the toxin rather than on treating the underlying dehydration. Furthermore, the word *toxicosis* was generally used to describe all severe diseases with cerebral symptoms and *toxicosis* could be both the name of a disease or it could be a symptom of many diseases, including gastroenteritis, meningitis, encephalitis, sepsis, and malignant hyperventilation.

Finkelstein (see p. 140, Fig. 3) used the word *toxicosis* in his textbook on diseases in infancy in 1912, to describe severe forms of nutritional disorders, and in the 1938 edition (21) he has a whole chapter on "Der Toxische Symptomen Komplex (Intoxikation. Coma Dyspepticum)." This included 12 clinical symptoms, of which at least nine should be present to make the diagnosis of toxicosis. The most important were diarrhea, stupor, and weight loss. The multifactorial etiology of toxicose-exsiccose is well illustrated in Fig. 3 (22).

The different names and conditions are confusing and an excellent description of these complicated terms and conditions was given in Kerpel-Fronius' outstanding book (23) reviewed in "Marasmus" (see p. 219). The need for bicarbonate in cholera patients was first shown by Sellards (24), a doctor from the United States in Manila, who in 1911 wrote a paper entitled "Indication of acid intoxication in Asiatic Cholera." He treated his patients with 30–90 grams of sodium bicarbonate and showed that this quantity was necessary to make the urine alkaline. The fact that children with severe gastroenteritis also had acidosis was first shown by Howland (see p. 268, Fig. 1) and Marriott (p. 141, Fig. 4) in 1916 (25). The same year, Ylppö (26) also published a paper on the importance of acidosis in the newborn.

Marriott later advanced the theory that all symptoms in severe dehydration or *an-*

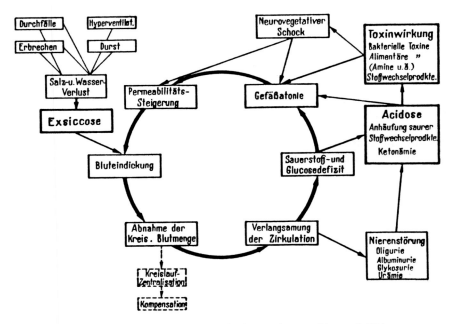

FIG. 3. Pathogenesis of intoxication-exsiccose. (From ref. 22.)

hydremia could be explained by the physiological effect of dehydration and a marked decrease of blood volume combined with hemoconcentration, low blood pressure, and decreased peripheral circulation, renal insufficiency with final shock and lethargy increasing to unconsciousness and death.

In spite of the fact that knowledge of dehydration and associated changes in water and electrolyte metabolism was available, it was not generally understood. The honor of achieving this general level of understanding must go to Gamble (27) (see pages 113 and 189). In carefully planned experiments he gave the answers to basic clinical problems related to water and electrolyte metabolism; furthermore, he knew how to present his results in simple conceptual diagrams that everybody could understand. By the late 1940s, treatment of dehydration with intravenous fluids had become a sign of advanced medical knowledge, and the importance of also giving potassium by the intravenous route, as shown by Darrow (28) (see p. 115, Fig. 2), was rapidly gaining acceptance. What Marriott did to emphasize the importance of changes in plasma volume, Gamble did to emphasize changes in the extracellular fluid, and Darrow, in the intracellular fluid.

In the early post-Second World War period, isotopes of water and electrolytes became available and made feasible the in vivo measurement of body composition, including total body water, extra- and intracellular fluid volume, and total body exchangeable potassium and sodium (see p. 249). The pioneer in this work was Moore (29), and similar measurements were carried out by the author in children in order to study the changes in body water compartments during growth (30). A general understanding of acid-base balance was finally achieved by the widespread use of the Astrup Micromethods and the Siggård Andersen and Engle diagram for measuring standard base excess, as recently described in *The History of Blood Gases, Acids and Bases* by Astrup (5).

It took 20 years or more to introduce the worldwide use of simple oral rehydration fluids, thereby making treatment available for the thousands of children suffering from gastroenteritis in developing countries. Such a rehydration fluid is simply made by using boiled water, sodium chloride, and cane sugar. Better still, UNICEF Rehydration Salts are provided as small paper bags containing sodium chloride, potassium chloride, sodium bicarbonate, and glucose. This salt mixture, together with mass vaccination programs, may very well be the major contribution of pediatrics to the general health of children throughout the developing world.

FLUID INTAKE OF PREMATURE INFANTS

This short summary of the history of dehydration and rehydration would not be complete without a brief account of water metabolism in premature infants. Foremost in this field was Budin (31) of the Maternité Hospital in Paris. Faced by the birth of large numbers of premature infants and by high mortality rates, he started to publish papers on premature infants in 1888, and his lectures to students were published in 1900. La Maternité and Clinic Tarnier because the first centers for clinical research and teaching of premature infant care.

In Germany, Finkelstein became director of the new children's hospital, Kinder Asyl, in Berlin in 1902. He also became interested in the problems of prematurity. In 1909, the new Kaiserin Auguste Victoria Haus in Berlin became a teaching center for the prevention of infant mortality under the direction of Professor Langstein. Best known from this period is the work of Ylppö (Fig. 4), who worked as a staff member and participated in research from 1912–1920 (32).

Human milk has been used since the earliest time for the feeding of premature infants, and also for general treatment. In 1828, Meissner (33) advised that in addition to being fed mother's milk, the congenitally debilitated infant should be given enemas of milk and at least two milk baths daily. In 1897, Biedert (34) claimed that casein was the indigestible element of cow's milk, for which reason he recommended dilution of the milk with three or four parts of water to keep the protein under 1%. Thus by dilution the content of fat and protein came closer to that of human milk. In 1920, Reuss (35) recommended that 20–50 ml of saline or Ringer's solution, be injected subcutaneously into premature infants for the first 2 or 3 days. As gavage feeding often resulted in vomiting and aspiration followed by fatal pneumonias, it became accepted practice to give premature infants nothing by mouth for the first hours and days of life. In 1947, Steward Clifford (36) from Children's Hospital in Boston wrote, ''we have been convinced on purely clinical grounds that infants with

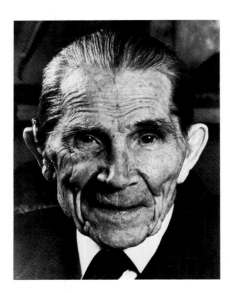

FIG. 4. Arvo Ylppö (b. 1887). (Courtesy of CNRC Archives; gift of J.K. Visakorpi.)

edema should not receive fluid until they have absorbed their subcutaneous fluid, even though this means withholding fluids for 4 to 5 days from even the smallest babies." In 1954, the *Manual of The American Academy of Pediatrics* stated, "It has been demonstrated that feeding of the smaller and more edematous infants may be delayed as long as four days. If the infant's condition is precarious, early feeding introduces extra hazards of vomiting and/or aspiration. Therefore a delay of at least 24 hours is justifiable and, by present knowledge, longer delays appear to be safe."

This regimen was described by Clement Smith (37) in his 1957 paper, "Reasons for Delaying the Feeding of Premature Infants:" He wrote, "There has been no increase in mortality following initial starvation. On the contrary our figures have been better and a negative balance for water and electrolytes thus seems to be unavoidable and so does a temporary period of negative balance of calories since this seems to us a less critical problem than that of water." Not everybody agreed and in 1954 Ylppö (26) wrote "Both vomiting and edema which are the starting points for this hunger therapy are ambiguous phenomena attributable in their etiology to very many reasons. I do not consider them sufficiently justified premises for such a radical method of feeding as 2–4 days complete fast. I feel further that many premature infants continuously supplied during the fetal period with both food and plenty of water and growing rapidly must suffer in a special manner from a sudden complete break in administration of fluid and food."

He compared clinically two methods of feeding newborn premature babies. In one, the infants were kept in a full fast, and in the other they were fed from the very first day of life. The mortality in both groups was practically the same, and he concluded that "vomiting and edema cannot be prevented by a complete fast; indeed on the basis of all that has been said I am of the opinion that we must try to arrange to feed the premature immediately after birth in conformity with nature and the conditions of the fetal period.''

This was the start of ''early feeding'' of premature infants. The concept was further supported by the work of Usher (38), who was the first to treat infants suffering from the respiratory distress syndrome of prematurity with sodium bicarbonate and glucose intravenously, but even this regimen gave rise to complications. In a study by Bell and colleagues (39) it was shown that too liberal an administration of fluid to small premature infants increases the risk of complications such as patent ductus arteriosus and retrolental fibroplasia.

At last it seems that most, if not all, of the major practical and theoretical problems of water and electrolyte metabolism have been elucidated after 150 years of study, mistakes, and progress.

REFERENCES

1. Peiper A. *Chronik Der Kinderheilkunde*. Leipzig: Thieme, 1955:116,118.
2. Berzelius JJ. *Föreläsninger över Djurkemien*. Stockholm: Marquard, 1808.
3. LeCanu LR. De l'Hematosine, ou matière colorante du sang. *Ann Chim Phys* 1830;45:5–27.
4. Clanny WR. Description of apparatus and experiments for determining the composition of blood in health and disease. *Edinburgh Med Surg J* 1829;32:40–3.
5. Astrup P, Severinghaus JW. *The history of blood gases, acids and bases*. Copenhagen: Munksgaard, 1986.
6. O'Shaughnessy WB. Experiments on the blood in cholera. *Lancet* 1830–31;i:490.
7. Clanny WR. Composition of healthy and of cholera blood. *Lancet* 1831–32;ii:232.
8. O'Shaughnessy WB. Poisoned confectionery; detection of gamboge, lead, copper, mercury, and chromate of lead in various articles of sugar confectionery. *Lancet* 1830–31;i–ii:366, 490.
9. Latta T. Malignant cholera. *Lancet* 1831–32;ii:274, 370, 490.
10. Stevens W. *Observations on the healthy and diseased properties of the blood*. London: Murray, 1832.
11. Stevens W. *Anviisning til Den asiatiske Choleras Behandling*. Copenhagen: Græbe, 1833.
12. Stevens W. Observations on the treatment of cholera. Copenhagen: Græbe, 1833.
13. Stevens W. Observations of the theory of respirations. *Phil Trans R Soc Lond* 1835;345–54.
14. Gamble JL. Early history of fluid replacement therapy. *Pediatrics* 1953;11:554–67.
15. Stevens W. *Observations on the nature and the treatment of the Asiatic cholera*. London: H Bailliére, 1853.
16. Geill T. *William Stevens. En dansk-vetindisk læge med verdensry*. Copenhagen: Dansk Medicinsk Historisk Årbog, 1976;8–39.
17. Cantani A. Cholerabehandlung. *Berlin Klin Wochenschr* 1892;29:913–24.
18. Bernard C. *Leçons sur les propriétés physiologiques et les alterations pathologiques des liquids de l'organisme*. Paris: J-B Baillière and Son, 1857.
19. Henderson LJ. *The fitness of the environment*. New York: Macmillan, 1913.
20. Hasselbalch KA. Die Berechnung der Wasserstoffzahle des Blutes aus der freien und gebundenen Kohlensäure desselben und die Sauerstoff-bindung der Blutes als Funktion des Wasserstoffzahl. *Biochem Z* 1917;78:112.
21. Finkelstein H. *Säuglingskrankheiten*. Amsterdam: Elsevier, 1938.
22. Ewerbeck H. *Der Säugling*, Berlin: Springer-Verlag, 1962:309.
23. Kerpel-Fronius E. *Pathologie und Klinik des salz- und wasser-haushaltes*. Budapest: Verlag der Ungarischen Akademie der Wissenschaften, 1959.
24. Sellars AW. Tolerance for alkalies in Asiatic cholera. *Philippine J Sci Sect B* 1910;5:363.
25. Howland J, Marriott W McK. Acidosis occurring with diarrhea. *Am J Dis Child* 1916;11:309–25.
26. Ylppö A. Premature children. Should they fast or be fed in the first days of life? *Ann Pediatr Fenn* 1954;1:99–104.

27. Gamble JL. *Companionship of water and electrolytes in organisation of body fluids* (Lane Medical Lecture). Stanford University Press, 1951.
28. Darrow DC. Body fluid-physiology: the role of potassium in clinical disturbance of body water and electrolytes. *N Eng J Med* 1950;242:978–83,1014–8.
29. Moore FD. The use of isotopes in surgical research. *Surg Gyn Obst* 1948;86:120–47.
30. Friis-Hansen B. Changes in body water compartments during growth. *Acta Paediatr Scand* 1956; suppl 110.
31. Budin P. Translation of *Le Nourrisson* (Paris, Doin 1900) London: Caxton, 1907.
32. Perheentupa J, Arvo Ylppö, 100 Years, Oct. 27, 1987. *Acta Paediatr Scand* 1987;76:849–50.
33. Meissner FL, Peiper LA. *Fest.* Leipzig, 1828.
34. Biedert Ph. Die Kinderernährung im Säuglingsalter. Stuttgart: F. Enke, 1880.
35. Reuss A. Translation of *Die Krankheiten des Neugeborenen*. London: John Bale, Sons & Danielsson, 1920.
36. Clifford SH. Management of emergencies. *Am J Dis Child* 1947;73:706–12.
37. Smith CA. Reasons for delaying the feeding of premature infants. *Ann Paediatr Fenn* 1957;3: 261–8.
38. Usher R. The respiratory distress syndrome of prematurity, *Pediatrics* 1959;24:562–76.
39. Bell EF, Warburton D, Stonestreect BS, Oh W. Effect of fluid administration on the development of symptomatic patent ductus arteriosus and congestive heart failure in premature infants. *N Engl J Med* 1980;302:598–604.

DISCUSSION

Dr. Udall: What was the thinking in the 1800s about the histological appearances in the intestine in cholera? I have the impression that it was thought that the disease was caused by architectural changes in the small intestine.

Dr. Friis-Hansen: The descriptions of autopsies in children that I have seen showed, as you suggest, widespread necrosis in the gut and enlargement of the liver. These probably represented postmortem changes or ischemic lesions taking place in the last stages of dehydration. However, at the time they were described as toxic lesions.

Dr. Waterlow: When did physicians in Europe first start giving intravenous fluids to children with dehydration?

Dr. Friis-Hansen: As far as I know the honor goes to Latta in 1832. In 1884, Cantanni started to treat cholera cases with fluids in Naples.

Dr. Ballabriga: I do not know of any earlier references. Sellars used intravenous fluid and electrolytes to treat cholera in Manila in 1912, followed later by Rogers in India.

History of Pediatrics 1850–1950, edited by
B.L. Nichols, A. Ballabriga, and N. Kretchmer.
Nestlé Nutrition Workshop Series, Vol. 22. Nestec
Ltd., Vevey/Raven Press, Ltd., New York © 1991.

Dedication of the Howland Auditorium

Buford L. Nichols, Jr.

*USDA/ARS Children's Nutrition Research Center, Departments of Pediatrics and
Physiology, Baylor College of Medicine, Houston, Texas 77030, USA*

The origins in Europe and America of pediatrics as an academic discipline, and
pediatric nutrition as a science, formed the basis for discussion on the first day of the
Nestlé History of Pediatrics workshop. A name that recurred throughout the discussion was that of Dr. John Howland (Fig. 1). Dr. Howland served at the Johns Hopkins University Medical School as the first full-time chairman of a pediatric
department in the United States, and he has been credited with introducing quantitative analytical techniques into pediatrics (Fig. 2) in the United States. He was also
first author of several quantitative clinical investigations concerning acidosis and
rickets.

Dr. Howland was well known in Europe. He worked in Germany and Austria in
1901, and with Czerny in Germany in 1910. Figure 3 is a photograph of Dr. and
Mrs. Howland (the former Susan M. Sanford) on their departure for Europe in
1926. During that journey, Dr. Howland died of complications of liver disease. A
bas-relief, originally located in the Howland Amphitheater at the Harriet Lane
Home of Johns Hopkins University Hospital, recognized Howland as the man who
introduced quantitative research into pediatrics in the United States. Although the
Harriet Lane Home was demolished, the bas-relief panel (Fig. 4) was saved and is
now displayed at the Children's Medical Center of Johns Hopkins University Hospital. The cherubs on either side of Howland represent the Spirits of Chemistry and
Physics. Representations of elements from the original sculptural relief were used in
a new bas-relief of Howland (Fig. 5) designed for the auditorium of the United
States Department of Agriculture/Agricultural Research Service, Children's Nutrition Research Center at Baylor College of Medicine. The sculpture was unveiled at
a ceremony during the Nestlé History of Pediatrics workshop in which the auditorium was dedicated to the memory of Dr. John Howland.[1]

Three photographs illustrate the scientific heritage that links the Children's Nutrition Research Center to Dr. Howland. Figure 6 shows Dr. Howland as Chairman of
Pediatrics at the Johns Hopkins University Medical School. Among his associates in

---

[1]Dr. Elihu S. Howland, his wife Joan, and their son John were present at the dedication of the Howland Auditorium. Elihu Howland, a retired psychiatrist who lives in suburban Chicago, is the son of John
Howland.

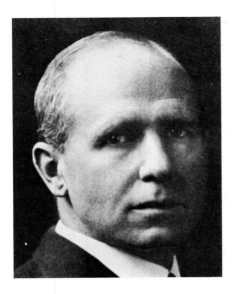

FIG. 1. John Howland was born February 3, 1873, in New York and died June 20, 1926, in London.

this photograph are many who pioneered the development of children's nutrition research in the United States: Joseph, Park, Powers, Gamble, Blackfan, Tisdall, and Shipley. During the 1930s, for example, Dr. Grover Powers served as chairman of the Department of Pediatrics at Yale University School of Medicine. In Fig. 7, Dr. Powers, Dr. Harold Harrison, and Dr. Darrow are pictured among the other house staff and faculty of the 1936 Department of Pediatrics at Yale. These three men are prominent figures in the history of American pediatrics. In Fig. 8, photographed at

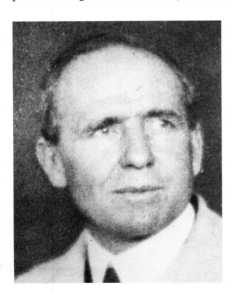

FIG. 2. John Howland in the laboratory at the Harriet Lane Home of the Johns Hopkins University Hospital, Baltimore, Maryland.

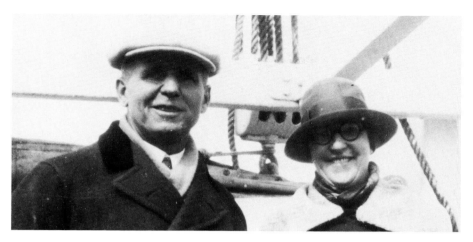

FIG. 3. Dr. and Mrs. John Howland were photographed in 1926 on a trip to Europe. (James L. Gamble, photographer.)

Yale in 1964, Dr. Powers, now the emeritus Chairman of Pediatrics, is pictured at center with Dr. Milton Sinn to his left and Dr. Dav Cook on his right. This photograph, in which I also appear, documents the lineage from Dr. John Howland, through Dr. Grover Powers, to the Children's Nutrition Research Center, which I currently direct. I would like to close this dedication ceremony with an excerpt from the 1952 John Howland Award Address given by Edwards A. Park (1):

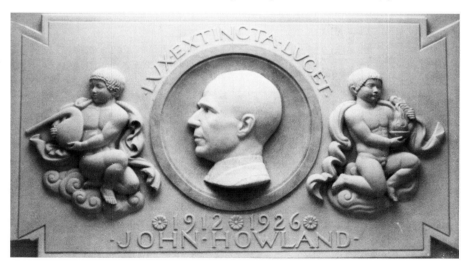

FIG. 4. Bas-relief of Howland sculpted by Paul Manship. This sculpture was originally displayed in the Howland Amphitheater of the Harriet Lane Home. Today it is displayed in the Children's Medical and Surgical Center of the Johns Hopkins University Hospital, Baltimore, Maryland.

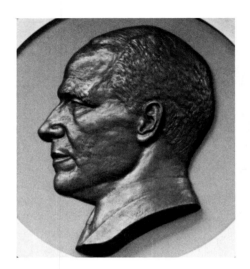

FIG. 5. Bas-relief of Howland sculpted by Joe Paderewski. The sculpture is displayed in the Howland Auditorium of the United States Department of Agriculture/Agricultural Research Service Children's Nutrition Research Center at Baylor College of Medicine, Houston, Texas.

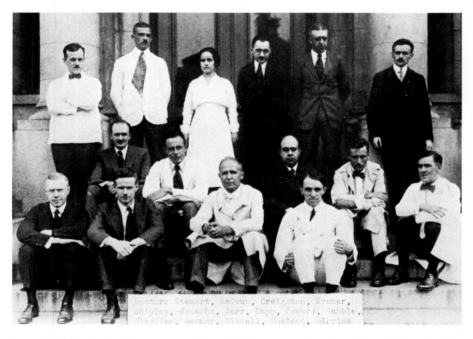

FIG. 6. John Howland and the members of the Department of Pediatrics of Johns Hopkins University School of Medicine. The original photograph is displayed in the Children's Medical and Surgical Center, Johns Hopkins University Hospital, Baltimore, Maryland.

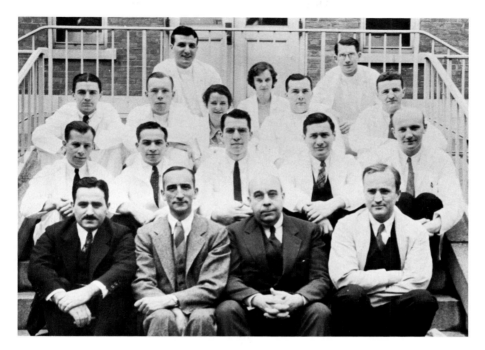

FIG. 7. The house staff and faculty at the Department of Pediatrics at the Yale University School of Medicine in 1936. Seated in the front row are Collatta, Trask, Powers, and Darrow. Harold Harrison, who participated in the Nestlé History of Pediatrics workshop, is seated behind and to the right of Trask. The photograph is a gift from Nelson Ordway to the Historical Archives of the Children's Nutrition Research Center.

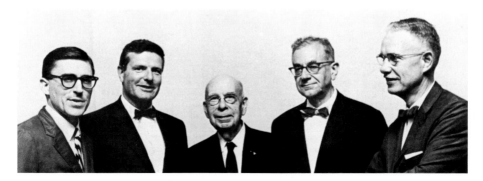

FIG. 8. Faculty members in the Department of Pediatrics, Yale University School of Medicine, in 1964: Nichols, Cook, Powers, Senn, and Ordway.

I now come to the concluding question: What has been John Howland's influence? What will be his place in pediatric history? These are my impressions concerning the verdict of time: Abraham Jacobi was the pioneer. He was a man of remarkable personality, far better educated medically and culturally, when he came to this country from Austria, than his American colleagues. He had great influence in raising the level of American medicine, particularly in New York City. But in pediatrics, so far as I can tell, his merit is limited to his having been the pioneer. He was the first, I might say, officer, to wear the pediatric uniform. If he has left a permanent imprint on pediatrics, I do not know what it is.

The case of Dr. Holt is very different. Holt established pediatrics in this country as a special branch of medicine, defining it and putting it in order and he made it include the welfare of the child in health as well as in disease. It was a big revolutionary conception, the idea that the physician is also charged with keeping the child well, coming at a time when physicians in general thought that their duties began and ended with sickness. When we say that pediatrics more than any other branch of medicine is directed toward preventive medicine, we must feel grateful to Dr. Holt for having started its flow that way. John Howland modernized pediatrics. He changed the course of pediatrics to what we know it now by substituting for bedside observation and conjecture the study of disease through laboratory methods and experiments. He caused pediatrics to become a dynamic, rapidly expanding subject. He accomplished this, not by scattering ideas which caused others to act, but by example. The example lay in the development of a model clinic, model from the point of view of administration, medical care, teaching, research, spirit—the Harriet Lane Home—known all over the world and in this country extensively copied just as he left it. Moreover, he created and sent out missionaries, his pupils, filled with his ideas and spirit.

ACKNOWLEDGMENTS

This work is a publication of the USDA/ARS Children's Nutrition Research Center, Department of Pediatrics, Baylor College of Medicine and Texas Children's Hospital, Houston, Texas. This project has been funded in part with federal funds from the U.S. Department of Agriculture, Agricultural Research Service under Cooperative Agreement number 58-7MN1-6-100. The contents of this publication do not necessarily reflect the views or policies of the U.S. Department of Agriculture, nor does mention of trade names, commercial products, or organizations imply endorsement by the U.S. Government.

REFERENCES

1. Park EA. John Howland Award Address. *Pediatrics* 1952;10:107.

History of Pediatrics 1850–1950, edited by
B.L. Nichols, A. Ballabriga, and N. Kretchmer.
Nestlé Nutrition Workshop Series, Vol. 22. Nestec
Ltd., Vevey/Raven Press, Ltd., New York © 1991.

Dedication of the Rubner Library

Buford L. Nichols, Jr.

*USDA/ARS Children's Nutrition Research Center, Departments of Pediatrics and
Physiology, Baylor College of Medicine, Houston, Texas 77030, USA*

The United States Department of Agriculture/Agricultural Research Service Children's Nutrition Research Center (CNRC) at Baylor College of Medicine, Houston, Texas, is devoted to the study of the nutritional needs of children and their mothers. The tenth anniversary of the CNRC was celebrated in a new building designed expressly to support its research. In dedicating the new building, we wished to recognize pioneers in the study of pediatrics and pediatric nutrition. We chose, therefore, to name the CNRC library in honor of Max Rubner, who was the first basic scientist to participate in nutritional investigations of children (1). The Rubner Library at the Children's Nutrition Research Center was dedicated February 21, 1989, at a ceremony during the Nestlé History of Pediatrics workshop. During the ceremony, an original plaster bust of Max Rubner (Fig. 1), sculpted in 1910 by Fritz Schaper, was unveiled. The bust was a gift to the library from Rubner's granddaughter, Elisabeth Peer.[1]

Rubner (Fig. 2) was born in Munich on June 2, 1854, and died in Berlin on April 27, 1932. He and Mrs. Rubner (the former Helene Leimbach) are pictured in Figure 3. As pioneers in the study of pediatric nutrition, Rubner and Otto Heubner in Berlin measured the heat production of young infants in a calorimeter, and their results were reported in *Zeitschrift für Biologie* in 1898 and 1899 (2,3). Earlier, Rubner had found that carbohydrate and fat were interchangeable in nutrition based upon their energy equivalents. He developed an energy doctrine based upon his discoveries that stated that (1) energy expenditure is obligatory during life and (2) the energy expended is replaced by energy liberated through the oxidative cleavage of organic molecules (1).

Rubner was also a skilled watercolorist. The CNRC is fortunate to have three of his water colors on exhibit in the Rubner Library.

Graham Lusk (see p. 52, Fig. 2) was Rubner's close friend and fellow student (4). Lusk became a professor of physiology at Cornell University Medical College in 1912 and developed a respiration calorimeter to study metabolism in infants. He collaborated with John Howland (see p. 268, Fig. 1), a pediatrician, in the first

---

[1]Ms. Elisabeth M. Peer, granddaughter and biographer of Max Rubner, was present for the unveiling of the Rubner bust. The bust had previously been kept in her home in Austria.

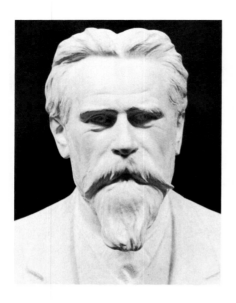

FIG. 1. Plaster bust of Max Rubner created in 1910 by Fritz Schaper. The only other copy of the bust was destroyed during the bombing of Berlin in World War II.

measurements of the energy expenditure of infants in the United States (5,6). The teamwork of Lusk and Howland in the United States followed the tradition of collaboration between basic scientist and clinical investigator that Max Rubner and Otto Heubner had begun in Germany.

Lusk eulogized Max Rubner, the man and the scientist, with these words: ''Great men are very rare. They are worth knowing. They give impulse and stimulus to

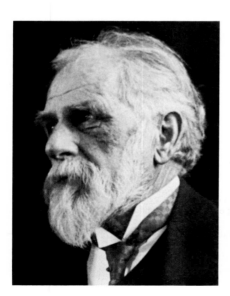

FIG. 2. Max Rubner (1854–1932) was the first scientist to participate in quantitative nutritional investigations in normal and marasmic infants. The photograph is a gift to the Children's Nutrition Research Center Historical Archives from Elisabeth Peer.

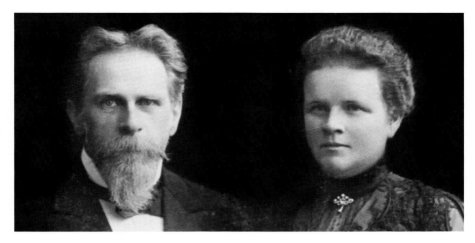

FIG. 3. Dr. and Mrs. Max Rubner. The photograph is a gift to the Children's Nutrition Research Center Historical Archives from Elisabeth Peer.

lesser men. They make the world more worthwhile for others to live in because of their presence in it. Max Rubner was the greatest man I ever knew.''

ACKNOWLEDGMENTS

This work is a publication of the USDA/ARS Children's Nutrition Research Center, Department of Pediatrics, Baylor College of Medicine and Texas Children's Hospital, Houston, Texas. This project has been funded in part with federal funds from the U.S. Department of Agriculture, Agricultural Research Service under Cooperative Agreement number 58-7MN1-6-100. The contents of this publication do not necessarily reflect the views or policies of the U.S. Department of Agriculture, nor does mention of trade names, commercial products, or organizations imply endorsement by the U.S. Government.

REFERENCES

1. Lusk G. Contributions to the science of nutrition. A tribute to the life and work of Max Rubner. *Science* 1932;76:129–35.
2. Rubner M, Heubner O. Die natürliche Ernährung eines Säuglings. *Z Biol* 1898;36:1–55.
3. Rubner M, Heubner O. Die künstliche Ernährung eines normalen und eines atrophischen Säuglings. *Z Biol* 1899;38:315–98.
4. Lusk G. The elements of the science of nutrition. 4th ed [reprint]. New York: Johnson Reprint Corporation, 1976.
5. Lusk G. Calorimetric observations. *Med Rec* 1912;Nov:1–11.
6. Howland J. The fundamental requirements of an infant's nutrition. *Trans Am Pediatr Soc* 1911;23:12–9.

History of Pediatrics 1850–1950, edited by
B.L. Nichols, A. Ballabriga, and N. Kretchmer.
Nestlé Nutrition Workshop Series, Vol. 22. Nestec
Ltd., Vevey/Raven Press, Ltd., New York © 1991.

Summary and Conclusion

Norman Kretchmer

*Department of Nutritional Sciences, University of California, Berkeley,
California 94720, USA*

There is a contemporary book in the United States entitled *The Rise and Fall of the Great Powers,* by Paul Kennedy. It predicted that the USA had reached a zenith. In general, the people of the United States did not enjoy that prediction, although a number of people in the audience have experienced this type of phenomenon in their countries.

A similar set of events has occurred in pediatric medicine. We have seen rises and falls in the power of medicine, starting with the Greeks, then the Arabs, and then the Europeans. During the past three days, the discussions have given insight into the growth of pediatrics in the United States, France, and Mexico and the rise of pediatrics in Europe and the United Kingdom. In this workshop, we specifically discussed Germany, the Austro-Hungarian Empire, and the United Kingdom.

One aspect of the history of medicine that needs to be explained is why the wave of medicine moved from place to place. As with other social events, it moved with war, with industry, and with social upheaval. The events after World War I brought about many changes in medicine in Europe; the disaster of Nazi Germany was greatly detrimental to medical advance in Germany.

Ballabriga quoted Goethe, who said: "To know the present, one must know the past." The future should be built on knowledge and experiences of the past. Some people desire to rediscover the wheel. It is easier to rediscover than to take advantage of what we have learned in the past and build on that store of information.

Another aspect of this conference that has impressed me is the repetition of names. A group of basic scientists kept reappearing: Liebig, Virchow, Rokitansky, and Bernard, and then the famous names in pediatrics: Finkelstein has been mentioned by almost everyone who came to this platform, and Czerny and Schlossman. Names from the United States that have been repeated are Rotch, Howland, Gamble, and Darrow.

In this conference we covered a period of 100 years of social upheaval and concomitant growth in pediatrics. That is the aspect of our field I would like to discuss, and I would like to borrow from the past to learn about the future.

We started our workshop at 1850. The subsequent changes described were remarkable. At that time pediatrics was descriptive, and we have quoted many people, starting with Rosenstein. We admired the linguistic beauty with which they described specific diseases and applied words, names to them—*codes* is the term that Waterlow used—specific codes so that physicians could understand the descriptions.

Pediatrics as an art has not changed over the subsequent years. We are trained to alleviate the problems of the ill child, but what has changed has been the availability of information. This has burgeoned so that we now have difficulty in handling the suffocating plethora of scientific information. During the late nineteenth century, science entered into pediatric medicine with new vigor, not only from basic anatomy, biochemistry, chemistry, and organic chemistry, but from general medicine, sufficiently for it to be suggested that there should be specialization within the field. Osler, who was a president of the American Pediatric Society, cautioned against specialization in his presidential speech in 1892. He thought ''specialism'' might destroy the field of general medicine. He was worried lest pediatrics would leave the fold of general medicine to become a specialty. However, in his later years as Regis Professor at Oxford, he specialized exclusively in internal medicine and left pediatrics. Thus by the beginning of the twentieth century, pediatrics had become a specialty and started borrowing directly from the scientific ideas of the other disciplines that were basic to children's concerns.

The first and most obvious pediatric problem was the bio-social condition that still persists in many parts of the world, that is, malnutrition. The problems facing pediatricians at the beginning of the century were infection and malnutrition: dirty milk, children left on the street, and shanty towns. We noted the writings of Dickens as a major influence in exposing how Victorian children could be abused and ignored by society. The problem of the disregard of the child still persists.

In the early years of the twentieth century, the science of nutrition bloomed. We heard about the discovery of new vitamins, amino acids, and protein requirements. From all over the world there were contributions to nutritional science as it related to children. At the same time, infection became understood from the work of Pasteur, Koch, and Ehrlich.

In the 1920s, nutrition reigned. Science was growing rapidly. Pediatrics was becoming a strong clinical specialty. Departments were tightly organized. At the same time, we have heard how people like Howland, who was perhaps the most prominent, brought basic scientists into pediatrics to answer specific clinical problems. Levine worked with Lusk and Dubois. There were examples of these cooperative activities between pediatrics and basic science all over the world. I remember Winnicka telling me about the advances in biochemistry conducted by Parnas in Poland, and I was shocked to discover that I knew so little about some of the early important work in carbohydrate metabolism.

Scientific information was growing. Departments of pediatrics proliferated. In 1950, there was an additional explosion of science with increasing understanding of metabolism. With these additions to the pool of knowledge, departments of pediatrics became immersed in basic science. This phenomenon was probably observed in the United States more than in any other place because of the availability of federal funding for research in the 1960s. Also, the United States had the advantage in that we attracted from Europe and Asia some of the most able scientists in the world. From 1933 to 1940, the Nazis forced many of the best minds out of Germany and from much of the rest of Europe. The United States benefited from these tragic social events, as evidenced in the expansion and vigor of biology, medicine, and physics. Now the immigration of brilliant minds into the United States derives mainly from Asia.

In 1959, I became the head of the Department of Pediatrics at Stanford. I had 25 faculty members in the department by 1969. All of them were trained in basic science. Thirty years later, there are more than 60 faculty members in the department, and there has not been a major increase in the patient population. The pediatric department here at Baylor College of Medicine has about 450 faculty members with 120 house officers.

With the explosion of science, information, and resources, pediatrics has grown and, as a consequence, has become fractured into subspecialties. On an academic level the pediatric generalists in this country are disappearing. The generalists still exist in other countries, but I am sure you will eventually emulate our pattern. The field of pediatrics has become so large, and the information has increased so greatly that we now have seven accredited subspecialties in pediatrics in the United States. In many areas of the USA today, if a person has a medical complaint and wants care, he should probably call for a family physician.

What is going to be the future of pediatrics? Can we borrow a lesson from the past? We have to accept that we are going to fragment into more specialties because the accrual of information has become so immense. In the biological fields, there are many unresolved problems. There is intrauterine development that includes many of the things that were mentioned under the heading of teratology. There is immunologic disease, a problem of huge scope in this country and the world. Pediatric antecedents to adult degenerative disease are exceedingly important and serve as a basis for the preventive medicine of tomorrow. There are recommendations that we determine cholesterol on all infants at birth so we can prevent heart disease in old age. These problems invade the realm of the pediatrician because that is where the physician can have a lifelong impact. Regulation and adaptation are biological mechanisms we do not fully understand. Major problems still remain for resolution in the social and behavioral pediatric field. We return to issues outlined by Dickens. There are homeless children in major cities throughout the world. There is the problem of drug abuse in the developed countries. There is social and economic unrest. Although there is no major war, there are many small wars, and wars affect children the most. Throughout history, children have always been drastically debilitated by war.

Malnutrition still exists in almost every part of the world, including the United States. To classify malnutrition as kwashiorkor or marasmus is not the real problem. What we must concern ourselves with as physicians and as citizens are the social and political conditions that lead to such childhood disaster. That is the real problem to be solved in the future. We must be active, as were Virchow and Jacobi, and our other forebears.

Pediatricians have unsolved problems to face. We have cured many diseases. We have established a tradition of general pediatrics, but scientific pediatrics is now fractured. This is useful, and the way it should be. As scientific information accrues, we observe this continuing fractionation.

I end my discussion with one point, and that is a comment on basic research and clinical research. I am a traditionalist. Like Marriott, I started my career in biochemistry, and I casually went to medical school, and casually became a pediatrician under the tutelage of Sam Levine and Henry Barnett. But research has an intellectual base, whether it be basic or clinical. Clinical research is much more difficult to accomplish than basic research because it involves a greater bureaucracy and more variables. Clinical research is becoming more and more difficult to carry on. It is increasingly difficult to derive answers to the practical clinical questions. I do not differentiate research into two areas. I call both "good science."

After these two-and-a-half days, we can all conclude that we came from a great tradition, and we have to carry on this tradition, but we must also realize what is happening to pediatrics and modernize. We must take advantage of our history as we move into the future.

History of Pediatrics 1850–1950, edited by
B.L. Nichols, A. Ballabriga, and N. Kretchmer.
Nestlé Nutrition Workshop Series, Vol. 22. Nestec
Ltd., Vevey/Raven Press, Ltd., New York © 1991.

Appendix

John C. Waterlow

Pediatric journals and their first year of publication. (Journals in parentheses have ceased publication.)

(Jahrbuch für Kinderheilkunde [Berlin][1]	Germany	1868)
(Archiv für Kinderheilkunde [Stuttgart][2]	Germany	1880)
(Archives of Pediatrics [became Clinical Pediatrics]	USA	1884)
(Zentralblatte für Kinderheilkunde [Leipzig]	Germany	1887)
(La Pediatria [Naples]	Italy	1893)
(Archives de Médecine des Enfants [Paris][3]	France	1897)
(Bulletin de la Societé de Pédiatrie [Paris][3]	France	1899)
(Abhandlung aus der Kinderheilkunde [Berlin][4]	Germany	1899)
(Revista de Clinica Pediatrica [Firenze]	Italy	1902)
Monatschrifte für Kinderheilkunde [Berlin]	Germany	1904
(British Journal of Children's Diseases[5]	UK	1904)
Ergebnisse der Inneren Medizin und Kinderheilkunde [Berlin]	Germany	1908
(Zeitschrift für Kinderheilkunde [Berlin][6]	Germany	1911)
American Journal of Disease of Children	USA	1911
(Bibliographie der Gesamten Kinderheilkunde [Berlin]	Germany	1912)
(Pediatria Española	Spain	1912)
(Jahrsbericht Kinderheilkunde [Berlin]	Germany	1916)
Acta Paediatrica Scandinavica	Sweden	1921
(Oriental Journal of Diseases of Children	Japan	1925)
(Pediatria [Napoli] [became Archivos di Patologia e Clinica Pediatrica]	Italy	1925)
Archives of Disease in Childhood	UK	1926

[1]Later became Annales Paediatrici in 1938 then Pediatric Research.
[2]Became Klinische Pädiatrie in 1971.
[3]Amalgamated in 1942 to become Archives Francaises de Pédiatrie.
[4]Became Bibliotheca Pediatrica in 1937.
[5]No longer exists.
[6]Became European Journal of Pediatrics.

(La Pediatrica del Medico Practico [Turin][7]	Italy	1926)
(Archivos de Pediatria [Rio de Janeiro]	Brazil	1928)
(Boletin de la Sociedad Catalana de Pediatria	Spain	1929)
(Archivos de Pediatria de Uruguay	Uruguay	1929)
(Boletin de la Sociedad Cubana de Pediatria	Cuba	1929)
(Il Lattante [Parma]	Italy	1929)
(Archivos Argentinos de Pediatria	Argentina	1930)
Kinderärtzliche Praxis [Leipzig]	Germany	1930
Maandschrift [now Tijdschrift] voor Kindergene-eskunde (Amsterdam)	Netherlands	1931
(Revista Mexicana de Pediatria	Mexico	1931)
Revista Chilena de Pediatria	Chile	1931
(Archivio Italiano de Pediatria e Puericultura [Bologna]	Italy	1932)
(Boletin Instituto Puericultura del Univ. Brazil	Brazil	1932)
Journal of Pediatrics	USA	1932
(Arch. Méd. Infantil del Hosp. Universitario	Cuba	1932)
(Jornal da Pediatria	Brazil	1934)
Annales de Pédiatrie	France	1934
(Archivos Venezolanos de Pediatria	Venezuela	1938)
(Revista de Pediatria de Cordova	?Argentina	1939)
Pediatriya	USSR	1941
(Revista Peruana de Pediatria	Peru	1941)
Archives Francaises de Pédiatrie[3]	France	1942
Advances in Pediatrics	USA	1942
Acta Pediatrica Española	Spain	1943
Helvetica Pediatrica Acta	Switzerland	1945
Pédiatrie	France	1945
Revista Española de Pediatria	Spain	1945
Revista Soc. Colombiana de Pediatria y Puericultura	Colombia	1945
Ceskoslovenska Pediatria	Czechoslovakia	1946
Österreichischer Zeitschrift fur Kinderheilkunde	Austria	1947
Acta Pediatrica Belgica [now European Journal of Pediatrics]	Belgium	1947
Revista del Soc. Boliviana de Pediatria	Bolivia	1947
Pediatrics	USA	1948
Acta Paediatrica Latina [Reggio Emilia]	Italy	1948
Minerva Pediatrica [Turin][7]	Italy	1949

---

[3]Amalgamated in 1942 to become Archives Francaises de Pédiatrie.
[7]Became Minerva Pediatrica.
Pediatric journals of unknown date of founding:

Paediatria Danubiana	Anales Espanoles de Pediatria
Pediatria Indonesica	Acta Paediatrica Japonica
Pediatria Medica e Chirurgica (Vicenza)	Ärztliche Jugendkunde (Leipzig)
Pediatria Polska	

Indian Journal of Child Health [now Indian Pediatrics]	India	1952
Annales Paediatricae Fenniae	Finland	1954
Pediatric Clinics of North America	USA	1954
Journal of Tropical Pediatrics [London]	UK	1955
Turkish Journal of Pediatrics	Turkey	1958
Acta Paediatrica Hungarica	Hungary	1960
Clinical Pediatrics	USA	1961
Pädiatrie und Grenzgebiete	E. Germany	1962
Revue de Pédiatrie	France	1965
Pädiatrie und Pädologie	Austria	1965
Australian Journal of Pediatrics	Australia	1965
Pediatric Clinics of India	India	1965
Pediatric Research	USA	1967

SUBJECT INDEX